Melanoma

Guest Editor

JEFFREY E. GERSHENWALD, MD, FACS

SURGICAL ONCOLOGY
CLINICS OF NORTH AMERICA

www.surgonc.theclinics.com

Consulting Editor

NICHOLAS J. PETRELLI, MD

January 2011 • Volume 20 • Number 1

SAUNDERS an imprint of ELSEVIER, Inc.

W.B. SAUNDERS COMPANY
A Division of Elsevier Inc.

1600 John F. Kennedy Boulevard • Suite 1800 • Philadelphia, PA 19103-2899

http://www.theclinics.com

SURGICAL ONCOLOGY CLINICS OF NORTH AMERICA Volume 20, Number 1
January 2011 ISSN 1055-3207, ISBN-13: 978-1-4557-0510-8

Editor: Jessica Demetriou

Surgical Oncology Clinics of North America (ISSN 1055-3207) is published quarterly by Elsevier Inc., 360 Park Avenue South, New York, NY 10010-1710. Months of publication are January, April, July, and October. Business and Editorial Offices: 1600 John F. Kennedy Blvd., Ste. 1800, Philadelphia, PA 19103-2899. Customer Service Office: 3251 Riverport Lane, Maryland Heights, MO 63043. Periodicals postage paid at New York, NY and additional mailing offices. Subscription prices are $241.00 per year (US individuals), $357.00 (US institutions) $119.00 (US student/resident), $277.00 (Canadian individuals), $444.00 (Canadian institutions), $171.00 (Canadian student/resident), $346.00 (foreign individuals), $444.00 (foreign institutions), and $171.00 (foreign student/resident). Foreign air speed delivery is included in all *Clinics* subscription prices. All prices are subject to change without notice. **POSTMASTER**: Send address changes to *Surgical Oncology Clinics of North America*, Elsevier Health Science Division, Subscription Customer Service, 3251 Riverport Lane, Maryland Heights, MO 63043. **Customer Service: 1-800-654-2452 (US and Canada). 314-447-8871 (outside U.S. and Canada). Fax: 314-447-8029. E-mail: journalscustomerservice-usa@elsevier.com** (for print support); **journalsonline support-usa@elsevier.com** (for online support).

Reprints. For copies of 100 or more, of articles in this publication, please contact the Commercial Reprints Department, Elsevier Inc., 360 Park Avenue South, New York, New York 10010-1710. Tel. 212-633-3813; Fax: 212-462-1935; E-mail: reprints@elsevier.com.

Surgical Oncology Clinics of North America is covered in *MEDLINE/PubMed (Index Medicus)* and *EMBASE/ Excerpta Medica, Current Contents/Clinical Medicine,* and *ISI/BIOMED.*

Printed and bound by CPI Group (UK) Ltd, Croydon, CR0 4YY

Transferred to Digital Print 2011

Contributors

CONSULTING EDITOR

NICHOLAS J. PETRELLI, MD
Bank of America Endowed Medical Director, Helen F. Graham Cancer Center at Christiana Care Health System, Newark, Delaware; Professor of Surgery, Thomas Jefferson University, Philadelphia, Pennsylvania

GUEST EDITOR

JEFFREY E. GERSHENWALD, MD, FACS
Professor, Department of Surgical Oncology; Professor, Department of Cancer Biology; and Medical Director, Melanoma and Skin Center, The University of Texas MD Anderson Cancer Center, Houston, Texas

AUTHORS

ROBERT L. ASKEW, MPH
Program Manager, Department of Surgical Oncology, The University of Texas MD Anderson Cancer Center, Houston, Texas

RUSSELL S. BERMAN, MD
Division of Surgical Oncology, Department of Surgery, New York University School of Medicine, NYU Cancer Institute, New York, New York

ABIGAIL S. CAUDLE, MD
Assistant Professor, Department of Surgical Oncology, The University of Texas MD Anderson Cancer Center, Houston, Texas

DANIEL G. COIT, MD
Attending Surgeon, Gastric and Mixed Tumor Service, Department of Surgery, Memorial Sloan-Kettering Cancer Center, New York, New York

JANICE N. CORMIER, MD, MPH
Associate Professor of Surgery and Biostatistics, Department of Surgical Oncology, The University of Texas MD Anderson Cancer Center, Houston, Texas

MICHAEL A. DAVIES, MD, PhD
Assistant Professor, Departments of Melanoma Medical Oncology and Systems Biology, The University of Texas MD Anderson Cancer Center, Houston, Texas

PAXTON V. DICKSON, MD
Fellow, Department of Surgical Oncology, The University of Texas MD Anderson Cancer Center, Houston, Texas

RYAN C. FIELDS, MD
Surgical Oncology Fellow, Department of Surgery, Memorial Sloan-Kettering Cancer Center, New York, New York

JEFFREY E. GERSHENWALD, MD, FACS
Professor, Department of Surgical Oncology; Professor, Department of Cancer Biology; and Medical Director, Melanoma and Skin Center, The University of Texas MD Anderson Cancer Center, Houston, Texas

RICARDO J. GONZALEZ, MD
Departments of Cutaneous Oncology and Sarcoma Oncology, H. Lee Moffitt Cancer Center and Research Institute; Assistant Professor, Department of Oncologic Sciences, University of South Florida College of Medicine, Tampa, Florida

JOSHUA C. GRIMM, BA
Department of Melanoma Medical Oncology, The University of Texas MD Anderson Cancer Center, Houston, Texas

JADE HOMSI, MD
Department of Melanoma Medical Oncology, The University of Texas MD Anderson Cancer Center, Houston, Texas

PATRICK HWU, MD
Department of Melanoma Medical Oncology, The University of Texas MD Anderson Cancer Center, Houston, Texas

RAGINI KUDCHADKAR, MD
Department of Cutaneous Oncology, H. Lee Moffitt Cancer Center and Research Institute; Assistant Professor, Department of Oncologic Sciences, University of South Florida College of Medicine, Tampa, Florida

PATRICK A. OTT, MD, PhD
Division of Medical Oncology, Department of Medicine, New York University School of Medicine, NYU Cancer Institute, New York, New York

VICTOR G. PRIETO, MD, PhD
Professor of Pathology and Dermatology, Departments of Pathology and Dermatology, The University of Texas MD Anderson Cancer Center, Houston, Texas

NIKHIL G. RAO, MD
Assistant Professor, Departments of Radiation Oncology and Cutaneous Oncology, H. Lee Moffitt Cancer Center, Tampa, Florida

AMANDA K. RAYMOND, MD
School of Medicine, Duke University, Durham, North Carolina

MERRICK I. ROSS, MD, FACS
Professor, Department of Surgical Oncology, The University of Texas MD Anderson Cancer Center, Houston, Texas

RICHARD A. SCOLYER, BMedSci, MBBS, MD, FRCPA, FRCPath
Senior Staff Specialist, Tissue Pathology and Diagnostic Oncology, Royal Prince Alfred Hospital; Clinical Professor, Discipline of Pathology, Central Clinical School, Sydney Medical School, The University of Sydney; Consultant Pathologist and Co-Director of Research, Melanoma Institute Australia, Sydney, New South Wales, Australia

VERNON K. SONDAK, MD
Professor and Chair, Department of Cutaneous Oncology, H. Lee Moffitt Cancer Center and Research Institute; Professor, Departments of Oncologic Sciences and Surgery, University of South Florida College of Medicine, Tampa, Florida

JOHN F. THOMPSON, MD, FACS
Melanoma Institute Australia, North Sydney; and Professor of Melanoma and Surgical Oncology, the University of Sydney, Sydney, New South Wales, Australia

ANDREA TROTTI III, MD
Professor, Director of Clinical Trails, Departments of Radiation Oncology and Cutaneous Oncology, H. Lee Moffitt Cancer Center, Tampa, Florida

RYAN S. TURLEY, MD
Department of Surgery, Duke University, Durham, North Carolina

DOUGLAS S. TYLER, MD
Professor, Department of Surgery, Duke University, Durham, North Carolina

HSIANG-HSUAN M. YU, MD
Assistant Professor, Department of Radiation Oncology, H. Lee Moffitt Cancer Center, Tampa, Florida

Contents

Staging of cutaneous melanoma continues to evolve through identification and rigorous analysis of potential prognostic factors. In 1998, the American Joint Committee on Cancer (AJCC) Melanoma Staging Committee developed the AJCC melanoma staging database, an international integrated compilation of prospectively accumulated melanoma outcome data from several centers and clinical trial cooperative groups. Analysis of this database resulted in major revisions to the TNM staging system reflected in the sixth edition of the AJCC Cancer Staging Manual published in 2002. More recently, the committee's analysis of an updated melanoma staging database, including prospective data on more than 50,000 patients, led to staging revisions adopted in the seventh edition of the AJCC Cancer Staging Manual published in 2009. This article highlights these revisions, reviews relevant prognostic factors and their impact on staging, and discusses emerging tools that will likely affect future staging systems and clinical practice.

Histologic analysis remains the gold standard for diagnosis of melanoma. The pathology report should document those histologic features important for guiding patient management, including those characteristics on which the diagnosis was based and also prognostic factors. Pathologic examination of sentinel lymph nodes provides very important prognostic information. New techniques, such as comparative genomic hybridization and fluorescence in situ hybridization are currently being studied to determine their usefulness in the diagnosis of melanocytic lesions. Recent molecular studies have opened new avenues for the treatment of patients with metastatic melanoma (ie, targeted therapies) and molecular pathology is likely to play an important role in the emerging area of personalized melanoma therapy.

The surgical management of primary cutaneous melanoma, from the diagnostic biopsy through the wide local excision and nodal staging, must be carefully planned, and the biology of the melanoma, microstaging and primary tumor pathologic features of the melanoma, location on the body, patient preferences, and comorbidities must be considered. The treating surgeon must balance preservation of oncologic principles, with optimization of functional and aesthetic outcome. This article reviews the rationale behind the surgical approach in the patient with a primary melanoma.

The technique of lymphatic mapping and sentinel lymph node (SLN) biopsy was introduced 20 years ago as an important advance in the management of patients with stage I and II melanoma. After 2 decades of experience, SLN biopsy and the practice of selective lymphadenectomy represents a minimally invasive standard of care that facilitates the accurate staging of the clinically negative regional lymph node basin, provides durable regional disease control, and improves survival in node-positive patients.

For in-transit melanoma confined to the extremities, regional chemotherapy in the form of hyperthermic isolated limb perfusion and isolated limb infusion are effective treatment modalities carrying superior response rates to current standard systemic therapy. Despite high response rates, most patients will eventually recur, supporting the role for novel research aimed at improving durable responses and minimizing toxicity. Although the standard cytotoxic agent for regional chemotherapy is melphalan, alternative agents such as temozolomide are currently being tested, with promising preliminary results. Current strategies for improving chemosensitivity to regional chemotherapy are aimed at overcoming classic resistance mechanisms such as drug metabolism and DNA repair, increasing drug delivery, inhibiting tumor-specific angiogenesis, and decreasing the apoptotic threshold of melanoma cells. Concurrent with development and testing of these agents, genomic profiling and biomolecular analysis of acquired tumor tissue may define patterns of tumor resistance and sensitivity from which personalized treatment may be tailored to optimize efficacy. In this article rational strategies for treatment of in-transit melanoma are outlined, with special emphasis on current translational and clinical research efforts.

Adjuvant therapy is commonly used in melanoma because recurrence after surgery usually results in the patient's eventual death. Surgeons have a profound influence on patients' decisions regarding adjuvant therapy, beginning with providing a clear understanding of the risk of specific types of recurrence. This review summarizes the potential oncologic benefits and relevant toxicities of adjuvant systemic therapies for melanoma that are currently available and under investigation.

mutations. The challenges that must be overcome to achieve improved outcomes with targeted therapies in melanoma in the future are also discussed.

This article reviews the best evidence available to guide the follow-up of patients with melanoma, focusing on incidence of, and detection of, melanoma recurrence, frequency of follow-up visits, yield of, laboratory and radiographic tests, outcomes of patients with recurrent melanoma based on method of detection, detection of secondary melanomas, and stage-specific follow-up.

Assessment of patient-reported outcomes (PROs) provides important information to assist with clinical decision making. There has been significant progress in the field of PROs over the past 2 decades with the introduction of validated disease- and symptom-specific instruments. The Functional Assessment of Cancer Therapy-Melanoma (FACT-M) is a melanoma-specific module to accompany the FACT-General, which was validated to assess health-related quality of life for patients with all stages of melanoma. Melanoma-specific health state utilities also have been reported from a number of studies. Assessment of PROs should be incorporated into routine clinical practice to inform clinicians and researchers of the patient perspective for clinical decision making and to evaluate the effects of psychosocial and medical interventions.

VISIT THE CLINICS ONLINE!

Access your subscription at:
www.theclinics.com

Foreword

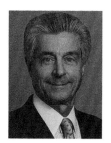

Nicholas J. Petrelli, MD
Consulting Editor

This edition of the *Surgical Oncology Clinics of North America* has been organized by Jeffrey Gershenwald, MD from the MD Anderson Cancer Center in Houston, Texas. Dr Gershenwald has brought together a core of outstanding authors with experience in the treatment of melanoma. This year, there will be approximately 68,000 new cases of melanoma in the United States. Approximately 38,000 will be diagnosed in males and 29,000 in females. In addition, there will be 8,700 deaths from this skin cancer. In our own state of Delaware with a population of 800,000 individuals, there will be approximately 200 cases of melanoma diagnosed in 2011. This is due to the beautiful beaches in the southern part of the state with sun exposure and its subsequent consequences to the skin. In 2010, melanoma was the fifth most common cancer in males and the seventh most common cancer in females.

Melanoma is an increasing public health problem both in the United States and globally. It has been increasing faster than any other cancer in the United States. Diagnosing melanoma in its early stage cannot be overstated. Accurate diagnosis in an early stage can lead to earlier treatment and result in successful management. It has been estimated that 90% of expenditures for melanoma therapy in the United States is related to advanced disease. In view of this, significant savings in health care cost can occur if melanoma can be detected in an early, more easily treatable, stage. Although biopsy followed by histopathologic examination is the key to rule out melanoma, the challenge lies in identifying skin lesions that have the highest probability of being melanoma. In 1985, investigators at New York University devised the ABCD acronym (**A**symmetry, **B**order irregularity, **C**olor variegation, **D**iameter of the lesion >6mm). These criteria were developed to be a simple tool that could be utilized by both lay persons and health care professionals to alert them to the clinical features of early melanoma. The ABCD criteria have been verified in multiple studies.

Instructing patients to perform regular skin self-examination is extremely important. Melanomas can indeed be detected by patients, and persons undergoing skin self-examination have been found to be more aware of melanoma and to have the lesions

Surg Oncol Clin N Am 20 (2011) xiii–xiv
doi:10.1016/j.soc.2010.10.002
1055-3207/11/$ – see front matter © 2011 Elsevier Inc. All rights reserved.

surgonc.theclinics.com

they detect be thinner when biopsied versus persons who did not practice this self-examination approach.

I would like to thank Dr Gershenwald and his colleagues for this edition of the *Surgical Oncology Clinics of North America* and encourage the authors to share this information with all of their trainees.

Nicholas J. Petrelli, MD
Helen F. Graham Cancer Center
4701 Ogletown-Stanton Road, Suite 1213
Newark, DE 19713, USA

E-mail address:
npetrelli@christianacare.org

Preface

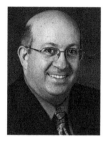

Jeffrey E. Gershenwald, MD
Guest Editor

Although melanoma is often curable if diagnosed and treated at its earliest stages, it remains among the most challenging malignancies to eradicate if distant metastases develop. Despite these challenges, improved insight into the biology of melanoma has led to significant advances in our understanding of the natural history, diagnosis, and treatment of this disease. This issue of *Surgical Oncology Clinics of North America* is devoted to a comprehensive review and discussion of advances in the field over the past two decades. It aims to provide the practicing surgical oncologist with information that will enhance their multidisciplinary care of the melanoma patient.

The development of an international collaborative melanoma database, coupled with an evidence-based analytic approach, has transformed our ability to stage patients with melanoma. Surgical strategies, including recommendations for primary tumor wide excision margins, widespread use of lymphatic mapping and sentinel lymph node biopsy in patients with intermediate- and high-risk primary cutaneous melanoma (the latter resulting from the truly pioneering efforts of Donald Morton), and more recently, innovative approaches to the treatment of in-transit disease and resectable distant metastasis, have significantly shaped the landscape for patients with melanoma. A recent randomized, prospective clinical trial in patients with advanced regional melanoma metastasis has shed light on the role of adjuvant radiation therapy. Remarkably, advances in our understanding of the immunology of metastatic melanoma have been translated into new treatments that target the immune system. Tremendous strides in our understanding of the molecular biology of melanoma have fostered development of promising new targeted therapies that specifically block aberrant cellular pathways resulting from specific mutations arising in melanoma tumors.

In the first article, Dr Paxton Dickson joins me in providing a contemporary overview of staging and prognosis of cutaneous melanoma. This overview highlights revisions to the recently updated AJCC melanoma staging system, reviews relevant prognostic factors and their impact on staging, and discusses emerging tools that will likely affect future staging systems and clinical practice, including the important concept of *individualized prognosis*. Drs Richard Scolyer and Victor Prieto follow with a state-of-the-art overview of clinically relevant issues in melanoma pathology. Drs Patrick Ott and Russell Berman very capably review the surgical approach to primary cutaneous melanoma.

Surg Oncol Clin N Am 20 (2011) xv–xvi
doi:10.1016/j.soc.2010.10.004
1055-3207/11/$ – see front matter © 2011 Elsevier Inc. All rights reserved.

surgonc.theclinics.com

Drs Merrick Ross and John Thompson join me in providing a "20th anniversary" critical assessment of the role of sentinel lymph node biopsy for melanoma. This issue will be published exactly 20 years after the first sentinel lymph node biopsy was performed at MD Anderson, just months after Dr Donald Morton's now landmark presentation at the Annual Meeting of the Society of Surgical Oncology in 1990. Following this review, Drs Ryan Turley, Amanda Raymond, and Douglas Tyler tackle the clinical problem of in-transit melanoma metastasis and provide a comprehensive overview of rational treatment strategies for this relatively unique manifestation of melanoma intralymphatic metastasis. Their overview focuses on regional chemotherapy in the form of hypothermic isolated limb perfusion and isolated limb infusion, with a special emphasis on current translational and clinical research efforts.

The discussion thematically evolves to address the important question of the role of adjuvant therapy for melanoma. Dr Vernon Sondak and his colleagues, Drs Ricardo Gonzalez and Ragini Kudchadkar, provide a surgical perspective of adjuvant therapy for melanoma, and Drs Nikhil Rao, Hsiang-Hsuan Yu, Andrea Trotti III, and Vernon Sondak discuss the role of radiation therapy.

Drs Abigail Caudle and Merrick Ross present an update on the evolving role of metastasectomy for stage IV melanoma. Following discussion of this important theme, Drs Jade Homsi, Joshua Grimm, and Patrick Hwu present an up-to-date review of the current status of immunotherapy for melanoma, with a focus on the recent promising results from using vaccines, cytotoxic T-lymphocyte antigen-4 antibodies, and adoptive cell therapy. Dr Michael Davies and I then lead a discussion regarding targeted therapy for melanoma, a critically important theme in view of our expanding knowledge base regarding activating mutations prevalent in melanoma and recent early-phase clinical trial evidence demonstrating that targeting aberrant cellular pathways can result in meaningful clinical response.

Rounding out this issue, Drs Ryan Fields and Daniel Coit review evidence-based follow-up for the melanoma patient. Drs Janice Cormier and Robert Askew comprehensively assess patient-reported outcomes, both particularly relevant contributions as the United States enters an era of heath care reform.

I would like to express my sincere gratitude to all of the authors for their enthusiastic support for and outstanding contributions to this issue. My sincere thanks also go to Ms Jessica Demetriou for dedicated editorial assistance, Ms LeighAnne Helfmann for efficiently navigating this project through production, and Dr Nicholas J. Petrelli for inviting me to serve as guest editor for this issue dedicated to melanoma.

I hope that this issue of Surgical Oncology Clinics of North America—representing the collective work of dedicated clinicians and clinician-scientists who are leaders in their respective fields—serves as a useful resource to educate those who care for patients with melanoma and to inspire further discovery as we strive to realize improved outcomes for patients with this disease.

Jeffrey E. Gershenwald, MD
Departments of Surgical Oncology and Cancer Biology
Melanoma and Skin Center
The University of Texas MD Anderson Cancer Center
Unit 444
1515 Holcombe Boulevard
Houston, TX 77030, USA

E-mail address:
jgershen@mdanderson.org

Staging and Prognosis of Cutaneous Melanoma

Paxton V. Dickson, MD, Jeffrey E. Gershenwald, MD*

KEYWORDS

• Melanoma • Staging • Prognosis

Formal staging of cancer is fundamental in providing clinicians and patients with prognostic information, developing treatment strategies, and directing and analyzing clinical trials. Staging of cutaneous melanoma continues to evolve through identification and rigorous analysis of potential prognostic factors. The first multivariate analyses of prognostic factors for melanoma were published more than 3 decades ago, and several well-designed reports have subsequently advanced our understanding of important prognostic indicators for this disease.[1–3] Despite these important efforts, the need for a unified melanoma staging system applicable to both clinical practice and research became evident.[4–6] In 1998, the American Joint Committee on Cancer (AJCC) Melanoma Staging Committee, which included experts from North America, Europe, and Australia, developed the AJCC melanoma staging database, a first-in-kind international integrated compilation of prospectively accumulated melanoma outcome data from several centers and clinical trial cooperative groups.[7] Analysis of this database resulted in major revisions to the Tumor-Node-Metastasis (TNM) staging system reflected in the sixth edition of the AJCC Cancer Staging Manual published in 2002. More recently, the committee's analysis of an updated melanoma staging database, including prospective data on more than 50,000 patients, led to staging revisions adopted in the seventh edition of the AJCC Cancer Staging Manual published in 2009.[8,9] This article highlights these revisions, reviews relevant prognostic factors and their impact on staging, and discusses emerging tools that will likely affect future staging systems and clinical practice.

This work was supported in part by The University of Texas MD Anderson Cancer Center Melanoma SPORE (P50 CA93459) and the Grossman Family Foundation.
The authors have nothing to disclose.
Department of Surgical Oncology, The University of Texas MD Anderson Cancer Center, 1515 Holcombe Boulevard, Unit 444, Houston, TX 77030, USA
* Corresponding author. Department of Cancer Biology, University of Texas MD Anderson Cancer Center, 1515 Holcombe Boulevard, Suite 444, Houston, TX 77030.
E-mail address: jgershen@mdanderson.org

doi:10.1016/j.soc.2010.09.007
1055-3207/11/$ – see front matter © 2011 Elsevier Inc. All rights reserved.

surgonc.theclinics.com

AJCC SEVENTH EDITION UPDATES AND HIGHLIGHTED CHANGES FROM THE SIXTH EDITION

Staging systems for melanoma continue to be refined as our understanding of the complex biology of this disease improves. In 2002, the sixth edition AJCC staging system included significant revisions to the prior system based on prognostic factor analysis of the original melanoma staging database.[10,11] These revisions included: new strata for primary tumor thickness, incorporation of primary tumor ulceration in the T and N classifications, the distinction of nodal tumor burden as a prognostic factor in patients with regional metastases, and new categories for stage IV disease. Analysis of an updated AJCC melanoma staging database was subsequently performed to provide further insight into the prognostic significance of several biologic factors and to refine the sixth edition. These updates are reflected in the seventh edition melanoma staging system of the AJCC Cancer Staging Manual published in 2009 (**Tables 1** and **2**).[8] While this most recent staging schema remains largely intact compared with the prior version, several noteworthy revisions are briefly highlighted here and are further detailed where appropriate throughout this article (**Table 3**).

A fundamental change to the new staging system is the addition of mitotic rate as a criterion for defining T1b primary melanoma. Mitotic rate of the primary tumor, defined as mitoses/mm^2, was included as a covariate in the staging analysis and was identified to have significant prognostic implications, further discussed below.

A second important change is the formal inclusion of immunohistochemical assessment, rather than just hematoxylin and eosin (H&E) staining, as acceptable in defining the presence of nodal metastases. Of importance, at least one melanoma-specific marker, such as HMB-45, Melan-A, or MART 1, should be used. Furthermore, unlike criteria used in breast cancer staging, there is no lower threshold of tumor burden used to define nodal micrometastases, reflecting the consensus that even small amounts of metastatic disease are potentially clinically relevant.

Historically, patients with melanoma with an unknown primary presenting with metastases arising in the skin, subcutaneous tissue, and/or lymph nodes have variably been classified as having either stage III or stage IV disease, provided that a staging evaluation does not reveal other sites of disease. However, recent studies focused on patients with melanoma of unknown primary with metastases to lymph nodes have demonstrated a survival profile similar (if not more favorable) to patients with regional nodal disease and a known primary melanoma.[12,13] In the updated staging system, metastatic melanoma to the skin, subcutaneous tissue, or lymph nodes with an unknown primary is classified as stage III disease. Accordingly, such patients should be offered surgical management and participation in adjuvant stage III trials.

LOCALIZED MELANOMA (STAGE I AND II)

The prognosis for patients with localized melanoma is generally favorable. In the sixth-edition AJCC melanoma staging system, tumor thickness and ulceration were identified as the dominant independent predictors of survival.[10] However, based on emerging data from several single institution studies reporting tumor mitotic rate as an adverse prognostic factor,[14–17] mitotic rate was included in the analysis of the updated AJCC melanoma staging database. Although some investigators predicted that ulceration would no longer maintain its prognostic significance for patients with localized disease, in fact, tumor thickness, mitotic rate, and the presence of ulceration were each found to be significant independent predictors of survival in this group of patients.[8,9] Furthermore, in the seventh edition AJCC melanoma staging system, these 3 factors were used to define T categories (see **Tables 1** and **2**).[8,9]

Table 1
TNM staging categories for cutaneous melanoma (seventh edition)

T Classification	Thickness	Ulceration Status
Tis	NA	NA
T1	≤1.00 mm	a: without ulceration and mitosis <1/mm^2 b: with ulceration or mitoses ≥1/mm^2
T2	1.01–2.0 mm	a: without ulceration b: with ulceration
T3	2.01–4.0 mm	a: without ulceration b: with ulceration
T4	>4.0 mm	a: without ulceration b: with ulceration

N Classification	# of Metastatic Nodes	Nodal Metastatic Burden
N0	0	NA
N1	1	a: micrometastasis[a] b: macrometastasis[b]
N2	2–3	a: micrometastasis[a] b: macrometastasis[b] c: in transit met(s)/satellite(s) without metastatic nodes
N3	4+ metastatic nodes, or matted nodes, or in transit metastases/satellites with metastatic nodes	

M Classification	Site	Serum LDH
M0	No distant metastases	NA
M1a	Distant skin, subcutaneous, or nodal metastases	Normal
M1b	Lung metastases	Normal
M1c	All other visceral metastases	Normal
	Any distant metastasis	Elevated

Abbreviations: NA, not applicable; LDH, lactate dehydrogenase.
[a] Micrometastases are diagnosed after sentinel lymph node biopsy.
[b] Macrometastases are defined as clinically detectable nodal metastases confirmed pathologically.
From Balch CM, Gershenwald JE, Soong S, et al. Final version of 2009 AJCC melanoma staging and classification. J Clin Oncol 2009;27(36):6200; with permission.

Primary tumor thickness was introduced as a prognostic factor by Alexander Breslow in 1970,[18] and has subsequently been validated in multiple studies.[1,19–21] At present, the AJCC staging system uses tumor thickness cut points of 1.0 mm, 2.0 mm, and 4.0 mm to define T-category strata based on their statistical significance and, importantly, their clinical utility in defining tumor thickness as thin (<1 mm), intermediate (1–4 mm), and thick (>4 mm) tumors.[4,22] In analysis of more than 27,000 patients from the AJCC melanoma staging database with stage I or II disease, as primary tumor thickness increased there was a significant decrease in survival (**Fig. 1**A and B).[9]

Ulceration is defined as the lack of an intact dermis overlying the primary tumor on histologic evaluation. Multiple studies demonstrate that the presence of ulceration

Table 2
Anatomic stage groupings for cutaneous melanoma (seventh edition)

	Clinical Staging[a]				Pathologic Staging[b]		
	T	N	M		T	N	M
0	Tis	N0	M0	0	Tis	N0	M0
IA	T1a	N0	M0	IA	T1a	N0	M0
IB	T1b	N0	M0	IB	T1b	N0	M0
	T2a	N0	M0		T2a	N0	M0
IIA	T2b	N0	M0	IIA	T2b	N0	M0
	T3a	N0	M0		T3a	N0	M0
IIB	T3b	N0	M0	IIB	T3b	N0	M0
	T4a	N0	M0		T4a	N0	M0
IIC	T4b	N0	M0	IIC	T4b	N0	M0
III	Any T	N > N0	M0	IIIA	T1–4a	N1a	M0
					T1–4a	N2a	M0
				IIIB	T1–4b	N1a	M0
					T1–4b	N2a	M0
					T1–4a	N1b	M0
					T1–4a	N2b	M0
					T1–4a	N2c	M0
				IIIC	T1–4b	N1b	M0
					T1–4b	N2b	M0
					T1–4b	N2c	M0
					Any T	N3	M0
IV	Any T	Any N	M1	IV	Any T	Any N	M1

[a] Clinical staging includes microstaging of the primary melanoma and clinical/radiologic evaluation for metastases. By convention, it should be used after complete excision of the primary melanoma with clinical assessment for regional and distant metastases.

[b] Pathologic staging includes microstaging of the primary melanoma and pathologic information about the regional lymph nodes after partial (ie, sentinel lymph node biopsy) or complete lymphadenectomy. Pathologic Stage 0 or Stage IA patients are the exception; they do not require pathologic evaluation of their lymph nodes.

From Balch CM, Gershenwald JE, Soong S, et al. Final version of 2009 AJCC melanoma staging and classification. J Clin Oncol 2009;27(36):6200; with permission.

represents a more aggressive tumor phenotype with a higher likelihood of metastasis and worse prognosis.[23,24] For patients with ulcerated melanomas, survival is significantly lower than for patients with nonulcerated tumors of equivalent depth. Moreover, analysis of the original AJCC melanoma staging database (published in the 2002 AJCC Cancer Staging Manual) demonstrated that survival outcomes for patients with ulcerated tumors were remarkably similar to those of patients with nonulcerated tumors of the next highest T category.[10] This finding was validated in the 2008 database analysis and is reflected in the 2009 AJCC melanoma staging system (see **Fig. 1**A and B).[8,9]

Primary tumor mitotic rate deserves special mention, as it represents a fundamental change in the revised melanoma staging system. This change is based on a body of data showing a significant correlation between increasing mitotic rate and decreased survival. Salman and Rogers[25] first suggested the prognostic importance of the

Table 3
Differences between the previous (2002) and the current (2009) versions of the AJCC melanoma staging system

Factor	2002 Criteria	2009 Criteria	Comments
Thickness	Primary determinant of T staging; thresholds of 1.0, 2.0, 4.0 mm	Same	Correlation of metastatic risk is a continuous variable
Level of invasion	Used only for defining T1 melanomas	No longer used	Clark levels IV or V may be used in rare instances as a criterion for defining T1b melanoma only if mitotic rate cannot be determined in a nonulcerated melanoma
Ulceration	Included as a second determinant of T and N staging	Same	Signifies a locally advanced lesion; dominant prognostic factor for grouping Stage I, II, and III
Mitotic rate per mm^2	Not used	Used for categorizing T1 melanoma	Mitosis ≥ 1/mm^2 used as a primary determinant for defining T1b melanoma
Satellite metastases	In N category	Same	Merged with in transit lesions
Immunochemical detection of nodal metastases	Not allowed	Allowed	Must include at least one melanoma-specific marker (eg, HMB-45, Melan-A, MART 1)
0.2 mm threshold of defined N-positive disease	Implied	No lower threshold of staging N-positive disease	
Number of nodal metastases	Dominant determinant of N staging	Same	Thresholds of 1 vs 2–3 vs >4 nodes
Metastatic "volume"	Included as a second determinant of N staging	Same	Clinically occult ("microscopic") vs clinically apparent ("macroscopic") nodal volume
Lung metastases	Separate category as M1b	Same	Has a somewhat better prognosis than other visceral metastases
Elevated serum LDH	Included as a second determinant of M staging	Same	Recommend a second confirmatory LDH if elevated
Clinical vs pathologic staging	Sentinel node results incorporated into definition of pathologic staging	Same	Large variability in outcome between clinical and pathologic staging; sentinel node staging encouraged for standard patient care and should be required before entry into clinical trials

From Balch CM. Melanoma of the skin. In: Edge SB, Byrd DR, Compton CC, et al, editors. AJCC cancer staging manual. 7th edition. New York: Springer Verlag; 2009. p. 327; with permission.

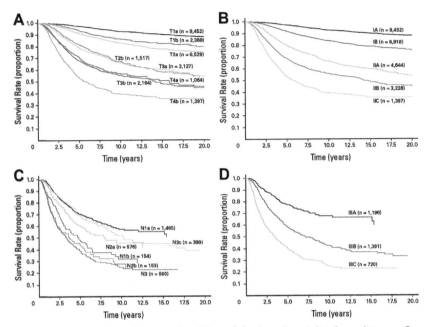

Fig. 1. Survival curves from the seventh edition of the American Joint Committee on Cancer melanoma staging database comparing (A) the different T categories and (B) the stage groupings for stages I and II melanoma. Note that survival outcomes for patients with ulcerated tumors were remarkably similar to those of patients with nonulcerated tumors of the next highest T category. For patients with stage III disease, survival curves are shown comparing (C) the different N categories and (D) the stage groupings. Note in particular the marked heterogeneity in survival among these patients with stage III disease. (*From* Balch CM, Gershenwald JE, Soong S, et al. Final version of 2009 AJCC melanoma staging and classification. J Clin Oncol 2009;27(36):6201; with permission.)

mitotic index of the primary tumor, identifying that it was associated with a higher rate of metastasis in patients with thin lesions. Several other investigators have subsequently confirmed tumor mitotic rate as an independent prognostic factor.[14–17] Multivariate analysis of 10,233 patients from the updated AJCC melanoma staging database with localized melanoma (stages I and II) revealed mitotic rate as the second most important predictor of survival, after tumor thickness, and was particularly pronounced among patients with T1 melanoma.[9] Accordingly, in a multivariate analysis of 4861 patients with T1 melanoma, tumor thickness, mitotic rate, and ulceration were all powerful predictors of survival; level of invasion was no longer statistically significant when mitotic rate and ulceration were included in the analysis.[9] The 10-year survival rate was 95% for nonulcerated T1 melanomas with a mitotic rate of less than $1/mm^2$, and dropped to 88% if the mitotic rate was $1/mm^2$ or more ($P<.0001$).[9] Although ulcerated T1 melanomas were associated with a mitotic rate of $1/mm^2$ or higher in 78% of patients, the 10-year survival rate was similar regardless of whether the mitotic rate was less than $1/mm^2$ or $1/mm^2$ or greater (85% vs 87%; $P = .41$). Based on these data, mitotic rate (operationally defined in the seventh-edition melanoma staging system as a dichotomous variable) replaced Clark level of invasion as a primary criterion for defining T1b melanoma.[8,9]

The mitotic rate of the primary melanoma should be assessed following biopsy. The suggested approach is detailed in the seventh edition of the AJCC Cancer Staging

Manual.[8] In brief, the recommended technique is to first find the area within the dermis containing the most mitotic figures, the so-called hot spot. After counting mitoses in the hot spot, the count is extended to adjacent fields until an area of 1 mm^2 is assessed. The count is then expressed as mitoses/mm^2. If no hot spot can be identified and mitoses are randomly scattered throughout the lesion, then a representative mitosis is chosen, and beginning with that field, the count is then extended until an area corresponding to 1 mm^2 is assessed. Individual microscopes should be calibrated for accurate recording. If the invasive area of a tumor is less than 1 mm^2, then the number of mitoses present in 1 mm^2 of dermal tissue that includes the tumor should be determined and recorded as mitoses/mm^2. Alternatively, in these tumors, the simple presence or absence of a mitosis can be designated as at least 1/mm^2 (ie, "mitogenic") or 0/mm^2 (ie, "nonmitogenic"), respectively.

Determining mitotic rate is important not only in providing prognostic information but also in discussing and planning extent of surgery. In the sixth edition of the AJCC Staging Manual, sentinel lymph node (SLN) biopsy was recommended for patients with T1b tumors, based on an approximately 10% incidence of identifying occult nodal metastasis in patients with thin melanomas that were either ulcerated or had Clark level IV invasion.[10] Although the updated AJCC melanoma staging database does not permit a precise estimation of predicting nodal micrometastasis in this cohort, others have demonstrated increased mitotic activity in the primary tumor to be a predictor of SLN positivity.[14–17,26] In a preliminary report based on a multivariate analysis of patients with T1 melanoma who underwent sentinel node biopsy, Caudle and colleagues[27] found that a mitotic rate of 1/mm^2 or more was an independent predictor of sentinel lymph node histologic status. Although this clinical question is not yet fully resolved, available data suggest that in addition to using other potential prognostic factors, consideration should be given to offering SLN biopsy in patients with thin ($\leq$1 mm) melanoma if the primary tumor mitotic rate is 1/mm^2 or more.

For years Clark level of invasion has been known to have prognostic significance, and has served as a criterion in several melanoma staging systems.[28] Nonetheless, several investigators have demonstrated that level of invasion is less reproducible among pathologists, and is less accurate in providing prognostic information than tumor thickness.[1,29–31] In the sixth edition AJCC melanoma staging system, Clark level of invasion of at least IV (or ulceration) was used to define T1b tumors. However, in the T1 category-specific AJCC multivariate analysis, level of invasion was no longer an independent predictor of survival relative to mitotic rate and ulceration.[9] In the seventh edition AJCC melanoma staging system, level of invasion is only to be used to define T1b tumors in the rare occurrence that mitotic rate cannot be accurately determined.

STAGE III MELANOMA

Patients with regional metastasis (ie, regional lymph node, satellite, and/or in-transit metastasis) represent a heterogeneous group with regard to staging and prognosis. It is well established that regional lymph nodes are the most common first site of metastasis in melanoma patients.[32] The sixth edition AJCC melanoma staging system identified the number of regional lymph nodes harboring metastatic disease, regional node tumor burden (empirically classified as microscopic vs macroscopic), and ulceration of the primary tumor as independent predictors of survival in this cohort.[10,11] Recent analysis of patients from the AJCC melanoma staging database used for the seventh edition melanoma staging system confirm these criteria as important prognostic factors, and includes long-term follow-up of patients staged in the era of SLN biopsy.

Regional Lymph Nodes

In previous staging systems, the size of metastasis-containing regional lymph nodes was the primary criterion used in stratifying stage III patients.[5] However, more recent analyses have demonstrated that in patients with regional metastasis, the number of nodes harboring metastatic disease is the most important predictor of survival.[4,10,11,33–36] The current AJCC N category stratifies patients according to number of nodes involved based on best statistical grouping: 1 (N1) versus 2 to 3 (N2) versus 4 or more (N3) nodes.[8]

Regional node tumor burden, empirically defined in the AJCC melanoma staging system as microscopic or macroscopic metastasis, was the second most important prognostic factor in patients with stage III disease in the AJCC database analysis. Microscopic disease refers to metastatic deposits detected on histologic analysis following elective lymph node dissection, or more commonly, SLN biopsy. Macroscopic disease refers to nodal metastases that are clinically or radiographically apparent and pathologically confirmed. Of importance, these definitions are based on method of detection, not the size or "visibility" of the nodal metastasis. This criterion is used to subcategorize the N classification in the current staging system. For example, N1a to N3a refers to patients with micrometastasis and N1b to N3b to patients with macrometastasis. Analysis of patients in the AJCC melanoma staging database demonstrated significant differences in survival when accounting for nodal tumor burden (see **Fig. 1C, D; Table 4**).[8,9]

Lymphatic mapping and sentinel node biopsy is now widely used as the standard method of staging patients deemed to have significant risk of clinically occult regional nodal metastasis. Most contemporary series reveal that the majority of patients with stage III disease present with micrometastasis, usually detected on SLN biopsy.[9,37–40] Recently, analysis of patients from the AJCC melanoma staging database with stage III disease was performed to identify and compare independent predictors of survival between those with micrometastases and macrometastases.[37] This investigation confirmed significant survival differences based on nodal tumor burden, and remarkable heterogeneity in survival among substages of patients with stage III disease. Multivariate analysis demonstrated differences in independent predictors of survival when

Table 4
Five-year survival rates for stage III (nodal metastases) patients stratified by number of metastatic nodes, primary tumor ulceration, and nodal tumor burden (microscopic or macroscopic) (N = 2313)

Primary Tumor Ulceration	No. of Nodal Micrometastases, % ± SE (n = 1872)			No. of Nodal Macrometastases, % ± SE (n = 441)		
	1	2–3	≥4	1	2–3	≥4
Absent	81.5 ± 1.9 (777)	73.2 ± 3.7 (246)	38.0 ± 8.5 (46)	51.6 ± 7.2 (75)	46.6 ± 7.9 (67)	45.4 ± 9.1 (50)
Present	56.6 ± 2.9 (531)	53.9 ± 4.2 (223)	34.0 ± 8.3 (49)	49.4 ± 6.2 (88)	37.7 ± 6.2 (93)	29.2 ± 6.7 (68)

From Balch CM, Gershenwald JE, Soong SJ, et al. Multivariate analysis of prognostic factors among 2313 patients with stage III melanoma: comparison of nodal micrometastases vs macrometastases. J Clin Oncol 2010;28:2454; with permission.

stage III patients were stratified by nodal tumor burden (**Table 5**).[37] In both groups, number of positive lymph nodes remained the most significant predictor of survival. In addition, older age was found to be an independent adverse prognostic factor, regardless of nodal tumor burden. However, in patients with nodal micrometastases, features of the primary tumor including thickness, mitotic rate, ulceration, and anatomic location were found to significantly affect survival. In contrast, these primary tumor

Table 5
Multivariate Cox regression analyses for nodal micrometastases and for nodal macrometastases with mitotic rate data available (N = 1338)

Variable	df	Nodal Micrometastases (n = 1070)			Nodal Macrometastases (n = 268)		
		Chi-Square (χ^2)	P value	Hazard Ratio	Chi-Square (χ^2)	P value	Hazard Ratio
No. of Positive Nodes	2	43.0	<.001		6.1	.0480	
1**	—	—	—	1.00	—	—	1.00
2–3	1	2.2	.1343	1.25	0.2	.6800	1.11
≥4	1	43.0	<.001	3.59	5.7	.0172	1.83
Thickness (mm)	3	21.4	<.001		5.7	.1267	
0–2.00**	—	—	—	1.00	—	—	1.00
2.01–4.00	1	7.0	.0083	1.62	0.8	.3842	0.74
4.01–6.00		4.3	.0380	1.58	0.3	.5811	1.22
>6.00	1	21.2	<.001	3.00	0.6	.4210	1.34
Ulceration	1	11.1	.001		2.8	.0959	
Absent**	—	—	—	1.00	—	—	1.00
Present	1	11.1	.001	1.59	2.7	.0959	1.45
Clark Level	1	0.003	.9597		0.4	.5140	
II/III**	—	—	—	1.00	—	—	1.00
IV/V	1	0.003	.9597	1.01	0.4	.5140	1.27
Mitotic Rate	2	23.4	<.001		2.71	.2582	
<1**	—	—	—	1.00	—	—	1.00
1–19.99	1	0.02	.8993	0.96	2.6	.1085	0.45
≥20	1	6.1	.0134	2.69	2.4	.1239	0.41
Age (years)	2	12.7	.0018		13.8	.0010	
<50**	—	—	—	1.00	—	—	1.00
50–69	1	2.5	.1160	1.26	1.6	.2121	0.75
≥70	1	12.6	.0004	1.83	6.3	.0118	1.92
Site	1	5.0	.0251		0.4	.5413	
Extremity**	—	—	—	1.00	—	—	1.00
Axial	1	5.0	.0251	1.36	0.4	.5413	1.13
Gender	1	1.1	.2959		0.9	.3435	
Male**	—	—	—	1.00	—	—	1.00
Female	1	1.1	.2959	0.86	0.9	.3435	0.79

** Reference for hazard ratio calculation.

From Balch CM, Gershenwald JE, Soong SJ, et al. Multivariate analysis of prognostic factors among 2,313 patients with stage III melanoma: comparison of nodal micrometastases vs macrometastases. J Clin Oncol 2010;28:2457; with permission.

features were not independent predictors in patients with nodal macrometastases (see **Table 5**). These results reveal important differences regarding prognosis based on nodal tumor burden (see **Fig. 1**C, D and **Table 4**), and provide the groundwork for further refinement in prognostic assessment of stage III patients, particularly, but not exclusively, among the dominant cohort with nodal micrometastases.

Primary tumor ulceration was first included as a stratification criterion for stage III melanoma in the sixth edition AJCC melanoma staging system based on data demonstrating its significance as an independent adverse predictor of survival in this cohort.[4,10,11,41] This criterion was upheld in the recently published seventh edition AJCC staging system (see **Tables 4** and **5**).[8,9] Similar to its impact on survival estimates for stage I and II melanoma, primary tumor ulceration is associated with decreased survival in stage III, essentially upstaging such a patient whose primary tumor is ulcerated to that of a patient with a nonulcerated primary who has a higher nodal tumor burden category (see **Fig. 1**C, D and **Table 4**). This criterion is therefore again used to define N-category substages (see **Table 2**).[8,9] For example, 5-year survival is 53.9% and 46.6%, respectively, in patients with 2 to 3 microscopically involved regional nodes and an ulcerated primary melanoma, versus 2 to 3 macroscopically involved lymph nodes in patients whose primary tumor is not ulcerated (see **Table 4**).[37]

The criteria discussed here revealed marked heterogeneity in the prognosis for patients with stage III disease, and are used to define stage III substages into IIIA, IIIB, and IIIC (see **Fig. 1**C, D, and **Tables 2** and **4**).[9] Future studies involving staging and management of patients with regional metastases, particularly those with microscopic nodal tumor burden, are likely to be better refined by incorporating other features of the primary tumor, including mitotic rate.

In-Transit and Satellite Disease

The final criterion for defining stage III disease is the presence of intralymphatic metastases in the form of either in-transit disease or satellite lesions. In both the previous and most recent editions of the AJCC melanoma staging system, a designation of N2c is given to patients with in-transit or satellite disease in the absence of nodal metastases, while patients with concomitant nodal metastases and in-transit and/or satellite lesions are classified as having N3 disease.[8–11] Based on current analyses of the AJCC melanoma staging database, patients with N2c disease have 5- and 10-year survival rates of 69% and 52%, respectively. These survival rates are actually higher than those of patients with N2a and N2b disease, and more favorable than in prior reports.[4,42–45] Nonetheless, the survival for patients with intralymphatic metastases (in the absence of nodal metastases) still fits best into the stage IIIB category (see **Tables 1** and **2**).

STAGE IV MELANOMA

The prognosis for patients with distant metastases is generally poor, with historical 5-year survival rates of less than 10%.[46–48] Several factors have been examined in attempt to better predict survival in this group.[3,48–50] Beginning with the sixth edition AJCC melanoma staging system, patients with stage IV melanoma were categorized as having M1a (metastasis to distant skin, subcutaneous tissues, and/or lymph nodes), M1b (metastasis to the lungs), and M1c (metastasis to any nonpulmonary visceral site) disease. In addition, patients with an elevated serum lactate dehydrogenase (LDH) were assigned to the M1c category, regardless of site of distant metastasis. Analysis of the updated database, including more than 8000 patients, validated these criteria as significant independent prognostic factors in patients with stage IV disease.[8,9]

Based on this most recent analysis, patients with metastasis to distant skin, subcutaneous tissues, and/or lymph node basins (M1a) have the highest 1-year survival rate (62%) among patients with stage IV disease. Patients with pulmonary metastasis (M1b) have an intermediate prognosis (1-year survival rate, 53%). Finally, patients with nonpulmonary visceral metastases and/or an elevated serum LDH (M1c) have the worst 1-year survival among stage IV patients (33%) (see **Table 2**; **Fig. 2**A, B).[8,9]

Serum markers are uncommonly used in staging solid tumors. However, multiple reports have consistently demonstrated an elevated serum LDH to represent a highly significant, independent adverse prognostic factor in patients with stage IV melanoma.[51–53] These findings were recapitulated in the seventh edition AJCC melanoma database analysis, and revealed that 1- and 2-year survival rates for stage IV patients with a normal LDH were 65% and 40%, respectively, compared with 32% and 18%, respectively, in those patients with an elevated LDH level (see **Fig. 2**A, B).[9] Although the exact pattern of elevated LDH isoforms is nonspecific in melanoma patients and the mechanism for LDH elevation is not fully understood, an overwhelming amount of clinical data supports its use as a prognostic factor in patients with stage IV disease. Accordingly, it is recommended that serum LDH levels are measured in all melanoma patients when diagnosed with distant metastasis (see **Table 2** and **Fig. 2**A, B).

Several studies have reported the number of distant metastases to be a relevant prognostic factor in patients with metastatic melanoma.[46,54,55] Although analysis of stage IV patients in the updated staging database confirms this finding,[8,9] the challenge of standardizing the diagnostic modalities used to identify and quantify distant disease makes it difficult to incorporate this as a formal criterion in the current staging system.

EMERGING THEMES FOR STAGING AND PROGNOSIS FOR CUTANEOUS MELANOMA: CONDITIONAL SURVIVAL ESTIMATES, ELECTRONIC PROGNOSTIC MODELS, AND MOLECULAR PROFILING
Conditional Survival Estimates

For staging purposes, survival estimates for melanoma patients are determined from the time of melanoma diagnosis and are typically reported using the methods of

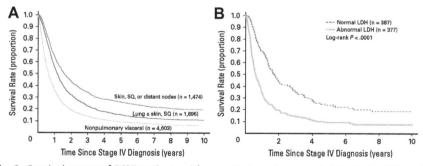

Fig. 2. Survival curves of 7635 patients with metastatic melanoma at distant sites (stage IV) subgrouped by (*A*) the site of metastatic disease and (*B*) serum lactate dehydrogenase (LDH) levels. LDH values are not used to stratify patients. Curves in (*A*) are based only on site of metastasis. The number of patients is shown in parentheses. SQ, subcutaneous. (*From* Balch CM, Gershenwald JE, Soong S, et al. Final version of 2009 AJCC melanoma staging and classification. J Clin Oncol 2009;27(36):6202; with permission.)

Kaplan and Meier. Although well-characterized, stage-specific 5-year and 10-year survival estimates based on analysis of large patient populations at time of initial melanoma diagnosis are informative, such traditional survival estimates become less relevant for patients surviving several years beyond diagnosis and treatment, as a patient's cancer-specific risk profile changes over time, particularly for patients with advanced disease at initial presentation. Over the past decade, the concept of conditional survival, that is, having survived "x" years since initial diagnosis, what is "my" predicted survival from that point forward?, has emerged as an important technique to estimate survival for cancer survivors. Conditional survival estimates have been published for a variety of malignancies.[56–63] Recently, analyses of patients with cutaneous melanoma have demonstrated that conditional survival estimates increase over time in patients with advanced disease.[64–66] For instance, in an analysis of melanoma patients using the SEER (Surveillance, Epidemiology, and End Results) database, 5-year conditional survival estimates in patients with stage II, III, and IV melanoma improved from 72% to 86%, 51% to 87%, and 19% to 84%, respectively, in which that latter estimate in each range corresponded to the subset of patients that survived 5 years following initial diagnosis.[66] Furthermore, among stage III patients treated at the University of Texas MD Anderson Cancer Center, 5-year conditional disease-specific survival estimates for patients with stage IIIA, IIIB, and IIIC improved from 78% to 90%, 54% to 79%, and 39% to 78%, respectively.[64]

Understanding that survival estimates are not static, but rather improve for melanoma survivors who initially present with advanced disease, provides an opportunity for more accurate prognostic assessment for patients and clinicians alike. Conditional survival estimates provide quantitative information that educates clinicians, may reduce patient anxiety about risk of cancer recurrence and death, and potentially serve as motivation for clinicians to continue to pursue aggressive treatment strategies in patients with advanced disease.

Beyond TNM-Based Staging

Despite the strong evidenced-based predictive capacity of the current AJCC melanoma staging system, it is de facto constrained by the rigorous structure inherent in its TNM-based design. AJCC database analyses demonstrate several important predictors of survival not included in the current staging system.[9] Variables such as age, gender, primary tumor site, extent of microscopic tumor burden, and number of sites of distant metastases have been shown to have prognostic relevance. Tools that allow clinicians to incorporate these demographic and clinicopathologic data for a specific patient can ultimately yield personalized and ever more accurate estimates of recurrence and survival. As our understanding of the biology of melanoma as well as stage-specific prognostic factors continues to expand, greater emphasis on development and implementation of individualized patient prognostic models is essential to continue to improve patient care. An ideal system would incorporate state-of-the-art prognostic factor analyses, permit health care providers to remotely enter relevant data, and provide real-time feedback.

Recently, the first electronic predictive tool for patients with localized melanoma based on the large AJCC melanoma staging database was published.[67] Based on this model, an individual patient's 1-, 2-, 5-, and 10-year survival with associated 95% confidence intervals are available. Refined risk stratification schemata to allow for treatment and surveillance planning, selection of patients appropriate for clinical trials, and comparison of effectiveness of therapies for well-defined patient subgroups within trials is possible. An initial version of this model is available on the Internet (http://www.melanomaprognosis.org). Following on-screen prompts, data for patients with localized melanoma, as well as those with regional metastases, are entered using drop-down menus, and survival estimates are immediately displayed. This model serves as a template for providing patients and clinicians with prognostic information and as a foundation on which to plan future individualized treatment studies.

Molecular-Based Profiling and Melanoma Biomarkers

In the future, it is likely that molecular profiling endeavors will provide additional information pertinent to staging and prognosis for cutaneous melanoma. Recent developments in targeted therapies for patients with metastatic melanoma are certainly based on an improved understanding of disease biology at the molecular level.[68–73] Furthermore, studies attempting to provide "genetic signatures" for individual patients are under way and are beginning to shed light on the potential use of these techniques in prognostic models and treatment planning.[74–76] Of note, the nascent phase II effort of the National Institutes of Health (NIH) Cancer Genome Atlas Project (TCGA) specifically includes melanoma and will, it is hoped, provide invaluable insight into the molecular biology of melanoma in years to come. Further information regarding this exciting initiative can be found at http://cancergenome.nih.gov.

Biomarkers for melanoma identification, prediction of disease progression, prognosis, and treatment planning are lacking. Although serum LDH is part of the current staging system, it is nonspecific and cannot readily be used to evaluate response to therapy. Although a discussion of emerging melanoma biomarkers is beyond the scope of this article, identification of relevant biomarkers will likely contribute to enhanced prognostic assessment and potentially hasten clinical trial development and evaluation. It is hoped that this area of intense investigation will yield meaningful surrogates for selecting future therapies, for monitoring treatment response, and add to individualized prognostic modeling.

SUMMARY

The AJCC melanoma staging database forms the foundation for the current melanoma staging system; future analyses based on this robust platform will likely continue to serve as a foundation for future improvements in melanoma staging. As our understanding of the biology of this complex tumor system continues to evolve, both clinical and molecular factors that may have significant prognostic implications will undoubtedly be unveiled. Notable updates to melanoma staging published in the seventh edition of the AJCC melanoma staging system include: incorporation of mitotic rate into T1 criteria; inclusion of immunohistochemical detection of nodal micrometastases; and categorization of patients with melanoma of an unknown primary (ie, metastatic melanoma arising in the skin, subcutaneous tissue, or regional lymph nodes in a patient whose staging evaluation does not reveal other sites of disease) as stage III, rather than stage IV.

Based on the results of the AJCC melanoma staging database analysis, studies on future prognostic factors should evaluate the formal impact of mitotic rate across all stages of disease, further assess the influence of microscopic nodal tumor burden in patients with stage III disease in this era of SLN biopsy, and continue to refine staging and prognosis for patients with stage IV melanoma. Moreover, it is hoped that continued development and application of conditional survival estimates in melanoma patients, increased use of prognostic tools that incorporate relevant criteria beyond the scope of TNM-based staging, molecular profiling endeavors (including, for example, lessons learned from the nascent and ongoing NIH-sponsored TCGA, which specifically includes melanoma), and identification of melanoma-specific biomarkers will provide opportunities for more accurate staging and individualized prognosis for melanoma patients in the future.

REFERENCES

1. Balch CM, Murad TM, Soong SJ, et al. A multifactorial analysis of melanoma: prognostic histopathological features comparing Clark's and Breslow's staging methods. Ann Surg 1978;188:732.
2. Eldh J, Boeryd B, Peterson LE. Prognostic factors in cutaneous malignant melanoma in stage I. A clinical, morphological and multivariate analysis. Scand J Plast Reconstr Surg 1978;12:243.
3. Van Der Esch EP, Cascinelli N, Preda F, et al. Stage I melanoma of the skin: evaluation of prognosis according to histologic characteristics. Cancer 1981;48:1668.
4. Buzaid AC, Ross MI, Balch CM, et al. Critical analysis of the current American Joint Committee on Cancer staging system for cutaneous melanoma and proposal of a new staging system. J Clin Oncol 1997;15:1039.
5. Gershenwald JE, Buzaid AC, Ross MI. Classification and staging of melanoma. Hematol Oncol Clin North Am 1998;12:737.
6. Ross M. Modifying the criteria of the American Joint Commission on Cancer staging system in melanoma. Curr Opin Oncol 1998;10:153.
7. Thompson JF, Shaw HM, Hersey P, et al. The history and future of melanoma staging. J Surg Oncol 2004;86:224.
8. Balch CM. Melanoma of the skin. In: Edge SB, Byrd DR, Compton CC, et al, editors. AJCC cancer staging manual. 7th edition. New York: Springer Verlag; 2009. p. 325–44.
9. Balch CM, Gershenwald JE, Soong SJ, et al. Final version of 2009 AJCC melanoma staging and classification. J Clin Oncol 2009;27:6199.
10. Balch CM, Buzaid AC, Soong SJ, et al. Final version of the American Joint Committee on Cancer staging system for cutaneous melanoma. J Clin Oncol 2001;19:3635.
11. Balch CM, Soong SJ, Gershenwald JE, et al. Prognostic factors analysis of 17,600 melanoma patients: validation of the American Joint Committee on Cancer melanoma staging system. J Clin Oncol 2001;19:3622.
12. Cormier JN, Xing Y, Feng L, et al. Metastatic melanoma to lymph nodes in patients with unknown primary sites. Cancer 2006;106:2012.
13. Lee CC, Faries MB, Wanek LA, et al. Improved survival after lymphadenectomy for nodal metastasis from an unknown primary melanoma. J Clin Oncol 2008; 26:535.
14. Azzola MF, Shaw HM, Thompson JF, et al. Tumor mitotic rate is a more powerful prognostic indicator than ulceration in patients with primary cutaneous melanoma: an analysis of 3661 patients from a single center. Cancer 2003; 97:1488.
15. Barnhill RL, Katzen J, Spatz A, et al. The importance of mitotic rate as a prognostic factor for localized cutaneous melanoma. J Cutan Pathol 2005;32:268.
16. Busam KJ. The prognostic importance of tumor mitotic rate for patients with primary cutaneous melanoma. Ann Surg Oncol 2004;11:360.
17. Gimotty PA, Elder DE, Fraker DL, et al. Identification of high-risk patients among those diagnosed with thin cutaneous melanomas. J Clin Oncol 2007; 25:1129.
18. Breslow A. Thickness, cross-sectional areas and depth of invasion in the prognosis of cutaneous melanoma. Ann Surg 1970;172:902.

19. Balch CM, Soong S, Ross MI, et al. Long-term results of a multi-institutional randomized trial comparing prognostic factors and surgical results for intermediate thickness melanomas (1.0 to 4.0 mm). Intergroup melanoma surgical trial. Ann Surg Oncol 2000;7:87.

20. Breslow A, Cascinelli N, van der Esch EP, et al. Stage I melanoma of the limbs: assessment of prognosis by levels of invasion and maximum thickness. Tumori 1978;64:273.

21. Shaw HM, Balch CM, Soong SJ, et al. Prognostic histopathological factors in malignant melanoma. Pathology 1985;17:271.

22. Buttner P, Garbe C, Bertz J, et al. Primary cutaneous melanoma. Optimized cutoff points of tumor thickness and importance of Clark's level for prognostic classification. Cancer 1995;75:2499.

23. Balch CM, Wilkerson JA, Murad TM, et al. The prognostic significance of ulceration of cutaneous melanoma. Cancer 1980;45:3012.

24. McGovern VJ, Shaw HM, Milton GW, et al. Ulceration and prognosis in cutaneous malignant melanoma. Histopathology 1982;6:399.

25. Salman SM, Rogers GS. Prognostic factors in thin cutaneous malignant melanoma. J Dermatol Surg Oncol 1990;16:413.

26. Sondak VK, Taylor JM, Sabel MS, et al. Mitotic rate and younger age are predictors of sentinel lymph node positivity: lessons learned from the generation of a probabilistic model. Ann Surg Oncol 2004;11:247.

27. Caudle AS, Ross MI, Prieto VG, et al. Mitotic rate predicts sentinel lymph node involvement in melanoma: impact of the 7th edition AJCC melanoma staging system. In: Society of surgical oncology 63rd annual cancer symposium. St. Louis (MO); 2010. p. S8.

28. Clark WH Jr, From L, Bernardino EA, et al. The histogenesis and biologic behavior of primary human malignant melanomas of the skin. Cancer Res 1969;29:705.

29. Breslow A. Tumor thickness in evaluating prognosis of cutaneous melanoma. Ann Surg 1978;187:440.

30. Morton DL, Davtyan DG, Wanek LA, et al. Multivariate analysis of the relationship between survival and the microstage of primary melanoma by Clark level and Breslow thickness. Cancer 1993;71:3737.

31. Vollmer RT. Malignant melanoma. A multivariate analysis of prognostic factors. Pathol Annu 1989;24(Pt 1):383.

32. Gershenwald JE, Hwu P. Melanoma. In: Hong WK, Bast RC, Halit WN, et al, editors. Cancer medicine. 8th edition. Shelton (CT): People's Medical Publishing House-USA; 2010. p. 1459–86.

33. Buzaid AC, Anderson CM. The changing prognosis of melanoma. Curr Oncol Rep 2000;2:322.

34. Gershenwald JE, Colome MI, Lee JE, et al. Patterns of recurrence following a negative sentinel lymph node biopsy in 243 patients with stage I or II melanoma. J Clin Oncol 1998;16:2253.

35. Gershenwald JE, Fischer D, Buzaid AC. Clinical classification and staging. Clin Plast Surg 2000;27:361.

36. White RR, Stanley WE, Johnson JL, et al. Long-term survival in 2,505 patients with melanoma with regional lymph node metastasis. Ann Surg 2002;235:879.

37. Balch CM, Gershenwald JE, Soong SJ, et al. Multivariate analysis of prognostic factors among 2,313 patients with stage III melanoma: comparison of nodal micrometastases versus macrometastases. J Clin Oncol 2010;28:2452.

38. McMasters KM, Noyes RD, Reintgen DS, et al. Lessons learned from the sunbelt melanoma trial. J Surg Oncol 2004;86:212.
39. Morton DL, Thompson JF, Cochran AJ, et al. Sentinel-node biopsy or nodal observation in melanoma. N Engl J Med 2006;355:1307.
40. Scolyer RA, Murali R, Satzger I, et al. The detection and significance of melanoma micrometastases in sentinel nodes. Surg Oncol 2008;17:165.
41. Balch C, Soong S, Murad T, et al. A multifactorial analysis of melanoma: prognostic factors in melanoma patients with lymph node metastases (stage II). Ann Surg 1981;193:377.
42. Cascinelli N, Bufalino R, Marolda R, et al. Regional nonnodal metastases of cutaneous melanoma. Eur J Surg Oncol 1986;12:175.
43. Day CL Jr, Harrist TJ, Gorstein F, et al. Malignant melanoma. Prognostic significance of "microscopic satellites" in the reticular dermis and subcutaneous fat. Ann Surg 1981;194:108.
44. Leon P, Daly JM, Synnestvedt M, et al. The prognostic implications of microscopic satellites in patients with clinical stage I melanoma. Arch Surg 1991;126:1461.
45. Pawlik TM, Ross MI, Thompson JF, et al. The risk of in-transit melanoma metastasis depends on tumor biology and not the surgical approach to regional lymph nodes. J Clin Oncol 2005;23:4588.
46. Barth A, Wanek LA, Morton DL. Prognostic factors in 1,521 melanoma patients with distant metastases [see comment]. J Am Coll Surg 1995;181:193.
47. Manola J, Atkins M, Ibrahim J, et al. Prognostic factors in metastatic melanoma: a pooled analysis of Eastern Cooperative Oncology Group trials. J Clin Oncol 2000;18:3782.
48. Unger JM, Flaherty LE, Liu PY, et al. Gender and other survival predictors in patients with metastatic melanoma on Southwest Oncology Group trials. Cancer 2001;91:1148.
49. Eton O, Legha SS, Moon TE, et al. Prognostic factors for survival of patients treated systemically for disseminated melanoma. J Clin Oncol 1998;16:1103.
50. Ryan L, Kramar A, Borden E. Prognostic factors in metastatic melanoma. Cancer 1993;71:2995.
51. Bedikian AY, Johnson MM, Warneke CL, et al. Prognostic factors that determine the long-term survival of patients with unresectable metastatic melanoma. Cancer Invest 2008;26:624.
52. Keilholz U, Martus P, Punt CJ, et al. Prognostic factors for survival and factors associated with long-term remission in patients with advanced melanoma receiving cytokine-based treatments: second analysis of a randomised EORTC Melanoma Group trial comparing interferon-alpha2a (IFNalpha) and interleukin 2 (IL-2) with or without cisplatin. Eur J Cancer 2002;38:1501.
53. Sirott MN, Bajorin DF, Wong GY, et al. Prognostic factors in patients with metastatic malignant melanoma. A multivariate analysis. Cancer 1993;72:3091.
54. Balch CM. Cutaneous melanoma: prognosis and treatment results worldwide. Semin Surg Oncol 1992;8:400.
55. Staudt M, Lasithiotakis K, Leiter U, et al. Determinants of survival in patients with brain metastases from cutaneous melanoma. Br J Cancer 2010;102:1213.
56. Choi M, Fuller CD, Thomas CR Jr, et al. Conditional survival in ovarian cancer: results from the SEER dataset 1988-2001. Gynecol Oncol 2008;109:203.
57. Fuller CD, Wang SJ, Thomas CR Jr, et al. Conditional survival in head and neck squamous cell carcinoma: results from the SEER dataset 1973-1998. Cancer 2007;109:1331.

58. Henson DE, Ries LA, Carriaga MT. Conditional survival of 56,268 patients with breast cancer. Cancer 1995;76:237.
59. Kato I, Severson RK, Schwartz AG. Conditional median survival of patients with advanced carcinoma: surveillance, epidemiology, and end results data. Cancer 2001;92:2211.
60. Merrill RM, Bird JS. Effect of young age on prostate cancer survival: a population-based assessment (United States). Cancer Causes Control 2002;13:435.
61. Merrill RM, Henson DE, Ries LA. Conditional survival estimates in 34,963 patients with invasive carcinoma of the colon. Dis Colon Rectum 1998;41:1097.
62. Wang SJ, Emery R, Fuller CD, et al. Conditional survival in gastric cancer: a SEER database analysis. Gastric Cancer 2007;10:153.
63. Wang SJ, Fuller CD, Emery R, et al. Conditional survival in rectal cancer: a SEER database analysis. Gastrointest Cancer Res 2007;1:84.
64. Bowles TL, Xing Y, Hu CY, et al. Conditional survival estimates improve over 5 years for melanoma survivors with node-positive disease. Ann Surg Oncol 2010;17:2015.
65. Rueth NM, Groth SS, Tuttle TM, et al. Conditional survival after surgical treatment of melanoma: an analysis of the surveillance, epidemiology, and end results database. Ann Surg Oncol 2010;17:1662.
66. Xing Y, Chang GJ, Hu CY, et al. Conditional survival estimates improve over time for patients with advanced melanoma: results from a population-based analysis. Cancer 2010;116:2234.
67. Soong SJ, Ding S, Coit D, et al. Predicting survival outcome of localized melanoma: an electronic prediction tool based on the AJCC melanoma database. Ann Surg Oncol 2010;17:2006.
68. Hingorani SR, Jacobetz MA, Robertson GP, et al. Suppression of BRAF(V599E) in human melanoma abrogates transformation. Cancer Res 2003;63:5198.
69. Jiang X, Zhou J, Yuen NK, et al. Imatinib targeting of KIT-mutant oncoprotein in melanoma. Clin Cancer Res 2008;14:7726.
70. Sumimoto H, Miyagishi M, Miyoshi H, et al. Inhibition of growth and invasive ability of melanoma by inactivation of mutated BRAF with lentivirus-mediated RNA interference. Oncogene 2004;23:6031.
71. Bollag G, Hirth P, Tsai J, et al. Clinical efficacy of a RAF inhibitor needs broad target blockade in BRAF-mutant melanoma. Nature 2010;467:596–9.
72. Flaherty KT, Puzanov I, Kim KB, et al. Inhibition of mutated, activated BRAF in metastatic melanoma. N Engl J Med 2010;363:809.
73. Hodi FS, Friedlander P, Corless CL, et al. Major response to imatinib mesylate in KIT-mutated melanoma. J Clin Oncol 2008;26:2046.
74. Jonsson G, Busch C, Knappskog S, et al. Gene expression profiling-based identification of molecular subtypes in stage IV melanomas with different clinical outcome. Clin Cancer Res 2010;16:3356.
75. Philippidou D, Schmitt M, Moser D, et al. Signatures of microRNAs and selected microRNA target genes in human melanoma. Cancer Res 2010;70:4163.
76. Rother J, Jones D. Molecular markers of tumor progression in melanoma. Curr Genomics 2009;10:231.

Melanoma Pathology: Important Issues for Clinicians Involved in the Multidisciplinary Care of Melanoma Patients

Richard A. Scolyer, BMedSci, MBBS, MD, FRCPA, FRCPath[a,b,c,*],
Victor G. Prieto, MD, PhD[d,e]

KEYWORDS

- Diagnosis • Melanoma • Pathology • Prognosis
- Sentinel node, Staging • Biopsy • B-RAF
- Molecular pathology • Mutation

Pathology is a key aspect in the multidisciplinary care of patients with melanoma. The initial definitive diagnosis of primary melanoma is usually established by pathologic examination of a tissue biopsy. The pathologic assessment of various tumor parameters enables the most accurate estimation of prognosis in early clinical stages and determines the most appropriate next stages of further clinical management.[1–4] Pathologic assessment of any potential or likely metastasis is also critical.[5–9] To both reduce the risk of diagnostic error and to facilitate optimal patient management, it is important that clinicians are aware of potential pitfalls and limitations of pathologic

Sources of support: Professor Scolyer is a Cancer Institute New South Wales Clinical Research Fellow.
The investigators declare no conflicts of interest.
[a] Tissue Pathology and Diagnostic Oncology, Royal Prince Alfred Hospital, Missenden Road, Camperdown, Sydney, NSW 2050, Australia
[b] Discipline of Pathology, Central Clinical School, Sydney Medical School, The University of Sydney, Sydney, NSW 2006, Australia
[c] Melanoma Institute Australia, 40 Rocklands Road, North Sydney, NSW 2060, Australia
[d] Department of Pathology, University of Texas MD Anderson Cancer Center, 1515 Holcombe Boulevard, Unit 85, Houston, TX 77030, USA
[e] Department of Dermatology, University of Texas MD Anderson Cancer Center, 1515 Holcombe Boulevard, Unit 85, Houston, TX 77030, USA
* Corresponding author. Tissue Pathology and Diagnostic Oncology, Royal Prince Alfred Hospital, Missenden Road, Camperdown, Sydney NSW 2050, Australia.
E-mail address: richard.scolyer@sswahs.nsw.gov.au

assessment. In the past decade, new insights into the molecular pathogenesis of melanoma have been obtained and these are now being harnessed clinically to improve patient management.[10] For example, molecular pathology is now used to enhance melanoma diagnosis, classification, prognostication, and to predict responsiveness to novel promising selective targeted therapies for melanoma.

PATHOLOGIC DIAGNOSIS OF MELANOMA

Although melanoma may be strongly suspected from the clinical features of the tumor, definitive diagnosis requires pathologic examination of a tissue biopsy. Melanoma can usually be diagnosed accurately, rapidly, and reproducibly by routine pathology.[11,12] Pathologic diagnosis rests on balancing at least 20 architectural and cytologic features together with those of any host response and must be correlated with clinical features such as the age of the patient and anatomic site of the lesion.[13] A credible diagnosis requires accurate pathologic assessment, awareness of potential pitfalls, and the ability to make a logical and reasoned judgment from all the information available.

Accurate assessment and documentation of important pathologic variables critically influence the management of patients with melanoma.[14] However, of even greater importance is the need to accurately determine whether a cutaneous melanocytic lesion is benign or malignant (ie, a nevus or a melanoma).[15] For this reason, pathology reports of melanocytic lesions should (1) document the key criteria on which the diagnosis was based, and (2) provide the pathologic prognostic and other parameters important for patient management (**Box 1**).

Although the pathologic diagnosis of most melanocytic lesions is straightforward, there is a troublesome subset of cases for which it may be difficult to obtain a uniformly agreed diagnosis, even amongst melanoma pathology experts. Such diagnostically problematic melanocytic tumors include melanomas resembling Spitz nevi,[16–19] blue nevi,[20,21] deep penetrating nevi,[11] and combined nevi.[22,23] Also, there is a group of melanomas that display many features of standard, commonly acquired, or dysplastic benign nevi, the so-called nevoid melanoma, that often cause diagnostic problems.[11,24]

HOW TO BIOPSY A SUSPICIOUS PIGMENTED LESION: THE PATHOLOGISTS' PERSPECTIVE (INCLUDING THE LIMITATIONS OF PARTIAL BIOPSIES)

It is usually recommended that when a biopsy is taken from a primary skin lesion to confirm or exclude a diagnosis of melanoma, that an excision biopsy with narrow (2 mm) margins be performed, unless clinical reasons dictate otherwise.[4] Other types of biopsies, such as shave or punch biopsies, are not usually recommended because they are associated with an increased risk of misdiagnosis, primarily as a result of unrepresentative sampling of a heterogeneous lesion.[25] For example, melanoma may develop focally within a preexisting nevus (**Fig. 1A, B**). Thus, analysis of a partial biopsy of such a lesion that does not include the melanoma will inevitably be unable to diagnose malignancy. Furthermore, a partial biopsy may not provide sufficient tissue for adequate assessment of the pathologic criteria necessary to permit correct diagnosis. For instance, some of the important pathologic diagnostic criteria include features at the peripheral and deep aspects of the tumor (eg, circumscription, pattern of growth, and pagetoid upward migration at the periphery of the lesion), which may not be available in an incomplete biopsy.

Obviously, clinical features must also be taken into account when determining the most appropriate biopsy technique. For example, an excision biopsy may not be recommended for large lesions occurring on cosmetically or functionally sensitive anatomic sites such as the face, palms, or soles particularly when the clinical diagnosis is not certain (eg, in melanocytic lesions not appearing pigmented clinically or when the clinical suspicion of melanoma is very low). In such instances, partial biopsies may be the most appropriate method of establishing a diagnosis of melanoma. Similarly, punch biopsies may be used to map the extent of large melanocytic lesions (eg, on the face, digits, palms, or soles) to facilitate surgical planning for wide local excision. However, given the limitations of the specimen, it should be recognized that melanoma cannot be excluded by a negative partial biopsy and, if the clinical suspicion is high, a repeat biopsy may be indicated. Furthermore, if the pathologist considers that the specimen does not contain enough histologic evidence for a straightforward diagnosis of nevus or melanoma, a descriptive diagnosis of atypical melanocytic proliferation may be made, usually followed by a comment stating if a benign or malignant diagnosis is favored.

Highlighting the importance of the method of performing biopsies in melanocytic lesions, a recent study showed that histopathologic misdiagnosis is more common for melanomas that have been assessed with punch and shave biopsy than with excision biopsy.[26] Adverse outcomes caused by misdiagnosis were more commonly associated with punch biopsy than with shave and excision biopsy (odds ratio 16.6, $P<0.001$).[26]

Even when such incomplete biopsies allow a correct diagnosis of melanoma, they may provide inaccurate assessment of important pathologic features, such as Breslow thickness (**Fig. 2**). Accurate assessment of pathologic features of a primary melanoma allows prognosis to be reliably estimated; it also guides selection of appropriate management (width of excision margins, appropriateness of sentinel node biopsy, and so forth); thus inaccurate pathologic assessment can lead to inappropriate therapy.

Despite the problems and limitations of partial biopsies of melanocytic tumors, it should be emphasized that performing a suboptimal (partial) biopsy of a suspicious melanocytic tumor, although not ideal, at least allows an opportunity for a melanoma to be diagnosed at an earlier clinical stage of disease than if no biopsy was performed.

CLINICOPATHOLOGIC CORRELATION IMPROVES DIAGNOSTIC ACCURACY

The accuracy of the pathologic report may depend on the amount of tissue provided and the availability of relevant clinical details. It is particularly important to record factors that may induce atypical pathologic features in melanocytic nevi (eg, previous biopsy, trauma, surface irritation, pregnancy, topical treatment, and recent prolonged sunlight exposure) and may lead to a misdiagnosis of melanoma.[11] Other clinical factors relevant to diagnosis include patient age and sex, and the site of the lesion.[27]

Following lesional trauma, biopsy, irritation or topical treatment, melanocytic nevi may display many histologic features that commonly occur in melanomas (including pagetoid epidermal invasion, cytologic atypia, occasional dermal mitotic figures, and HMB-45 positivity) (**Fig. 3**).[28] Such regenerating nevi have been termed pseudomelanomas and are prone to over diagnosis as melanomas. Changes typically occur within 6 months of a previous injury, and the pathologic changes are confined to the area affected by the inciting agent. This may be a portion of a nevus in the case of trauma/irritation/biopsy, but it may also be the entire lesion in the case of topical treatment (or even trauma/irritation). Because the histologic changes of nevi or melanoma recurring after trauma may be similar, it is essential that the previous biopsy be reviewed. Another important consequence of trauma is that it may result in ulceration. Therefore, in most cases of reexcision of melanoma, it is difficult to determine if such

---

Box 1
Example of a synoptic or structured melanoma pathology report

Diagnostic summary

Excision of skin lesion from right arm: melanoma, AJCC (2010) pT3b, pNX, margins clear

Supporting information

Clinical

    Site and laterality: right arm

    Clinical diagnosis:? melanoma arising in a dysplastic nevus

    Specimen type: excision biopsy

    Previous treatment/trauma: nil known

    Previous melanoma: nil

    Distant metastasis: nil known

    Other medical history: none relevant

    Comment: suspicious area marked by suture

Macroscopic

    Size of specimen: 35 mm × 15 mm

    Description: an ellipse of skin, 35 mm × 15 mm, bearing an irregularly pigmented plaque 14 mm × 11 mm. This shows irregular margins with central ulceration. A central 3-mm area of increased pigmentation has been marked by a suture. The lesion is 2 mm from the nearest superficial margin.

    Other lesions: N/A

Microscopic

    Diagnosis: primary melanoma, invasive

    Tumor thickness: 2.3 mm

    Excision margins:

        Invasive, clear, 3.7 mm

        In situ, clear, 1.4 mm

        Deep, clear, 5.0 mm

    Ulceration (mm diameter): present (2.0 mm)

    Mitotic rate (/mm^2): 6

    Microsatellites: absent

    Level of invasion (Clark): IV

    Lymphovascular invasion: absent

    Tumor-infiltrating leucocytes:

        Distribution: focal

        Density: sparse

    Intermediate/late regression: absent

    Desmoplasia: absent

    Neurotropism: absent

    Associated benign nevus: dysplastic compound nevus

    Intraepidermal growth: mixed lentiginous and pagetoid

Subtype: superficial spreading

Description: the sections show skin and underlying subcutis with an asymmetric compound melanocytic tumor. The epidermal component shows lentiginous and focally nested growth of large epithelioid melanocytes with variable intracytoplasmic pigment. There is focal single-cell and nested pagetoid epidermal invasion by large atypical cells mainly in the central part of the tumor. The dermal component shows expansile asymmetrical growth, variable, mostly poor maturation and composed of cells with similar cytologic characteristics to those of the epidermal component. Multiple mitoses are present in dermal melanocytes including 2 mitoses near the deep edge of the tumor. There is an associated dysplastic compound nevus.

ulceration is spontaneous and should therefore be considered as a negative prognostic factor, or else be ignored (see also section on evaluation of reexcision specimens).

Nevi occurring on certain sites (including the palms, sole, fingers and toes, flexural sites, genitalia, the breast, and ear) often display irregular architecture (ie, asymmetry, single-cell growth, focal pagetoid migration) that would be considered evidence favoring melanoma in melanocytic tumors occurring on other sites.[27]

Excision specimens should be oriented if the status of specific surgical margins is critical in determining the need for, or extent of, further surgery. Specimen orientation may be indicated with marking sutures or other techniques. If a specimen is oriented, the orientation should be indicated on the specimen request form (and this may be facilitated by the use of a diagram).

Any clinically or dermatoscopically identified suspicious areas should be examined histopathologically, because they may represent melanoma (see **Fig. 1**). As an example, a long-standing lesion with a recent change in color or texture may suggest a melanoma developing within a preexisting nevus. Such areas should be identified, documented and marked for sectioning (eg, with a suture or by superficially scoring the epidermis and superficial dermis around the area of concern, using a suitably sized punch or other technique) to allow identification at the time of processing the tissue and reviewing the slides.

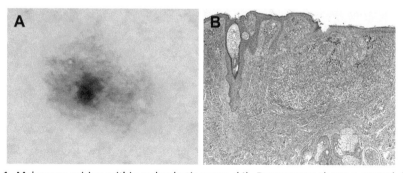

Fig. 1. Melanoma arising within a dysplastic nevus. (*A*). Dermoscopy shows a central dark focus (which represents the melanoma) within a variegated pigmented lesion (which represents a dysplastic nevus). (*Courtesy of* Professor Scott Menzies, Sydney, Australia.) (*B*). Histopathology shows the focus of melanoma (larger darkly pigmented cells involving the epidermis and dermis on the right-hand side of the image) with an underlying lymphoid infiltrate and adjacent nevus cells (smaller nonpigmented dermal cells on the left-hand side of the image).

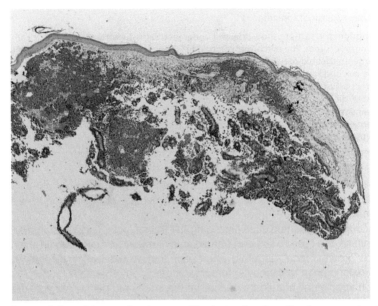

Fig. 2. Disrupted shave biopsy of melanoma. The lesion involves the deep margin of resection and thus an accurate Breslow thickness cannot be determined.

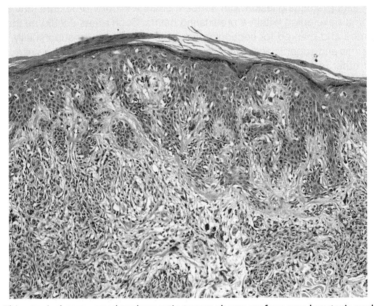

Fig. 3. This atypical compound melanocytic tumor shows surface parakeratosis and hyperkeratosis, which is suggestive of superficial irritation. There is also some upwards migration of melanocytes in the epidermis (pagetoid epidermal invasion). Although the latter is often a feature of melanoma, in this case it is most likely a reactive phenomenon secondary to surface irritation of a dysplastic compound nevus.

Clinical or other diagnostic imaging (eg, dermoscopy or confocal microscopy) or a diagram should be included with the clinical request form if this information is useful to direct the pathologist to areas of particular clinical concern in the specimen, or to improve clinicopathologic correlation. Photography can also be helpful when assessing clinically or dermoscopically heterogeneous lesions to direct the pathologist to areas of particular clinical concern.

TISSUE BANKING

In many melanoma treatment centers with active translational research programs, tissue samples from fresh specimens may be used for tissue banking or other research purposes. The decision to provide tissue should only be made if it is certain that the diagnostic process and pathologic evaluation will not be compromised. After close examination, the pathologist, in consultation with the clinician, is the most appropriate person to make this decision. As a safeguard, research use of the specimen should be deferred until the diagnostic process is complete. If there are any diagnostic problems (eg, it is difficult to determine whether a lesion is nevus or melanoma), the portion of the specimen that had been reserved for research can be retrieved and used for diagnostic purposes.

MELANOMA HISTOPATHOLOGIC PROGNOSTIC FACTORS

The histologic analysis of primary melanoma provides important prognostic information that is also critically important in directing patient further management such as the width of further excision margins and the appropriateness of sentinel lymph node (SLN) biopsy. The prognosis for a patient with clinically localized primary cutaneous melanoma is principally correlated with its vertical depth of tumor growth (Breslow thickness) (**Fig. 4**).[1,2] However, other factors are also important such as its dermal

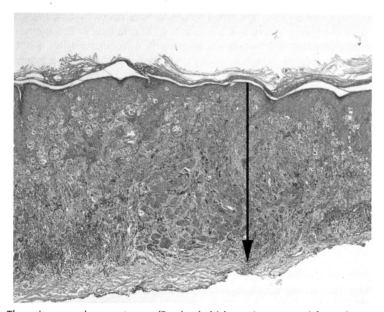

Fig. 4. The primary melanoma tumor (Breslow) thickness is measured from the top of the epidermal granular layer to the deepest dermal invasive cell (*arrow*).

mitotic rate, the presence of ulceration, Clark level of invasion, and anatomic location, as well as patient characteristics, such as sex and age.[29–32] It is important that all relevant histologic features are described in the pathology report to allow the most accurate estimate of prognosis to be made and an appropriate management plan prepared. A structured or synoptic reporting format can facilitate this (see **Box 1**).[33–35]

HISTOLOGICALLY AMBIGUOUS OR BORDERLINE MELANOCYTIC TUMORS

Many histologic features are common to both nevi and melanomas.[36] Furthermore, no single pathologic criterion is generally diagnostic of either a nevus or melanoma. For these reasons, in some instances, as discussed earlier, it may not be possible for a pathologist to be certain from histologic assessment of a tissue biopsy whether a melanocytic tumor is benign or malignant. Such lesions are sometimes referred to as histologically ambiguous or borderline melanocytic tumors because they display some features favoring nevus and others favoring melanoma. Some pathologists report these lesions as melanocytic tumor of uncertain malignant potential (MELTUMP). Although this is not a diagnosis per se, it is a useful term for conveying the diagnostic uncertainty to both the treating clinician and the patient.

Probably the most common and well-documented example of histologically ambiguous melanocytic tumors are those displaying some, but not all, features of Spitz nevus (**Fig. 5**A, B). The lack of consensus regarding the diagnosis of such difficult cases and the difficulty in predicting their biologic behavior from histopathologic assessment are well documented in the literature.[16–18]

Our recommended approach to the histopathologic reporting of histologically ambiguous melanocytic tumors is to present the evidence in favor of and against a particular diagnosis, and to render a preferred diagnosis, while acknowledging the degree of uncertainty. It is also probably prudent to seek opinions from 1 or more experienced colleagues. Analysis of the primary tumor by molecular techniques such as comparative genomic hybridization (CGH) or fluorescence in situ hybridization (FISH) has the potential to provide useful additional information that may assist in classifying it as a melanoma if multiple chromosomal aberrations or melanoma-specific mutations are detected.[37–40] However, at present, molecular testing is not always definitive and the lack of detection of any chromosomal or genetic abnormalities is

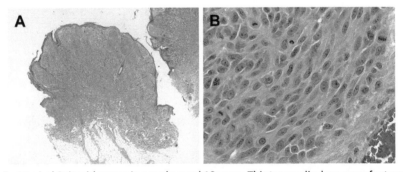

Fig. 5. Atypical Spitzoid tumor in a male aged 16 years. This tumor displays some features of a benign tumor and other features raising the possibility of melanoma. It is not possible to predict with certainty how it will behave clinically purely from its histologic features. (*A*) The low-power silhouette of the lesion shows a symmetric polypoid nodule (a feature usually associated with benign melanocytic tumors). (*B*) At high magnification the tumor includes numerous mitoses.

not conclusive evidence that a lesion is benign. Furthermore, these tests require further independent validation and are not widely available at present.

Complete excision of ambiguous lesions is probably mandatory, but plans for further management should be formulated on case-by-case basis. Although the safest course of action will usually be to manage the tumor as if it were a melanoma (taking into account the tumor's thickness and other prognostic variables), this may not always be appropriate, particularly if it is located in a cosmetically sensitive site such as the face. In some cases, it may be appropriate for the surgical oncologist to convey the diagnostic uncertainty to patients and to present them with management choices so that they can decide whether they wish to be managed aggressively (as for a melanoma) or conservatively. An SLN biopsy (see also later discussion) may be recommended from the primary tumor characteristics, but the clinical significance of lymph node involvement for these tumors is not yet clear, and it may not have the same prognostic implications as nodal involvement from an unequivocal conventional melanoma.[16,41–45] In patients with apparently clinically localized primary cutaneous MELTUMPs, identifying the SLNs by lymphoscintigraphy for subsequent close monitoring by clinical examination and ultrasound may offer an alternative, noninvasive strategy that may allow early detection of growing metastases.[46]

PATHOLOGIC ASSESSMENT OF WIDE EXCISION SPECIMENS

When a diagnosis of melanoma is established, it usually requires a reexcision to ensure that the entire lesion is removed, primarily with the intention of reducing the risk of local recurrence. The extent of the subsequent excision varies according to the diagnosis (ie, dysplastic nevus, melanoma in situ, invasive melanoma). In general, most authorities recommend a 0.5 cm margin (measured clinically) from the periphery of the lesion for melanoma in situ, a 1 cm margin for invasive melanoma less than 1.0 mm in thickness, a 1- to 2-cm margin for melanomas 1 to 2 mm in thickness, and a 2-cm margin for melanomas greater then 2.0 mm in thickness.[47] However, it is important to emphasize that these margins are merely recommendations, because the surgery should be tailored to a particular patient balancing the risk of recurrence with the likely surgical morbidity/cosmetic sequelae. For instance, a thin melanoma on the face close to the eyelid may be most appropriately managed with a margin less than 1 cm (see also article by Berman elsewhere in this issue).

The skin surface and cut surfaces of wide excision specimens should be examined for macroscopic evidence of residual tumor, and then serially sectioned into 2- to 3-mm slices. If the melanoma was completely excised and had no unusual features (eg, desmoplasia or neurotropism) in the original biopsy, and there is no suspicion of residual tumor on visual inspection, then it is probably sufficient to submit only 1 or 2 slices from the center of the scar for microscopic examination. Another option is to submit entirely the scar area and only sample the margins. It is our experience that both methods provide similar rates of additional histologic findings in reexcision specimens.[33]

If the melanoma includes a desmoplastic component or shows neurotropism, the entire scar area should be blocked for microscopic examination. The evaluation of surgical margins and identification of residual desmoplastic melanoma in reexcision specimens can be very difficult. As desmoplastic melanomas are typically characterized by a relatively hypocellular proliferation of mildly atypical cells, small clusters of tumor cells may be difficult to distinguish from myofibroblastic cells in scar tissue. Furthermore, they can show very subtle perineural involvement. In such cases, immunohistochemical studies may be very helpful because the areas of tumor will usually strongly express S-100 protein in most cells, in contrast with scar tissue, in which only a few spindle cells (Schwann cells, dendritic cells, and possibly some myofibroblasts) will express S-100 protein.[48] Desmoplastic melanomas are almost invariably negative for more specific melanoma markers such as HMB-45 or melanA/MART-1, and hence these immunostains are generally unhelpful in this clinical setting.

The histologic examination of the reexcision specimen requires analysis of surgical margins and detection of residual melanoma. At our institutions, in order to avoid possible errors in interpretation, the pathology report may not contain a full pathology template but rather the presence or absence of melanoma, its Breslow thickness, the margin status, and any pathology findings worse than those seen in the original biopsy; for example, mitotic index if the reexcision specimen has a higher value than the original specimen, presence of perineural invasion if this was not seen in the original biopsy.

SLNs

Since the early 1990s, many clinicians have been routinely evaluating SLNs for the early staging of several solid malignancies, including melanoma.[49] For pathologic assessment of SLNs, most techniques usually use multiple formalin-fixed, paraffin-embedded sections for both routine histology and immunohistochemistry (**Fig. 6**A, B), although some research protocols have used additional techniques such as polymerase chain reaction (PCR) to detect melanoma-associated tumor products or antigens.[44,50] Approximately 20% of patients with cutaneous melanoma who undergo SLN biopsy are found to harbor metastasis in their SLN.[45]

From the point of view of pathologists, an important advantage of SLN biopsy is that it allows a more intense examination of a single or small number of SLNs, in a manner that would not be feasible to perform for all the lymph nodes retrieved in a routine, regional lymphadenectomy specimen (the latter is usually examined with a single hematoxylin and eosin (H&E) stained slide per cassette compared with the multiple H&E and immunohistochemically stained sections examined for SLNs). Some current studies are evaluating the possible therapeutic value of removal of positive SLN in patients with cutaneous melanoma.[51] At the present time, most authorities accept that detection of a positive SLN conveys an impaired prognosis and thus helps in more accurately staging patients with melanoma and providing more accurate risk stratification for patients groups in clinical trials.[45,51,52]

Criteria for Recommendation of Sentinel Lymphadenectomy

Most protocols recommend SLN examination in patients with melanoma with Breslow thickness of 1 mm or more, or if less than 1 mm, if the primary tumor is ulcerated, or

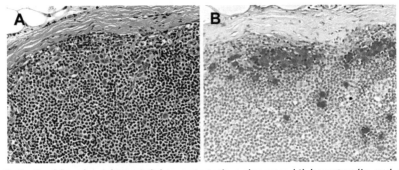

Fig. 6. Sentinel lymph node containing metastatic melanoma: (A) hematoxylin and eosin stain; (B) S-100 protein immunostain.

shows Clark level IV invasion.[51] The latter criterion has been replaced in the seventh edition (2010) of the American Joint Committee on Cancer (AJCC) staging system in favor of mitotic rate (see also article by Gershenwald and Dickson in this issue). At our institutions, other clinicopathologic elements that have been incorporated into the decision-making process on whether to perform SLN biopsy include vertical growth phase (in particular those cases with dermal mitotic figures), vascular invasion (particularly highlighted with anti-D2-40),[53] satellitosis and patient age less than 40 years old. Paucity of lymphocytic infiltrate may be associated with a higher positivity rate of SLN but it is unclear if regression correlates with higher rate of positive SLN. Pure desmoplastic melanomas are associated with a very low SLN metastatic risk[54] (in contrast to mixed-type desmoplastic melanomas, which have an SLN risk similar to nondesmoplastic melanoma). As a consequence, pure desmoplastic melanomas are not considered for SLN biopsy in some melanoma treatment centers.[55] (For additional discussion, see the article by Ross elsewhere in this issue).

Processing of SLNs

Frozen sections usually provide suboptimal morphology and may lack the subcapsular region of the lymph node (the area most likely involved in small metastases).[56,57] Also, processing of the frozen tissue requires additional sectioning and micrometastases may be lost in the discarded unexamined sections. Therefore, for SLNs from patients with melanoma, most protocols consider the examination of routinely processed material (formalin-fixed, paraffin-embedded) as the gold standard.[58] A possible alternative is touch preparations/cytologic specimens and these seem to provide accurate and cost effective SLN assessment in some specialized centers.[43]

Regarding the grossing technique of SLN, it was initially recommended that SLNs be bivalved through the hilum because it was suggested the metastases were more likely to occur in the peripheral sinuses of the central meridian of the SLN.[59,60] At our institutions, we now recommend bread-loafing of the SLN to allow examination of a larger area of the subcapsular region. Pathologists should examine multiple H&E and immunohistochemically stained sections from each SLN, but it is unclear from the currently available evidence what constitutes the most appropriate sectioning and staining protocol. Relevant factors to consider include the accuracy of the procedure, the time, labor, and costs involved, and clinical follow-up data, which are likely to vary between institutions; hence individual protocols should be developed locally by pathologists in consultation with their surgical colleagues. Most current protocols require more than 1 H&E section, usually with the addition of immunohistochemistry. The optimal number of sections to examine and the interval/depth/distance between them is not uniformly agreed at the present time. However, it is well documented that immunohistochemistry for melanoma-associated antigens such as S-100 protein, HMB-45, anti-MART1, and anti-tyrosinase, increases the detection of melanoma metastases and most protocols recommend using a combination of these antibodies.[44] To increase sensitivity, some clinical trials use a portion of the SLN for PCR analysis to try to detect mRNA associated with melanocytic differentiation.

Microscopic Features

Metastatic melanoma cells may display a large variety of morphologies (ie, epithelioid or spindled, pigmented or amelanotic),[61–63] but most commonly, metastatic melanoma cells resemble the cells of the primary tumor.[64] Although the pathologic diagnosis of melanoma SLN metastasis is usually straightforward, in some problematic cases in which there is uncertainty as to whether or not a melanoma metastasis is present it may be very helpful to study the original primary melanoma, to compare the morphologic features with any suspicious cells seen in the SLN.

In general, melanoma cells in the SLN are most commonly located in the subcapsular sinus of the SLN, as single cells, small nests, or large expansile clusters. Less frequently, the metastasis is intraparenchymal and such metastases may occur with or without subcapsular deposits. In less than 5% of cases there is extracapsular extension into the perinodal fibroadipose tissues. Immunohistochemical studies are helpful when trying to detect small metastatic deposits and sometimes to differentiate metastasis from benign, capsular nevus cells.[65]

SLN Tumor Burden

We recommend that the pathology report should document the number of positive nodes and the total number of SLNs removed, both spelled out and as numbers to avoid possible typographical errors (eg, melanoma metastasis in one of three lymph nodes [1/3]) (**Table 1**).

Quantification of melanoma metastasis size in SLN correlates with subsequent involvement of non-SLNs from the same anatomic region and with prognosis.[66–69] If there are only a few metastatic cells in the subcapsular sinus of the sentinel node, the prognosis is good and the chance of finding additional metastatic disease in a completion lymph node dissection (CLND) specimen is extremely small.[70,71] If, on the other hand, there are multiple large foci of tumor that extend deeply into the central part of the SLN, the prognosis is much worse, and the chance of finding metastases in non-SLNs in a CLND specimen is high.[68,69,72] However, it remains unclear which particular method of assessment of SLN tumor burden or other micromorphometric parameters of melanoma deposits in SLNs accurately predict the probability of non-SLN involvement and prognosis. Some investigators recommend measuring the so-called tumor penetrative depth (measurement of the distance between the capsule and the most deeply located deposit).[67,72] Other important measures of tumor burden in the SLN

Table 1	
An example of a template for the microscopic pathology reporting of positive sentinel nodes in melanoma patients	
Feature	**Description**
Anatomic site of sentinel node	Left axilla
No. of tumor foci	2
Intranodal compartment(s) involved by tumor	Subcapsular sinus and parenchyma
Maximum dimension of largest deposit (mm)	2.65
Maximum tumor penetrative depth (mm)	0.57
% cross-sectional area of sentinel node involved by tumor	15
Extranodal spread	Absent
Immunophenotype of tumor	
S-100	+++ (nuclear and cytoplasmic)
HMB-45	++ (patchy)
MelanA	+++ (strong and diffuse)
Nodal nevus cells	Present (capsular)
Other comments	Nil

Abbreviations: +++, strong positivity; ++, moderate positivity.

include the size of the largest tumor deposit (in 2 dimensions, in millimeters), the location (subcapsular vs other), and presence or absence of extracapsular extension (see **Table 1**).[67,68,72] It is controversial whether there is a minimal tumor burden below which melanoma patients can be safely spared further treatment.[70,71] Unlike breast carcinomas, in which SLN with tumor deposits smaller than 0.2 mm are not considered positive by some investigators, it seems likely that even melanoma metastases less than 0.2 mm in maximum size may be associated with an adverse clinical outcome in some patients.[73,74]

Regarding additional techniques, some studies have indicated that PCR detection of melanocytic mRNA in SLN correlates with decreased survival but other studies have not found such a correlation.[75–80] A possible explanation for these differences may be the presence of nodal nevi in some SLN, because these deposits could result in positive PCR results. Therefore, unless mRNA specific for melanoma cells is available, it seems likely that histologic examination will remain the gold standard for detecting melanoma metastasis in SLN.

MOLECULAR PATHOLOGY

The role of molecular pathology in diagnosis and management of melanoma patients has rapidly expanded in recent years and is likely to become even more important as an era of personalized medicine evolves. As discussed earlier, molecular techniques such as CGH and FISH have the potential to assist in the classification of histologically ambiguous primary melanocytic tumors.[37,39,40] With the recent development and testing of new promising targeted therapies for patients with metastatic melanoma, molecular pathology mutation testing for BRAF and c-KIT has become common in many melanoma treatment centers.[81–83]

CGH and FISH Analysis of Primary Melanocytic Tumors

Recent studies evaluating chromosomal aberrations of melanocytic tumors using CGH have shown that melanomas usually harbor numerous chromosomal aberrations, whereas such aberrations are rare in nevi.[37] In view of these findings, attempts have been made to use CGH to assist in accurate classification of melanocytic tumors, particularly for primary cutaneous melanocytic tumors in which the histopathologic features alone do not permit clear characterization as benign or malignant. However, because CGH is a laborious and time-consuming technique that requires expensive technology, at the present time it is only readily accessible as an approved supplementary diagnostic method in a few specialized centers.

An alternative technique for the study of chromosomal aberrations in tumors that can be more readily used in routine pathologic practice is FISH. In contrast to CGH, in which the DNA is extracted from tumor samples and analyzed, FISH allows direct visualization of quantitative genetic alterations within individual tumor cells, and thereby permits the pathologist to analyze a pure tumor population. Results validating the use of this technique both to distinguish between nevi and melanomas and to classify histologically problematic melanocytic tumors have been reported recently.[39,40,84–87] Once validated in larger studies, this technique may become a supplementary diagnostic test in the assessment of problematic melanocytic tumors.

Mutation Testing

Molecular testing of melanocytic tumors also has the potential to identify subgroups of tumors with specific genetic signatures that may accurately predict their likely clinical course and/or response to treatment.

An interesting finding of recently reported molecular studies is the confirmation that the long-used traditional clinicopathologic classification of melanomas (ie, lentigo maligna, superficial spreading, and acral lentiginous melanomas) correlates with the genetic findings.[88] Thus, lesions with prominent solar damage (lentigo maligna) commonly harbor NRAS and sometimes c-KIT mutations,[89] whereas superficial spreading melanomas from intermittently sun-exposed areas often have BRAF mutations. Furthermore, these finding have important clinical repercussions for targeted therapy (see the next paragraph, and for additional discussion, see the article by Davies and Gershenwald elsewhere in this issue).

Activation of the mitogen-activated protein kinase pathway is present in most melanomas, and pharmacologic inhibition, especially of oncogenic BRAF, is a promising strategy for treating melanoma.[81,90–92] In phase I/II trials of highly specific mutant-BRAF inhibitors, partial and complete responses were seen in 80% of patients with mutant-BRAF metastatic melanoma, with a progression-free survival of 8 months.[81] Although much less common, activating c-KIT mutations or amplifications in melanomas (usually occurring in mucosal or acral lentiginous primary melanomas) have been identified that have also been associated with dramatic therapeutic responses to c-KIT inhibitors in patients with widespread metastases.[91,93] This exciting field of pathology promises to expand exponentially and will likely result in additional therapies.

ACKNOWLEDGMENTS

The authors gratefully acknowledge the support of their colleagues at Melanoma Institute Australia, Tissue Pathology and Diagnostic Oncology, Royal Prince Alfred Hospital, Sydney, Australia and the Departments of Pathology, Dermatology, Surgical Oncology, and Medical Oncology, University of Texas MD Anderson Cancer Center, Houston, TX, USA. Critical review of the manuscript by Dr Jeffrey Gershenwald and accompanying helpful suggestions were also much appreciated.

REFERENCES

1. Balch CM, Gershenwald JE, Soong SJ, et al. Final version of 2009 AJCC melanoma staging and classification. J Clin Oncol 2009;27:6199.
2. Gershenwald JE, Soong SJ, Balch CM. 2010 TNM staging system for cutaneous melanoma and beyond. Ann Surg Oncol 2010;17:1475.
3. Soong SJ, Ding S, Coit D, et al. Predicting survival outcome of localized melanoma: an electronic prediction tool based on the AJCC Melanoma Database. Ann Surg Oncol 2006;17.
4. Thompson JF, Scolyer RA, Kefford RF. Cutaneous melanoma. Lancet 2005;365:687.
5. Doubrovsky A, Scolyer RA, Murali R, et al. Diagnostic accuracy of fine needle biopsy for metastatic melanoma and its implications for patient management. Ann Surg Oncol 2008;15:323.
6. Murali R, Doubrovsky A, Watson GF, et al. Diagnosis of metastatic melanoma by fine-needle biopsy: analysis of 2,204 cases. Am J Clin Pathol 2007;127:385.
7. Murali R, Loughman NT, McKenzie PR, et al. Cytologic features of metastatic and recurrent melanoma in patients with primary cutaneous desmoplastic melanoma. Am J Clin Pathol 2008;130:715.
8. Murali R, Loughman NT, McKenzie PR, et al. Cytological features of melanoma in exfoliative fluid specimens. J Clin Pathol 2009;62:638.

9. Murali R, Thompson JF, Uren RF, et al. Fine-needle biopsy of metastatic melanoma: clinical use and new applications. Lancet Oncol 2010;11:391.
10. Thompson JF, Scolyer RA, Kefford RF. Cutaneous melanoma in the era of molecular profiling. Lancet 2009;374:362.
11. McCarthy SW, Scolyer RA. Melanocytic lesions of the face: diagnostic pitfalls. Ann Acad Med Singapore 2004;33:3.
12. Shea CR, Prieto VG. Recent developments in the pathology of melanocytic neoplasia. Dermatol Clin 1999;17:615.
13. Scolyer RA, McCarthy SW, Elder DE. Frontiers in melanocytic pathology. Pathology 2004;36:385.
14. Thompson JF, Scolyer RA. Cooperation between surgical oncologists and pathologists: a key element of multidisciplinary care for patients with cancer. Pathology 2004;36:496.
15. Scolyer RA, Thompson JF, Stretch JR, et al. Pathology of melanocytic lesions: new, controversial, and clinically important issues. J Surg Oncol 2004;86:200.
16. Busam KJ, Murali R, Pulitzer M, et al. Atypical spitzoid melanocytic tumors with positive sentinel lymph nodes in children and teenagers, and comparison with histologically unambiguous and lethal melanomas. Am J Surg Pathol 2009;33:1386.
17. Crotty KA, Scolyer RA, Li L, et al. Spitz naevus versus Spitzoid melanoma: when and how can they be distinguished? Pathology 2002;34:6.
18. Dahlstrom JE, Scolyer RA, Thompson JF, et al. Spitz naevus: diagnostic problems and their management implications. Pathology 2004;36:452.
19. Paradela S, Fonseca E, Pita S, et al. Spitzoid melanoma in children: clinicopathological study and application of immunohistochemistry as an adjunct diagnostic tool. J Cutan Pathol 2009;36:740.
20. Barnhill RL, Argenyi Z, Berwick M, et al. Atypical cellular blue nevi (cellular blue nevi with atypical features): lack of consensus for diagnosis and distinction from cellular blue nevi and malignant melanoma ("malignant blue nevus"). Am J Surg Pathol 2008;32:36.
21. Murali R, McCarthy SW, Scolyer RA. Blue nevi and related lesions: a review highlighting atypical and newly described variants, distinguishing features and diagnostic pitfalls. Adv Anat Pathol 2009;16:365.
22. Murali R, McCarthy SW, Thompson JF, et al. Melanocytic nevus with focal atypical epithelioid components (clonal nevus) is a combined nevus. J Am Acad Dermatol 2007;56:889.
23. Scolyer RA, Zhuang L, Palmer AA, et al. Combined naevus: a benign lesion frequently misdiagnosed both clinically and pathologically as melanoma. Pathology 2004;36:419.
24. Harris GR, Shea CR, Horenstein MG, et al. Desmoplastic (sclerotic) nevus: an underrecognized entity that resembles dermatofibroma and desmoplastic melanoma. Am J Surg Pathol 1999;23:786.
25. Scolyer RA, Thompson JF, McCarthy SW, et al. Incomplete biopsy of melanocytic lesions can impair the accuracy of pathological diagnosis. Australas J Dermatol 2006;47:71.
26. Ng JC, Swain S, Dowling JP, et al. The impact of partial biopsy on histopathologic diagnosis of cutaneous melanoma: experience of an Australian tertiary referral service. Arch Dermatol 2010;146:234.
27. Khalifeh I, Taraif S, Reed JA, et al. A subgroup of melanocytic nevi on the distal lower extremity (ankle) shares features of acral nevi, dysplastic nevi, and melanoma in situ: a potential misdiagnosis of melanoma in situ. Am J Surg Pathol 2007;31:1130.

28. Adeniran AJ, Prieto VG, Chon S, et al. Atypical histologic and immunohistochemical findings in melanocytic nevi after liquid nitrogen cryotherapy. J Am Acad Dermatol 2009;61:341.

29. Azzola MF, Shaw HM, Thompson JF, et al. Tumor mitotic rate is a more powerful prognostic indicator than ulceration in patients with primary cutaneous melanoma: an analysis of 3661 patients from a single center. Cancer 2003;97:1488.

30. Francken AB, Shaw HM, Thompson JF, et al. The prognostic importance of tumor mitotic rate confirmed in 1317 patients with primary cutaneous melanoma and long follow-up. Ann Surg Oncol 2004;11:426.

31. Murali R, Hughes MT, Fitzgerald P, et al. Interobserver variation in the histopathologic reporting of key prognostic parameters, particularly Clark level, affects pathologic staging of primary cutaneous melanoma. Ann Surg 2009; 249:641.

32. Scolyer RA, Shaw HM, Thompson JF, et al. Interobserver reproducibility of histopathologic prognostic variables in primary cutaneous melanomas. Am J Surg Pathol 2003;27:1571.

33. Frishberg DP, Balch C, Balzer BL, et al. Protocol for the examination of specimens from patients with melanoma of the skin. Arch Pathol Lab Med 2009;133:1560.

34. Haydu LE, Holt PE, Karim RZ, et al. Quality of histopathological reporting on melanoma and influence of use of a synoptic template. Histopathology 2010; 56:768.

35. Karim RZ, van den Berg KS, Colman MH, et al. The advantage of using a synoptic pathology report format for cutaneous melanoma. Histopathology 2008;52:130.

36. Rothberg BE, Moeder CB, Kluger H, et al. Nuclear to non-nuclear Pmel17/gp100 expression (HMB45 staining) as a discriminator between benign and malignant melanocytic lesions. Mod Pathol 2008;21:1121.

37. Bastian BC. Molecular cytogenetics as a diagnostic tool for typing melanocytic tumors. Recent Results Cancer Res 2002;160:92.

38. Bauer J, Bastian BC. Distinguishing melanocytic nevi from melanoma by DNA copy number changes: comparative genomic hybridization as a research and diagnostic tool. Dermatol Ther 2006;19:40.

39. Gerami P, Jewell SS, Morrison LE, et al. Fluorescence in situ hybridization (FISH) as an ancillary diagnostic tool in the diagnosis of melanoma. Am J Surg Pathol 2009;33:1146.

40. Morey AL, Murali R, McCarthy SW, et al. Diagnosis of cutaneous melanocytic tumours by four-colour fluorescence in situ hybridisation. Pathology 2009;41:383.

41. Mandal RV, Murali R, Lundquist KF, et al. Pigmented epithelioid melanocytoma: favorable outcome after 5-year follow-up. Am J Surg Pathol 2009;33:1778.

42. Murali R, Sharma RN, Thompson JF, et al. Sentinel lymph node biopsy in histologically ambiguous melanocytic tumors with spitzoid features (so-called atypical spitzoid tumors). Ann Surg Oncol 2008;15:302.

43. Murali R, Thompson JF, Scolyer RA. Sentinel lymph node biopsy for melanoma: aspects of pathologic assessment. Future Oncol 2008;4:535.

44. Scolyer RA, Murali R, McCarthy SW, et al. Pathologic examination of sentinel lymph nodes from melanoma patients. Semin Diagn Pathol 2008;25:100.

45. Scolyer RA, Murali R, Satzger I, et al. The detection and significance of melanoma micrometastases in sentinel nodes. Surg Oncol 2008;17:165.

46. Sanki A, Uren RF, Moncrieff M, et al. Targeted high-resolution ultrasound is not an effective substitute for sentinel lymph node biopsy in patients with primary cutaneous melanoma. J Clin Oncol 2009;27:5614.

47. Sladden MJ, Balch C, Barzilai DA, et al. Surgical excision margins for primary cutaneous melanoma. Cochrane Database Syst Rev 2009;4:CD004835.
48. Ivan D, Prieto VG. Use of immunohistochemistry in the diagnosis of melanocytic lesions: applications and pitfalls. Future Oncol 2010;6(7):1163–75.
49. Thompson JF, Stretch JR, Uren RF, et al. Sentinel node biopsy for melanoma: where have we been and where are we going? Ann Surg Oncol 2004;11:147S.
50. Chakera AH, Hesse B, Burak Z, et al. EANM-EORTC general recommendations for sentinel node diagnostics in melanoma. Eur J Nucl Med Mol Imaging 2009;36:1713.
51. Morton DL, Thompson JF, Cochran AJ, et al. Sentinel-node biopsy or nodal observation in melanoma. N Engl J Med 2006;355:1307.
52. Rousseau DL Jr, Ross MI, Johnson MM, et al. Revised American Joint Committee on Cancer staging criteria accurately predict sentinel lymph node positivity in clinically node-negative melanoma patients. Ann Surg Oncol 2003;10:569.
53. Petersson F, Diwan AH, Ivan D, et al. Immunohistochemical detection of lymphovascular invasion with D2-40 in melanoma correlates with sentinel lymph node status, metastasis and survival. J Cutan Pathol 2009;36:1157.
54. Murali R, Shaw HM, Lai K, et al. Prognostic factors in cutaneous desmoplastic melanoma: a study of 252 patients. Cancer 2010;116:4130.
55. Pawlik TM, Ross MI, Prieto VG, et al. Assessment of the role of sentinel lymph node biopsy for primary cutaneous desmoplastic melanoma. Cancer 2006;106:900.
56. Prieto VG. Use of frozen sections in the examination of sentinel lymph nodes in patients with melanoma. Semin Diagn Pathol 2008;25:112.
57. Scolyer RA, Thompson JF, McCarthy SW, et al. Intraoperative frozen-section evaluation can reduce accuracy of pathologic assessment of sentinel nodes in melanoma patients. J Am Coll Surg 2005;201:821.
58. Prieto VG, Clark SH. Processing of sentinel lymph nodes for detection of metastatic melanoma. Ann Diagn Pathol 2002;6:257.
59. Cochran AJ, Balda BR, Starz H, et al. The Augsburg Consensus. Techniques of lymphatic mapping, sentinel lymphadenectomy, and completion lymphadenectomy in cutaneous malignancies. Cancer 2000;89:236.
60. Cochran AJ, Essner R, Rose DM, et al. Principles of sentinel lymph node identification: background and clinical implications. Langenbecks Arch Surg 2000;385:252.
61. Prieto VG, Kanik A, Salob S, et al. Primary cutaneous myxoid melanoma: immunohistologic clues to a difficult diagnosis. J Am Acad Dermatol 1994;30:335.
62. Prieto VG, Woodruff JM. Expression of HMB45 antigen in spindle cell melanoma. J Cutan Pathol 1997;24:580.
63. Ruhoy SM, Prieto VG, Eliason SL, et al. Malignant melanoma with paradoxical maturation. Am J Surg Pathol 2000;24:1600.
64. Plaza JA, Torres-Cabala C, Evans H, et al. Cutaneous metastases of malignant melanoma: a clinicopathologic study of 192 cases with emphasis on the morphologic spectrum. Am J Dermatopathol 2010;32:129.
65. Biddle DA, Evans HL, Kemp BL, et al. Intraparenchymal nevus cell aggregates in lymph nodes: a possible diagnostic pitfall with malignant melanoma and carcinoma. Am J Surg Pathol 2003;27:673.
66. Gershenwald JE, Andtbacka RH, Prieto VG, et al. Microscopic tumor burden in sentinel lymph nodes predicts synchronous nonsentinel lymph node involvement in patients with melanoma. J Clin Oncol 2008;26:4296.

67. Murali R, Cochran AJ, Cook MG, et al. Interobserver reproducibility of histologic parameters of melanoma deposits in sentinel lymph nodes: implications for management of patients with melanoma. Cancer 2009;115:5026.

68. Murali R, Desilva C, Thompson JF, et al. Non-sentinel node risk score (N-SNORE): a scoring system for accurately stratifying risk of non-sentinel node positivity in patients with cutaneous melanoma with positive sentinel lymph nodes. J Clin Oncol 2010;28:4441–9.

69. Wiener M, Acland KM, Shaw HM, et al. Sentinel node positive melanoma patients: prediction and prognostic significance of nonsentinel node metastases and development of a survival tree model. Ann Surg Oncol 1995;17.

70. Murali R, Thompson JF, Shaw HM, et al. The prognostic significance of isolated immunohistochemically positive cells in sentinel lymph nodes of melanoma patients. Am J Surg Pathol 2008;32:1106.

71. Scolyer RA, Murali R, Gershenwald JE, et al. Clinical relevance of melanoma micrometastases in sentinel nodes: too early to tell. Ann Oncol 2007;18:806.

72. Scolyer RA, Li LX, McCarthy SW, et al. Micromorphometric features of positive sentinel lymph nodes predict involvement of nonsentinel nodes in patients with melanoma. Am J Clin Pathol 2004;122:532.

73. Prieto VG. Sentinel lymph nodes in cutaneous melanoma. Surg Pathol Clin 2009; 3:553.

74. Scheri RP, Essner R, Turner RR, et al. Isolated tumor cells in the sentinel node affect long-term prognosis of patients with melanoma. Ann Surg Oncol 2007; 14:2861.

75. Kammula US, Ghossein R, Bhattacharya S, et al. Serial follow-up and the prognostic significance of reverse transcriptase-polymerase chain reaction–staged sentinel lymph nodes from melanoma patients. J Clin Oncol 2004;22:3989.

76. Kuo CT, Hoon DS, Takeuchi H, et al. Prediction of disease outcome in melanoma patients by molecular analysis of paraffin-embedded sentinel lymph nodes. J Clin Oncol 2003;21:3566.

77. McMasters KM, Noyes RD, Reintgen DS, et al. Lessons learned from the Sunbelt Melanoma Trial. J Surg Oncol 2004;86:212.

78. McMasters KM, Sondak VK, Lotze MT, et al. Recent advances in melanoma staging and therapy. Ann Surg Oncol 1999;6:467.

79. Mocellin S, Hoon DS, Pilati P, et al. Sentinel lymph node molecular ultrastaging in patients with melanoma: a systematic review and meta-analysis of prognosis. J Clin Oncol 2007;25:1588.

80. Scoggins CR, Ross MI, Reintgen DS, et al. Prospective multi-institutional study of reverse transcriptase polymerase chain reaction for molecular staging of melanoma. J Clin Oncol 2006;24:2849.

81. Flaherty KT, Puzanov I, Kim KB, et al. Inhibition of mutated, activated BRAF in metastatic melanoma. N Engl J Med 2010;363:809.

82. Flaherty KT, Smalley KS. Preclinical and clinical development of targeted therapy in melanoma: attention to schedule. Pigment Cell Melanoma Res 2009;22:529.

83. Smalley KS, Flaherty KT. Development of a novel chemical class of BRAF inhibitors offers new hope for melanoma treatment. Future Oncol 2009;5:775.

84. Gerami P, Mafee M, Lurtsbarapa T, et al. Sensitivity of fluorescence in situ hybridization for melanoma diagnosis using RREB1, MYB, Cep6, and 11q13 probes in melanoma subtypes. Arch Dermatol 2010;146:273.

85. Gerami P, Wass A, Mafee M, et al. Fluorescence in situ hybridization for distinguishing nevoid melanomas from mitotically active nevi. Am J Surg Pathol 2009;33:1783.

86. Newman MD, Lertsburapa T, Mirzabeigi M, et al. Fluorescence in situ hybridization as a tool for microstaging in malignant melanoma. Mod Pathol 2009;22:989.
87. Pouryazdanparast P, Newman M, Mafee M, et al. Distinguishing epithelioid blue nevus from blue nevus-like cutaneous melanoma metastasis using fluorescence in situ hybridization. Am J Surg Pathol 2009;33:1396.
88. Viros A, Fridlyand J, Bauer J, et al. Improving melanoma classification by integrating genetic and morphologic features. PLoS Med 2008;5:e120.
89. Torres-Cabala CA, Wang WL, Trent J, et al. Correlation between KIT expression and KIT mutation in melanoma: a study of 173 cases with emphasis on the acral-lentiginous/mucosal type. Mod Pathol 2009;22:1446.
90. Davies MA, Stemke-Hale K, Tellez C, et al. A novel AKT3 mutation in melanoma tumours and cell lines. Br J Cancer 2008;99:1265.
91. Hwang CS, Prieto VG, Diwan AH, et al. Changes in pERK1/2 and pAKT expression in melanoma lesions after imatinib treatment. Melanoma Res 2008;18:241.
92. Nazarian RM, Prieto VG, Elder DE, et al. Melanoma biomarker expression in melanocytic tumor progression: a tissue microarray study. J Cutan Pathol 2010; 37(Suppl 1):41.
93. Kim KB, Eton O, Davis DW, et al. Phase II trial of imatinib mesylate in patients with metastatic melanoma. Br J Cancer 2008;99:734.

Surgical Approach to Primary Cutaneous Melanoma

Patrick A. Ott, MD, PhD[a], Russell S. Berman, MD[b],*

KEYWORDS

• Melanoma • Biopsy • Excision • Margins • Recurrence

The incidence of melanoma is increasing throughout the world. This trend is mainly driven by the increased diagnosis of thin melanomas (<1 mm).[1–3] Surgical excision remains the primary treatment of biopsy-proven invasive melanoma at any site. Despite recent advances and considerable enthusiasm about novel systemic treatment approaches, such as PLX4032 (a specific inhibitor targeting the $BRAF^{V600E}$ mutation)[4] and ipilimumab (an antibody-mediating costimulatory blockade),[5] that exploit our better understanding of the molecular biology of melanoma and immunobiology in general, only a small proportion of patients have a durable complete response to systemic treatment of advanced disease. Therefore, early diagnosis and adequate surgical management provide the best prospect for cure from this aggressive tumor. The initial biopsy plays a critical role in the diagnosis and selection of the appropriate surgical strategy, including the determination of optimal surgical resection margins and the decision whether or not to perform sentinel lymph node biopsy (SLNB). These decisions are largely based on the thickness, ulceration status, and mitotic rate of the primary melanoma. Radiological imaging with chest radiography, computed tomography, or positron emission tomography are commonly used by clinicians for initial staging after the diagnosis of intermediately thick or thick melanomas, despite a lack of consensus about its usefulness.[6–9] This article focuses on the recommendations for the surgical management of primary melanoma, including biopsy techniques, selection of appropriate wide excision margins, SLNB, and surgical considerations for melanomas arising at specific sites.

The authors have nothing to disclose.

[a] Division of Medical Oncology, Department of Medicine, New York University School of Medicine, New York University Cancer Institute, 160 East 34th Street, 9th Floor, New York, NY 10016, USA

[b] Division of Surgical Oncology, Department of Surgery, New York University School of Medicine, New York University Cancer Institute, 160 East 34th Street, 9th Floor, New York, NY 10016, USA

* Corresponding author.

E-mail address: russell.berman@nyumc.org

Surg Oncol Clin N Am 20 (2011) 39–56

doi:10.1016/j.soc.2010.10.001

surgonc.theclinics.com

BIOPSY TECHNIQUES

An excisional biopsy is the preferred method to establish a definitive diagnosis of melanoma and to obtain appropriate microstaging[10] when a lesion is suspected to be a melanoma based on clinical appearance or history. The excision should be performed with narrow margins around the visible lesion and with a cuff of subdermal fat. Local anesthesia is usually sufficient for most excisional biopsies. This type of biopsy allows the dermatopathologist to review a specimen that represents the full thickness of the melanoma and to evaluate for residual tumor at the excision margins. In general, the orientation of the surgical excision should be guided by the lymphatic drainage of the surrounding skin and by the ability to optimize primary closure. On an extremity, the biopsy should typically be oriented parallel to the long axis of the extremity.

In some cases, an incisional biopsy is the only appropriate option. An example is when the patient presents with a large cutaneous melanoma, particularly in an anatomically and cosmetically difficult area such as the face. It may also be difficult to perform excisional biopsies on acral or mucosal sites. The limitations for histopathologic review of incisional biopsies are severalfold: (1) the biopsy specimen might not represent the full thickness of the melanoma (2) the number of mitoses may not be adequately assessed if the tumor is not available in its entirety and (3) the margins (both deep and lateral) may not be adequately assessed. Any limitation to the dermatopathologic review may affect both staging and the determination of optimal surgical management.

Shave biopsies are not recommended when the diagnosis of melanoma is suspected because these biopsies may limit the amount of specimen available for adequate pathologic assessment and adequate microstaging, especially the assessment of tumor thickness.

HISTOPATHOLOGIC EVALUATION

Essential components of primary tumor histopathologic evaluation include the Breslow thickness (in millimeters), presence or absence of ulceration, mitotic rate, Clark level of invasion, status of lateral and deep margins, and presence or absence of satellite lesions. Other features, such as the presence and extent of tumor-infiltrating lymphocytes, regression, angiolymphatic invasion, neurotropism, and histologic subtype, may also provide useful additional information.

WIDE LOCAL EXCISION: DETERMINATION OF APPROPRIATE RESECTION MARGINS FOR PRIMARY MELANOMA
Overview and Historical Perspective

Wide local excision (WLE) of the primary melanoma and the surrounding tissue is a critical part of potential curative therapy for melanoma. The surgical treatment approach has evolved considerably over the last several decades. One important element of the surgical excision is the extent of the margins, an issue that has been studied extensively over the last 4 decades. Until the 1970s, 3- to 5-cm margins were often recommended, without distinction by thickness of the tumor.[11] The routine use of such wide margins of resection frequently necessitated skin grafting to cover the defect and increased the morbidity of the resection. More than 100 years ago, Handley[12] published his treatment of locally advanced cutaneous melanoma with wide (up to 5 cm) margin excision, and the exclusive use of wide margin resection for all melanomas has been routinely, although not necessarily correctly, attributed to him. Decades later, pathologic findings of atypical melanocytes present at the periphery of melanomas, several centimeters away from the primary tumor, added to the belief that a minimum of 5-cm margin of excision was mandatory for adequate surgical treatment of melanoma.[13]

The indiscriminant use of wide resection margins for all melanomas was called into question starting in the late 1970s, when evidence emerged that narrower resection margins were associated with identical outcomes in patients with melanoma.[14] Because of the retrospective nature and the limited numbers of patients, the issue remained controversial for more than a decade until large, randomized, prospective studies investigating the issue were completed.[15,16] In the following section, evidence-based recommendations for primary melanoma resection margins are discussed.

Key Clinical Trials Assessing Surgical Resection Margins

In 1988, a randomized prospective trial by the World Health Organization (WHO) Melanoma Programme in which more than 600 patients with melanoma thickness less than or equal to 2 mm were randomized to resection with 1-cm versus 3-cm margins revealed no differences in the incidence of lymph node or distant metastases, disease-free survival (DFS), or overall survival (OS) between the 2 groups at a median follow-up of 90 months (**Table 1**).[17,18] A subgroup analysis of recurrence-free survival or OS in patients with a primary tumor thickness of 0.1 to 1.0 mm versus 1.1 to 2.0 mm revealed no difference between the groups. However, in the group that had a tumor thickness of 1.1 to 2.0 mm, there was a nonsignificant increase in local recurrences in those who underwent a 1-cm margin (n = 3) resection compared with those who underwent a 3-cm margin (n = 0) resection. Therefore, although the investigators felt that a 1-cm margin of excision was appropriate for melanomas less than 2 mm in thickness, others cited the local recurrence data to support their determination that a 1-cm margin was safe only for patients with a melanoma of up to 1 mm in thickness.

More than a decade later, the results of the WHO trial were confirmed by 2 large, randomized, prospective, multicenter European clinical trials. The Swedish Melanoma Study Group performed a phase 3 trial in which almost 1000 patients with a primary melanoma of the trunk or the extremities with a thickness greater than 0.8 mm and less than or equal to 2.0 mm were randomized to receive WLE with margins of either 2 or 5 cm.[19,20] No difference in OS was found at a median follow-up of 11 years. The local recurrence rate was low and was not increased in patients with resection margins of 2 cm after a median follow-up of 8 years. The French Cooperative Group conducted a phase 3 trial in which 337 patients with melanoma thickness less than or equal to 2 mm were enrolled over a period of 5 years at 9 European institutions.[21] Patients were randomized to undergo WLE with resection margins of either 2 or 5 cm, which were identical to the margins in the Swedish trial. The investigators concluded that the 10-year OS and local recurrence rates were not statistically different and that a surgical margin of 2 cm was sufficient for melanomas with thickness less than or equal to 2 mm.

Based on these trials, for melanomas with thickness less than 1 mm, resection margins should be 1 cm. However, for melanomas with thickness between 1 and 2 mm the recommendations are less clear. Based on the 3 randomized prospective trials discussed earlier, which collectively enrolled almost 2000 patients, a 2-cm resection margin is clearly sufficient for melanomas with thickness between 1 and 2 mm. However, the data from the WHO trial suggest that a 1-cm margin may be appropriate. Therefore, in general, a melanoma with thickness between 1 and 2 mm should be resected with radial margins between 1 and 2 cm. The decision whether to perform a 1- or 2-cm margin should be personalized taking into consideration primary tumor

Table 1
Randomized prospective trials assessing resection margins in primary melanoma

Trial	Number of Patients	Breslow Thickness	Margins Compared (cm)	Percentage of OS for Narrow Margin/ Wide Margin	Percentage of Nodal Metastases for Narrow Margin/ Wide Margin	Percentage of Distant Metastases for Narrow Margin/ Wide Margin	Comment	References
WHO Melanoma Trial	612	<2 mm	1 vs 3	89.6%/90.3% (8 y)	NR	NR	4 local recurrences in narrow-margin group only	17,18
Swedish Melanoma Study Group	989	>0.8 mm to ≤2 mm	2 vs 5	79%/76% (11 y)	15%/12% (8 y)	15%/14% (8 y)	—	19,20
French Cooperative Group Trial	336	≤2.0 mm	2 vs 5	87%/86% (10 y)	8.1%/6.7% (20 y)	2.5%/6.1% (20 y)	—	21
Intergroup Melanoma Trial	486	1–4 mm	2 vs 4	70%/77% (10 y)	2.1%/2.6% (local recurrence)	NR	Included nonrandomized group with head and neck or distal extremity melanomas receiving 2-cm margins, which had higher local recurrence rate (6.3%)	22–24
United Kingdom Melanoma Trial	900	>2 mm	1 vs 3	NR; HR, 1.07 (95% CI, 0.85–1.36); P = .6 (5 y)	33%/29% (5 y)	NR	No surgical nodal staging done	26

Abbreviations: CI, confidence interval; HR, hazard ratio; NR, not reported.

factors, patient factors, and the location of the melanoma, especially when it is located in anatomic areas where cosmetic deficits or functional problems are anticipated with wider margins, such as the face or distal extremities (fingers or weight-bearing portion of the foot). Primary tumor ulceration status was not comprehensively assessed in these trials but was balanced in the subgroup of patients for which data were available in the French trial.

A multi-institutional and international cooperative group trial (The Intergroup Melanoma Trial) was conducted to assess surgical resection margins for melanomas with intermediate thickness (1–4 mm). About 486 patients with trunk and proximal extremity melanomas were randomly assigned to receive either a 2-cm or 4-cm surgical resection margin around the melanoma biopsy site. The local recurrence rate was 2.1% for 2-cm margins and 2.6% for 4-cm margins ($P = .72$).[22-25] There use of skin grafts for wound closure in the group with 4-cm margins (46%) was significantly higher than that in those with 2-cm (11%) margins. Furthermore, 10-year OS rates (70% vs 77%) were not affected by the smaller resection margins.[24] The investigators concluded that 2-cm resection margins are appropriate for melanomas with a thickness of 1 to 4 mm.

The United Kingdom Melanoma Study Group assessed the effect of a 1-cm versus 3-cm excision margin in patients with high-risk cutaneous melanomas (>2 mm Breslow thickness) on the trunk or limbs in a multicenter, randomized, prospective trial, enrolling 900 patients.[26] None of these patients underwent any surgical staging procedure of the regional lymph node basins, including SLNB or elective lymph node dissection (ELND). Locoregional (local, in-transit, and nodal) recurrence was significantly more frequent in the group with 1-cm resection margins than in the group with 3-cm resection margins (168 vs 142, respectively, $P<.05$), whereas OS ($P = .06$) was similar in both groups. The investigators recommend that a surgical margin of 1 cm should be avoided in patients with melanoma thicker than 2 mm because of the significantly higher risk of locoregional recurrence in this group.

However, there are several considerations to take into account when considering this trial. Nodal failures accounted for the largest number of locoregional recurrences, with no significant differences between the 2 groups when only local and in-transit recurrences were addressed (nodal failure excluded from locoregional failure analysis and considered separately). It is possible that a 3-cm margin excises clinically significant microscopic disease that would eventually manifest as a locoregional recurrence if a smaller 1-cm margin of resection is performed. It is also possible that SLNB or ELND would have removed microscopic disease that would have ultimately progressed to a locoregional failure (especially considering the high nodal recurrence rate). However, because no nodal staging surgery was performed, the effect is unclear. Considering current practice for patients with primary melanomas thicker than 2 mm and clinically uninvolved nodes, SLNB would be offered to most of the patients in this trial. The difference in locoregional failure rates between the 2 groups did not translate into a difference in the OS. Although it is possible that this observation can be explained by too few locoregional failures to statistically affect OS, another possibility is that locoregional failure is not necessarily a precursor to distant disease.

Another trial from the Scandinavian group randomized 936 patients with melanomas with thickness greater than 2 mm to receive resection margins of 2 cm and 4 cm and reported no differences in local recurrence rate, DFS, or OS after 5 years of follow-up.[27] One retrospective study from The University of Texas MD Anderson Cancer Center assessed clinical outcome in 278 patients with melanomas thicker than 4 mm who had resection margins either smaller or larger than

2 cm. Of the melanomas evaluated, 60% were between 4.1 and 6.0 mm in thickness, while 68% of patients had ulcerated lesions and 28% had lymph node disease. Margins less than 2 cm were performed in 63% of patients, and 37% had margins larger than 2 cm. No differences in local recurrence rate or OS at 5 or 10 years were found and the investigators concluded that a 2-cm resection margin may be applied to this group of patients who were at high-risk for melanoma.[28]

Resection Margins: Meta-Analysis and Recommendations

The earlier-mentioned randomized trials, including the WHO Trial, the Intergroup Melanoma Trial, the Swedish Melanoma Study Group Trial, the United Kingdom Melanoma Study Group trial, and the French Cooperative Group, were assessed in a meta-analysis.[29] A total of 3313 participants, 1639 randomized to narrow excision margins (1–2 cm) and 1674 to wide excision margins (3–5 cm), were included. Overall there were 393 deaths in the groups with narrow excision margins and 403 in the groups with wide excision margins. The pooled odds ratio for death was 0.99 (95% confidence interval, 0.85–1.17; $P = .93$), and the investigators concluded that wide (3–5 cm) excision margins do not improve the overall mortality compared with narrow margins in the surgical treatment of primary cutaneous melanoma.

Based on the current evidence, the authors recommend that excision margins for melanomas with thickness less than 1 mm should be 1 cm. For melanomas with thickness between 1 and 2 mm, the recommendations are somewhat less clear; most guidelines advise margins between 1 and 2 cm. For melanomas with thickness greater than 2 mm, excision margins of 2 cm are appropriate (**Table 2**). It is recommended that the excision extends down to the muscular fascia. Deeper resections that include fascia have not improved outcomes.[30] Prospective randomized data are not available for margin recommendations in the case of melanomas in situ. In general, based on consensus panels, a 0.5- to 1.0-cm radial margin with a deep extension that includes subcutaneous fat is suggested.

The National Comprehensive Cancer Network guidelines recommend a 0.5-cm margin for melanomas in situ, 1 cm margins for melanomas with thickness less than or equal to 1 mm, 1- to 2-cm margins for melanomas with thickness between 1.01 and 2.00 mm, and 2-cm margins for melanomas with thickness greater than 2 mm (http://www.nccn.org/professionals/physician_gls/f_guidelines.asp). The clinical practice guidelines for the treatment of melanomas in Australia and New Zealand recommend a 0.5-cm margin for melanoma in situ, a 1-cm margin for melanomas with thickness lesser than 1 mm, 1- to 2-cm margins for melanomas with thickness between 1 and 4 mm, and a 2-cm margin for melanomas with thickness greater than 4 mm (http://www.nhmrc.gov.au/publications/synopses/cp111syn.htm).

Table 2
Recommended resection margins for primary melanoma

Breslow Thickness	Recommended Resection Margins (cm)	Comment
Melanoma in situ	0.5–1.0 cm	—
<1 mm	1 cm	—
1–2 mm	Between 1 and 2 cm	Recommended by most guidelines
>2 mm	2 cm	—

SURGICAL MANAGEMENT
Approach to WLE

A WLE is the standard therapeutic intervention used to address the primary melanoma site. The WLE is intended to remove the entire primary melanoma along with any microscopic melanoma cells that may be present in the adjacent tissue. However, in addition to these oncologic principles, the surgeon must consider the morbidity of the resection and its effect on both function and cosmetic outcome. The radial margin chosen for the WLE is determined by the Breslow thickness as described earlier. When all or part of the primary melanoma remains intact, the margin should be measured from the perimeter of the visible lesion. When the primary melanoma has been excised during the biopsy, the margin is measured from the periphery of the biopsy scar. The resulting defect is greater for a shave biopsy scar than for an usually linear scar after excisional biopsy. For most invasive melanomas, a full-thickness excision of skin and subcutaneous tissue is removed down to, but not including, the muscular fascia.[28] Thus, the depth of excision may be variable depending on the location of the primary tumor. From the patient's perspective, the length of the WLE scar can be longer than what they may have anticipated, and the authors, therefore, routinely draw out the proposed surgical excision and estimated scar length to better prepare the patient for surgery during preoperative assessment and consultation.

The planning of the surgical incision needs to take into consideration not only the required margin of excision but also the anatomic location of the melanoma and the nature of the local tissue. When the surgeon measures a 1- or 2-cm margin from the primary melanoma or biopsy site, an oval or circular defect is typically marked out for excision. However, for improved cosmetic outcome and when primary closure is planned, the defect is modified into an ellipse. This modification allows for a more gradual transition in wound contour and decreases the size of the "dog-ears" that persist at the poles of the incision. Although the ellipse is often described as requiring a length 3 to 4 times that of the width of the defect, a shorter excision may be cosmetically acceptable while decreasing morbidity.

Most 1-cm margin excisions and many 2-cm margin excisions can be excised and primarily closed using an elliptical excision. On the extremities, the ellipse is oriented parallel to the long axis of the limb (just as when planning an excisional biopsy). This orientation facilitates primary closure, maximizes excision of lymphatics that are at risk for tumor cell emboli, and may decrease subsequent lymphedema risk (**Fig. 1**). On the trunk, the incision should be oriented in a way that optimizes primary closure while ideally incorporating at-risk lymphatic tissue. At times, a modified ellipse may be necessary using a "hurricane" or "lazy S" incision.

The specimen should always be carefully oriented for the pathologist before being completely removed from the intact tissues. It is common, especially for 2-cm margins, to require the mobilization of full-thickness advancement flaps. Flaps are typically made above the level of the fascia with full-thickness advancement of tissue over the surgical defect. Closed-suction drainage may be used at the discretion of the surgeon if large flaps are made but are generally not required for most WLE reconstructions. Usually the complex closure involves 1 or 2 layers of deep absorbable sutures. Intradermal sutures placed in a buried fashion are typically used, but a deeper subcutaneous layer may also be reapproximated, at the surgeon's discretion, if tissue of appropriate strength is available. The skin closure may be accomplished in a variety of ways depending on tension, location, mobility of the area, and surgeon preference. A subcuticular closure may be accomplished using absorbable suture or a nonabsorbable pull

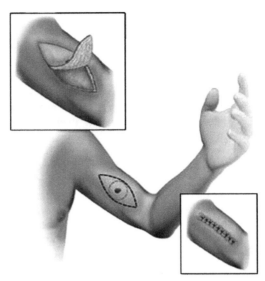

Fig. 1. WLE of primary melanoma. Appropriate radial margin marked schematically (*center, purple line*) along with proposed axially oriented elliptical incision to facilitate primary closure (*inset, bottom right*) after wide excision (*inset, top left*). (*Courtesy of* Jeffrey E. Gershenwald, MD, Houston, TX.)

through suture. Interrupted nonabsorbable sutures and skin staples may also be used. Dermal adhesives or adhesive bands may also be used at the surgeon's discretion.

It is not always possible to primarily close a WLE defect, especially on the distal extremities and in the head and neck region. Consideration, in these cases, must be given to either a skin graft or local flap technique. Skin grafts are relatively straightforward and allow for the careful monitoring of the primary excision site in patients with locally advanced melanomas. However, skin grafts have the potential for more significant morbidity, are considered more disfiguring, are insensate, and provide less protection to the underlying tissues. Split-thickness skin grafts are generally harvested from the posterior thigh. For a lower-extremity primary melanoma excision requiring a split-thickness skin graft, the graft is harvested from a donor site on the contralateral leg. Full-thickness skin grafts may be harvested from the inguinal groin crease, the lower neck region over the area of the clavicle, and behind the ear, depending on the ability to match color and texture of the skin. Full-thickness skin is harvested, and the donor site is closed primarily with dermal and subcuticular sutures. The decision to perform a skin graft or a local or rotational flap, however, must take numerous factors into account, including the location of the defect, stage of the primary melanoma, and patient comorbidities and preferences.

SLNB

The most important prognostic factor for the OS of patients with the American Joint Committee on Cancer stage I and II melanoma is the involvement of regional lymph nodes.[31] SLNB, initially described by Morton and colleagues[32] in 1992, is now widely performed for the initial staging of melanoma[33–37] and can accurately define the stage of the regional lymph node basin in approximately 97% of patients.[34,38,39] This technique is generally used for melanomas with thickness greater than or equal to 1 mm and has replaced ELND, which was previously a standard practice when nodes were clinically negative. The use of ELND, however, remained controversial because only 15% to 20% of patients have been shown to harbor metastatic disease in clinically negative nodes. Therefore, most patients who underwent ELND would not benefit from the surgery, which can cause debilitating postoperative lymphedema of the extremities. Furthermore, randomized trials demonstrated no benefit in OS from this procedure when all patients were considered.[40–44]

SLNB may also be used in thin melanomas (<1 mm thick). Although the likelihood of melanoma metastases in the sentinel node is less than 5% for melanomas with thickness lesser than or equal to 1 mm, the use of SLNB has been proposed by some investigators, especially when adverse primary pathologic features are present, including mitotic rate greater than zero, the presence of ulceration, shave biopsy to the base of the specimen, the presence of a vertical growth phase, and for melanomas with thickness greater than 0.75 mm.[45–49] Lymphoscintigraphy and intraoperative lymphatic mapping are standard elements of SLNB because lymphatic drainage cannot be predicted accurately by anatomy alone. Intradermal injection of ^{99m}Tc-labelled colloid around the primary melanoma or excisional biopsy site allows the localization of lymph node basins and assessment of the number of draining lymph node basins and potential sentinel nodes. Other tracers are available and used in other countries. The detection rate of the sentinel lymph node by SLNB is improved with the use of vital dye in addition to the radiolabeled tracer,[50] but dye is often not used in the head and neck area because of the risk of leaving a permanent tattoo in an exposed area. Although beyond the scope of this article, the pathologic analysis of the sentinel lymph node and the role of completion lymph node dissection (CLND) in patients with a positive sentinel node are discussed elsewhere in this issue (see the articles Pathologic Evaluation by Scolyer and colleagues and Sentinel Node Biopsy by Ross and colleagues elsewhere in this issue).

Recent attention has also focused on the use of ultrasonography (US) in combination with fine-needle aspiration cytology (FNAC) for the monitoring of regional lymph nodes and detection of metastases earlier than clinical examination only. In some centers, this technique has been reported to be associated with a high sensitivity and specificity in the follow-up of patients with melanoma.[51,52] Recent studies have shown that this technology might also be useful in the initial staging of melanoma. In a report from Germany, 65% of patients with positive sentinel lymph node metastases were detected using US and FNAC and patients could directly proceed to CLND in which the sentinel lymph node examined by fine-needle aspiration was histologically assessed as the gold standard.[53] Nevertheless, other groups have reported that US is not a substitute for SLNB and, although the technique has been incorporated in the initial staging of melanoma at some centers, it has not replaced SLNB as the standard of care.[54]

LOCAL RECURRENCE

True local recurrences are uncommon and are typically the result of incompletely or inadequately excised primary tumors. However, most of what are termed local recurrences after appropriately wide excision are a result of lymphatic tumor emboli and behave similar to in-transit and satellite disease, which is defined as recurrence in the dermis or subcutaneous tissue between the primary tumor and the draining regional basin as a result of intralymphatic tumor emboli.

SPECIAL MELANOMA SUBTYPES
Desmoplastic Melanoma

Desmoplastic melanoma, an uncommon subtype of melanoma, is histologically described as a collagen-producing spindle cell tumor. This melanoma is typically thicker at first presentation than nondesmoplastic cutaneous melanomas. As a result of different local growth and its unique tumor biology, desmoplastic melanoma has a higher tendency for local recurrence and resection margins need to be considered with extra caution.[55] In a large retrospective study it was shown that "pure" desmoplastic melanomas (without the presence of other common histologic subtypes) have a significantly lower incidence of positive sentinel lymph nodes than nondesmoplastic melanomas (2.2% vs 17.5%, respectively, P<.01).[56] This finding was corroborated by other groups,[57] and it was therefore suggested that SLNB may not be necessary for pure desmoplastic melanomas.

Lentigo Maligna

Lentigo maligna is a melanoma in situ that arises in sun-exposed areas, predominantly in the head and neck area, and has increased in incidence over the last several decades. Lentigo maligna melanoma is an invasive melanoma that has arisen from lentigo maligna and for which the standard recommendations for margin size, as discussed earlier, apply. The following discussion, including the description of Mohs surgery, applies strictly to the noninvasive lentigo maligna.

Recommended margins for melanomas in situ have traditionally been 0.5 cm in the United States, although several retrospective studies have shown recurrence rates of up to 20%, suggesting that a 5-mm margin might not always be sufficient.[58–62] In a recent study, assessing margins using Mohs micrographic surgery on 626 patients, the investigators concluded that 9-mm margins were necessary to achieve a tumor-free plane in most of them.[63] Similar results were reported in several additional studies, confirming that 5-mm margins are needed for most cases.[64–66] Because lentigo maligna occurs mainly in cosmetically and functionally challenging areas in the head and neck region, the achievement of adequate surgical margins can be a considerable challenge for the surgeon. Furthermore, the elderly population in whom lentigo maligna mainly occurs more frequently has comorbidities precluding extensive surgery. As a result, alternative approaches have been developed in recent years, including Mohs micrographic surgery. This procedure was originally performed mainly for basal cell and squamous cell carcinoma, but improved histopathologic technology, such as the use of immunoperoxidase staining technique for the processing of frozen tissue,[67] has allowed the application of this procedure to higher-risk lesions such as melanoma in situ. Because of the tangential nature of the tumor excision, Mohs surgery allows the assessment of the entire peripheral margin of a lesion. This comprehensive margin evaluation in combination with the tissue-sparing technique renders it a treatment option for lentigo maligna with its common occurrence in the head and neck region.

The main controversial issue surrounding Mohs surgery for melanoma in situ is the use of frozen tissue sections to identify malignant melanocytic cells.[68] The similarity of vacuolated keratinocytes and melanocytes and presence of dermal inflammatory cells and processing artifacts contribute to the difficulty of correctly assessing a frozen specimen for the presence of residual melanoma cells. Solutions to overcome these limitations and to increase the sensitivity for negative margins include the use of immunohistochemical staining[69] or rush permanent paraffin sections[70,71] or the incorporation of final assessment of permanent sections after the procedure has been completed. A recent prospective study reporting on 167 patients with melanoma in situ, 116 of them with lentigo maligna, demonstrated 95.7% clearance rate by Mohs surgery when margins were reassessed by dermatopathologic review on paraffin-embedded tissue sections.[72] At a median follow-up of 50 months, the cure rate was 99% in this patient group. Several retrospective studies using Mohs surgery have been reported. In a series of 331 patients with lentigo maligna followed up for a mean of 58 months, the 5-year local recurrence rate was 0% and the 5-year disease-specific survival rate was 99.7%.[63] Another retrospective study, which enrolled 184 patients with lentigo melanoma, 99.5% of whom were followed up for at least 5 years, showed a 5-year local recurrence rate of 0.5% and a 5-year survival rate of 99%.[73] A recent review of the literature confirmed the efficacy of Mohs surgery for treatment of melanoma in situ, reporting recurrence rates generally less than 1% after 3 to 5 years of follow-up.[74]

MELANOMA AT SPECIFIC SITES
Mucosal Melanoma

Primary melanoma originating from mucosal surfaces is a relatively rare subtype representing less than 2% of all melanoma cases.[75,76] Molecular differences between mucosal and cutaneous melanoma, such as the presence of c-kit mutations in approximately 20% of mucosal cases and the relatively rare occurrence (10% in mucosal as opposed to 50%–60% in cutaneous) of the BRAF[V600E] mutation, have been recognized recently and may play a significant role for the treatment of systemic disease.[77–80] (See also Targeted Therapy article by Drs Davies and Gershenwald elsewhere in this issue for further exploration of this topic.) These molecular differences are also present in certain acral melanomas and melanoma arising from sun-damaged skin. The most frequent sites of mucosal melanoma are the head and neck (mostly the sinonasal and oral cavities), constituting approximately 50% of all mucosal melanoma cases, as well as the female genital tract (20%) and the anogenital region (20%).[75,81]

Mucosal melanomas of the head and neck area

Mucosal melanomas of the head and neck area generally do not cause early symptoms, but even in the presence of symptoms, there is often a considerable delay in diagnosis, presumably because of the rarity of the disease and the similarity of the symptoms with benign conditions. The diagnosis requires a full-thickness biopsy of the lesion. For localized disease, wide surgical excision is the primary treatment approach; however, melanoma-free margins are difficult to achieve in many cases because of the close proximity of critical anatomic structures.[82,83] Another reason for the high local recurrence rate is the potentially aggressive behavior of mucosal melanoma in the sinonasal and oral cavities with satellite formation, multifocality, angiolymphatic invasion, and submucosal spread, often requiring radical surgical resection with reconstruction for even seemingly early-stage tumors.[84,85] In a retrospective analysis, adjuvant radiation therapy was shown to improve local control, but not OS.[86] Nevertheless, because of locally aggressive features, radiation is recommended by many investigators, even when melanoma-free margins have been achieved by WLE.[83,87,88] SLNB or prophylactic CLND are not routinely performed in head and neck mucosal melanomas.

Mucosal melanomas of the anorectal region

Most anorectal melanomas are located along the dentate line in the anal canal. Similar to anal carcinoma, the diagnosis is often delayed because the symptoms, such as pruritus or pain, can suggest the presence of a benign cause, such as hemorrhoids or a rectal polyp. Because up to 65% of anal melanomas are diagnosed when distant metastatic disease is present, the prognosis is poor with 5-year survival rates around 20%. Abdominoperineal resection (APR) has historically been advocated by some investigators,[89] whereas others have reported that sphincter-sparing WLE in conjunction with adjuvant radiotherapy is well tolerated and leads to successful locoregional control.[90] A recent retrospective study from the Memorial Sloan-Kettering Cancer Center documented that a shift in surgical approach from APR to local excision, which occurred in the late 1990s, did not result in a difference in outcome.[91] Because a significantly better survival outcome has never been shown with APR, WLE is the preferred approach by most surgeons to spare the patient unnecessary morbidity. APR with or without inguinal lymph node dissection should be reserved for patients with locally extensive disease, which is not amenable to local excision. Palliative surgery (such as local segmental resection or a diverting colostomy) along with systemic therapy is generally advocated for patients with advanced disease.

Melanoma of the Female Genital Tract

Most melanomas of the female genital tract are of vulvar origin. Presenting symptoms are similar to other gynecologic tumors. Although most patients present with localized disease, the prognosis is generally poor. In a study from Sweden, the 5-year survival was reported between 27% for disease with lymph node involvement and 65% for disease without lymph node involvement.[92] WLE with 1-cm margins for vulvar melanomas with thickness lesser than 1 mm and 2-cm margins for melanomas with thickness greater than or equal to 1 mm is the standard surgical approach.[93] Radical vulvectomy is associated with a much higher morbidity and has not demonstrated improved DFS or OS in several studies.[94–96]

Subungual Melanoma and Digital Melanoma

As with any melanoma excision, oncologic principles must be balanced with functional outcome and morbidity when considering melanomas on the skin of the fingers and toes or in the nail bed (subungual). Bones do not generally need to be resected for almost all melanomas, and, therefore, amputation is not an oncologic necessity. However, a straightforward amputation at the level of the metatarsophalangeal joint is usually performed for all but the great toe because there is minimal morbidity or resultant dysfunction. For nail bed and distal phalanx melanomas of the great toe and fingers, an amputation is often necessary to obtain appropriate oncologic margins. However, for melanomas of the proximal digits or web space, it may be possible to avoid amputation while maintaining oncologic principles. Skin grafts (typically full thickness), rotation flaps, or even more complex flaps for critical digits serve as reconstructive options for melanomas of the proximal digits and web space.

Cutaneous Melanoma of the Breast

Melanomas that arise in the skin of the breast should be treated with the same margins and surgical principles as outlined for cutaneous melanomas in other areas of the body. A mastectomy is not generally performed for primary cutaneous melanomas of the breast skin. The nipple-areolar complex can generally be spared for breast melanomas, unless the melanoma arises in the skin of the nipple-areolar complex itself.

Cutaneous Melanoma of the Ear

Although it is generally not oncologically necessary to resect the cartilaginous tissue of the ear for most melanomas, a full-thickness wedge excision of the skin and cartilage of the helix is usually amenable to primary closure and generally offers an acceptable cosmetic result. A skin graft may be necessary when a wedge excision is not a viable option.

Melanoma of the Foot

A comprehensive discussion of the management of foot melanomas is beyond the scope of this section. For most foot melanomas, primary closure after WLE is quite difficult. When the melanoma is present over a non–weight-bearing area of the plantar foot or on the dorsum of the foot, a split-thickness skin graft typically provides appropriate coverage. Melanomas on the plantar surface (especially the heel and over the weight-bearing metatarsal heads) of the foot are more challenging. The WLE is typically carried deep to the level of the plantar fascia, and split-thickness skin graft reconstruction may not provide durable coverage. A rotation flap, using full-thickness muscle and skin from a non–weight-bearing portion of the foot, may be mobilized to cover the defect in the weight-bearing portion of the foot. This flap provides a sensate and padded closure for the weight-bearing area of the foot. A skin graft is used to cover the non–weight-bearing donor site. On occasion, a free myocutaneous flap may be required to cover an extensive surgical defect. A temporary vacuum device may also be useful in this location, especially when there is doubt about adequate margins of resection. A delayed reconstruction with graft or flap may then be performed.

SUMMARY

The surgical management of primary melanoma, from diagnostic biopsy through the WLE and nodal staging, must be carefully planned and must take into consideration the biology of the melanoma, microstaging and primary tumor pathologic features of the melanoma, location on the body, patient preferences and comorbidities, as well as functional and aesthetic outcome. The balance of preserving oncologic principles while optimizing outcome must be personalized for each patient with melanoma, regardless of the extent of the disease. In this article, the authors discuss the surgical approach to primary cutaneous melanomas. The various pathologic variants and difficult anatomic locations as well as areas of controversy have been highlighted. Despite recent emergence of novel, more-efficacious agents for the treatment of systemic disease, the initial surgical approach likely remains the key treatment modality for patients with newly diagnosed melanoma.

REFERENCES

1. American Cancer Society. Cancer facts and figures 2008. Atlanta (GA): American Cancer Society; 2008.
2. de Vries E, Coebergh JW. Melanoma incidence has risen in Europe. BMJ 2005; 331:698.
3. Downing A, Yu XQ, Newton-Bishop J, et al. Trends in prognostic factors and survival from cutaneous melanoma in Yorkshire, UK and New South Wales, Australia between 1993 and 2003. Int J Cancer 2008;123:861–6.
4. Flaherty KT, Puzanov I, Kim KB, et al. Inhibition of mutated, activated BRAF in metastatic melanoma. N Engl J Med 2010;363:809–19.
5. Hodi FS, O'Day SJ, McDermott DF, et al. Improved survival with ipilimumab in patients with metastatic melanoma. N Engl J Med 2010;363(8):711–23.
6. Buzaid AC, Sandler AB, Mani S, et al. Role of computed tomography in the staging of primary melanoma. J Clin Oncol 1993;11:638–43.
7. Terhune MH, Swanson N, Johnson TM. Use of chest radiography in the initial evaluation of patients with localized melanoma. Arch Dermatol 1998;134:569–72.

8. Wagner JD, Schauwecker D, Davidson D, et al. Inefficacy of F-18 fluorodeoxy-D-glucose-positron emission tomography scans for initial evaluation in early-stage cutaneous melanoma. Cancer 2005;104:570–9.

9. Yancovitz M, Finelt N, Warycha MA, et al. Role of radiologic imaging at the time of initial diagnosis of stage T1b-T3b melanoma. Cancer 2007;110:1107–14.

10. Sober AJ, Chuang TY, Duvic M, et al. Guidelines of care for primary cutaneous melanoma. J Am Acad Dermatol 2001;45:579–86.

11. Goldman LI. The surgical therapy of malignant melanomas. Semin Oncol 1975;2:175–8.

12. Handley. The Hunterian lectures on the pathology of melanotic growths in relation to their operative treatment. Lancet 1907;1:927–53.

13. Petersen NC, Bodenham DC, Lloyd OC. Malignant melanomas of the skin. A study of the origin, development, aetiology, spread, treatment, and prognosis. Br J Plast Surg 1962;15:97–116.

14. Breslow A, Macht SD. Optimal size of resection margin for thin cutaneous melanoma. Surg Gynecol Obstet 1977;145:691–2.

15. Aitken DR, James AG, Carey LC. Local cutaneous recurrence after conservative excision of malignant melanoma. Arch Surg 1984;119:643–6.

16. Balch CM, Murad TM, Soong SJ, et al. Tumor thickness as a guide to surgical management of clinical stage I melanoma patients. Cancer 1979;43:883–8.

17. Veronesi U, Cascinelli N. Narrow excision (1-cm margin). A safe procedure for thin cutaneous melanoma. Arch Surg 1991;126:438–41.

18. Veronesi U, Cascinelli N, Adamus J, et al. Thin stage I primary cutaneous malignant melanoma. Comparison of excision with margins of 1 or 3 cm. N Engl J Med 1988;318:1159–62.

19. Cohn-Cedermark G, Rutqvist LE, Andersson R, et al. Long term results of a randomized study by the Swedish Melanoma Study Group on 2-cm versus 5-cm resection margins for patients with cutaneous melanoma with a tumor thickness of 0.8–2.0 mm. Cancer 2000;89:1495–501.

20. Ringborg U, Andersson R, Eldh J, et al. Resection margins of 2 versus 5 cm for cutaneous malignant melanoma with a tumor thickness of 0.8 to 2.0 mm: randomized study by the Swedish Melanoma Study Group. Cancer 1996;77:1809–14.

21. Khayat D, Rixe O, Martin G, et al. Surgical margins in cutaneous melanoma (2 cm versus 5 cm for lesions measuring less than 2.1-mm thick). Cancer 2003;97:1941–6.

22. Balch CM, Urist MM, Karakousis CP, et al. Efficacy of 2-cm surgical margins for intermediate-thickness melanomas (1 to 4 mm). Results of a multi-institutional randomized surgical trial. Ann Surg 1993;218:262–7 [discussion: 7–9].

23. Karakousis CP, Balch CM, Urist MM, et al. Local recurrence in malignant melanoma: long-term results of the multiinstitutional randomized surgical trial. Ann Surg Oncol 1996;3:446–52.

24. Balch CM, Soong SJ, Smith T, et al. Long-term results of a prospective surgical trial comparing 2 cm vs 4 cm excision margins for 740 patients with 1–4 mm melanomas. Ann Surg Oncol 2001;8:101–8.

25. Randomized trial of a resection margin of 2 cm versus 4 cm for cutaneous malignant melanoma with a tumor thickness of more than 2 mm. In: Proceedings 6th World Melanoma. 2005.

26. Thomas JM, Newton-Bishop J, A'Hern R, et al. Excision margins in high-risk malignant melanoma. N Engl J Med 2004;350:757–66.

27. Ringborg U, Brahme E, Drewiecki K. Randomized trial of a resection margin of 2 cm versus 4 cm for cutaneous malignant melanoma with a tumor thickness of more than 2 mm. In: World Congress on Melanoma. September 5–10,

Vancouver (BC): Canadian Melanoma Society, University of British Columbia, BC Cancer Agency; 2005.

28. Heaton KM, Sussman JJ, Gershenwald JE, et al. Surgical margins and prognostic factors in patients with thick (>4 mm) primary melanoma. Ann Surg Oncol 1998;5: 322–8.

29. Lens MB, Nathan P, Bataille V. Excision margins for primary cutaneous melanoma: updated pooled analysis of randomized controlled trials. Arch Surg 2007;142:885–91 [discussion: 91–3].

30. Kenady DE, Brown BW, McBride CM. Excision of underlying fascia with a primary malignant melanoma: effect on recurrence and survival rates. Surgery 1982;92: 615–8.

31. Balch CM, Buzaid AC, Soong SJ, et al. Final version of the American Joint Committee on Cancer staging system for cutaneous melanoma. J Clin Oncol 2001;19:3635–48.

32. Morton DL, Wen DR, Wong JH, et al. Technical details of intraoperative lymphatic mapping for early stage melanoma. Arch Surg 1992;127:392–9.

33. Balch CM, Morton DL, Gershenwald JE, et al. Sentinel node biopsy and standard of care for melanoma. J Am Acad Dermatol 2009;60:872–5.

34. Gershenwald JE, Thompson W, Mansfield PF, et al. Multi-institutional melanoma lymphatic mapping experience: the prognostic value of sentinel lymph node status in 612 stage I or II melanoma patients. J Clin Oncol 1999;17:976–83.

35. Morton DL, Thompson JF, Cochran AJ, et al. Sentinel-node biopsy or nodal observation in melanoma. N Engl J Med 2006;355:1307–17.

36. Morton DL, Thompson JF, Essner R, et al. Validation of the accuracy of intraoperative lymphatic mapping and sentinel lymphadenectomy for early-stage melanoma: a multicenter trial. Multicenter Selective Lymphadenectomy Trial Group. Ann Surg 1999;230:453–63 [discussion: 63–5].

37. Testori A, De Salvo GL, Montesco MC, et al. Clinical considerations on sentinel node biopsy in melanoma from an Italian multicentric study on 1,313 patients (SOLISM-IMI). Ann Surg Oncol 2009;16:2018–27.

38. Albertini JJ, Cruse CW, Rapaport D, et al. Intraoperative radio-lympho-scintigraphy improves sentinel lymph node identification for patients with melanoma. Ann Surg 1996;223:217–24.

39. Krag DN, Meijer SJ, Weaver DL, et al. Minimal-access surgery for staging of malignant melanoma. Arch Surg 1995;130:654–8 [discussion: 9–60].

40. Balch CM, Soong SJ, Bartolucci AA, et al. Efficacy of an elective regional lymph node dissection of 1 to 4 mm thick melanomas for patients 60 years of age and younger. Ann Surg 1996;224:255–63 [discussion: 63–6].

41. Cascinelli N, Morabito A, Santinami M, et al. Immediate or delayed dissection of regional nodes in patients with melanoma of the trunk: a randomised trial. WHO melanoma programme. Lancet 1998;351:793–6.

42. Sim FH, Taylor WF, Ivins JC, et al. A prospective randomized study of the efficacy of routine elective lymphadenectomy in management of malignant melanoma. Preliminary results. Cancer 1978;41:948–56.

43. Veronesi U, Adamus J, Bandiera DC, et al. Inefficacy of immediate node dissection in stage 1 melanoma of the limbs. N Engl J Med 1977;297:627–30.

44. Veronesi U, Adamus J, Bandiera DC, et al. Delayed regional lymph node dissection in stage I melanoma of the skin of the lower extremities. Cancer 1982;49: 2420–30.

45. Cecchi R, Buralli L, Innocenti S, et al. Sentinel lymph node biopsy in patients with thin melanomas. J Dermatol 2007;34:512–5.

46. Hershko DD, Robb BW, Lowy AM, et al. Sentinel lymph node biopsy in thin mela-noma patients. J Surg Oncol 2006;93:279–85.
47. Ranieri JM, Wagner JD, Wenck S, et al. The prognostic importance of sentinel lymph node biopsy in thin melanoma. Ann Surg Oncol 2006;13:927–32.
48. Wong SL, Brady MS, Busam KJ, et al. Results of sentinel lymph node biopsy in patients with thin melanoma. Ann Surg Oncol 2006;13:302–9.
49. Wright BE, Scheri RP, Ye X, et al. Importance of sentinel lymph node biopsy in patients with thin melanoma. Arch Surg 2008;143:892–9 [discussion: 899–900].
50. Brady MS, Coit DG. Sentinel lymph node evaluation in melanoma. Arch Dermatol 1997;133:1014–20.
51. Rossi CR, Seno A, Vecchiato A, et al. The impact of ultrasound scanning in the staging and follow-up of patients with clinical stage I cutaneous melanoma. Eur J Cancer 1997;33:200–3.
52. Voit C, Mayer T, Kron M, et al. Efficacy of ultrasound B-scan compared with phys-ical examination in follow-up of melanoma patients. Cancer 2001;91:2409–16.
53. Voit CA, van Akkooi AC, Schafer-Hesterberg G, et al. Rotterdam Criteria for sentinel node (SN) tumor burden and the accuracy of ultrasound (US)-guided fine-needle aspiration cytology (FNAC): can US-guided FNAC replace SN staging in patients with melanoma? J Clin Oncol 2009;27:4994–5000.
54. Sanki A, Uren RF, Moncrieff M, et al. Targeted high-resolution ultrasound is not an effective substitute for sentinel lymph node biopsy in patients with primary cuta-neous melanoma. J Clin Oncol 2009;27:5614–9.
55. Posther KE, Selim MA, Mosca PJ, et al. Histopathologic characteristics, recur-rence patterns, and survival of 129 patients with desmoplastic melanoma. Ann Surg Oncol 2006;13:728–39.
56. Pawlik TM, Ross MI, Prieto VG, et al. Assessment of the role of sentinel lymph node biopsy for primary cutaneous desmoplastic melanoma. Cancer 2006;106: 900–6.
57. Gyorki DE, Busam K, Panageas K, et al. Sentinel lymph node biopsy for patients with cutaneous desmoplastic melanoma. Ann Surg Oncol 2003;10:403–7.
58. Coleman WP 3rd, Davis RS, Reed RJ, et al. Treatment of lentigo maligna and len-tigo maligna melanoma. J Dermatol Surg Oncol 1980;6:476–9.
59. Osborne JE, Hutchinson PE. A follow-up study to investigate the efficacy of initial treatment of lentigo maligna with surgical excision. Br J Plast Surg 2002;55: 611–5.
60. Pitman GH, Kopf AW, Bart RS, et al. Treatment of lentigo maligna and lentigo maligna melanoma. J Dermatol Surg Oncol 1979;5:727–37.
61. Tsang RW, Liu FF, Wells W, et al. Lentigo maligna of the head and neck. Results of treatment by radiotherapy. Arch Dermatol 1994;130:1008–12.
62. Clinical practice guidelines in oncology: melanoma. 2009. Available at: http://www.nccn.org/professionals/physician_gls/PDF/melanoma.pdf. Accessed Sep-tember 1, 2010.
63. Bricca GM, Brodland DG, Ren D, et al. Cutaneous head and neck melanoma treated with Mohs micrographic surgery. J Am Acad Dermatol 2005;52:92–100.
64. Agarwal-Antal N, Bowen GM, Gerwels JW. Histologic evaluation of lentigo mali-gna with permanent sections: implications regarding current guidelines. J Am Acad Dermatol 2002;47:743–8.
65. Huilgol SC, Selva D, Chen C, et al. Surgical margins for lentigo maligna and len-tigo maligna melanoma: the technique of mapped serial excision. Arch Dermatol 2004;140:1087–92.

66. Zalla MJ, Lim KK, Dicaudo DJ, et al. Mohs micrographic excision of melanoma using immunostains. Dermatol Surg 2000;26:771–84.
67. El Tal AK, Abrou AE, Stiff MA, et al. Immunostaining in Mohs micrographic surgery: a review. Dermatol Surg 2010;36:275–90.
68. Dawn ME, Dawn AG, Miller SJ. Mohs surgery for the treatment of melanoma in situ: a review. Dermatol Surg 2007;33:395–402.
69. Erickson C, Miller SJ. Treatment options in melanoma in situ: topical and radiation therapy, excision and Mohs surgery. Int J Dermatol 2010;49:482–91.
70. Bub JL, Berg D, Slee A, et al. Management of lentigo maligna and lentigo maligna melanoma with staged excision: a 5-year follow-up. Arch Dermatol 2004;140: 552–8.
71. Clayton BD, Leshin B, Hitchcock MG, et al. Utility of rush paraffin-embedded tangential sections in the management of cutaneous neoplasms. Dermatol Surg 2000;26:671–8.
72. Bene NI, Healy C, Coldiron BM. Mohs micrographic surgery is accurate 95.1% of the time for melanoma in situ: a prospective study of 167 cases. Dermatol Surg 2008;34:660–4.
73. Zitelli JA, Brown C, Hanusa BH. Mohs micrographic surgery for the treatment of primary cutaneous melanoma. J Am Acad Dermatol 1997;37:236–45.
74. Clark GS, Pappas-Politis EC, Cherpelis BS, et al. Surgical management of melanoma in situ on chronically sun-damaged skin. Cancer Control 2008;15:216–24.
75. Chang AE, Karnell LH, Menck HR. The National Cancer Data Base report on cutaneous and noncutaneous melanoma: a summary of 84,836 cases from the past decade. The American College of Surgeons Commission on Cancer and the American Cancer Society. Cancer 1998;83:1664–78.
76. McLaughlin CC, Wu XC, Jemal A, et al. Incidence of noncutaneous melanomas in the U.S. Cancer 2005;103:1000–7.
77. Curtin JA, Busam K, Pinkel D, et al. Somatic activation of KIT in distinct subtypes of melanoma. J Clin Oncol 2006;24:4340–6.
78. Curtin JA, Fridlyand J, Kageshita T, et al. Distinct sets of genetic alterations in melanoma. N Engl J Med 2005;353:2135–47.
79. Davies H, Bignell GR, Cox C, et al. Mutations of the BRAF gene in human cancer. Nature 2002;417:949–54.
80. Gorden A, Osman I, Gai W, et al. Analysis of BRAF and N-RAS mutations in metastatic melanoma tissues. Cancer Res 2003;63:3955–7.
81. Patrick RJ, Fenske NA, Messina JL. Primary mucosal melanoma. J Am Acad Dermatol 2007;56:828–34.
82. Manolidis S, Donald PJ. Malignant mucosal melanoma of the head and neck: review of the literature and report of 14 patients. Cancer 1997;80:1373–86.
83. Stern SJ, Guillamondegui OM. Mucosal melanoma of the head and neck. Head Neck 1991;13:22–7.
84. Patel SG, Prasad ML, Escrig M, et al. Primary mucosal malignant melanoma of the head and neck. Head Neck 2002;24:247–57.
85. Tomicic J, Wanebo HJ. Mucosal melanomas. Surg Clin North Am 2003;83: 237–52.
86. Owens JM, Roberts DB, Myers JN. The role of postoperative adjuvant radiation therapy in the treatment of mucosal melanomas of the head and neck region. Arch Otolaryngol Head Neck Surg 2003;129:864–8.
87. Mendenhall WM, Amdur RJ, Hinerman RW, et al. Head and neck mucosal melanoma. Am J Clin Oncol 2005;28:626–30.

88. Wagner M, Morris CG, Werning JW, et al. Mucosal melanoma of the head and neck. Am J Clin Oncol 2008;31:43–8.
89. Brady MS, Kavolius JP, Quan SH. Anorectal melanoma. A 64-year experience at Memorial Sloan-Kettering Cancer Center. Dis Colon Rectum 1995;38:146–51.
90. Ballo MT, Gershenwald JE, Zagars GK, et al. Sphincter-sparing local excision and adjuvant radiation for anal-rectal melanoma. J Clin Oncol 2002;20:4555–8.
91. Yeh JJ, Shia J, Hwu WJ, et al. The role of abdominoperineal resection as surgical therapy for anorectal melanoma. Ann Surg 2006;244:1012–7.
92. Ragnarsson-Olding BK, Nilsson BR, Kanter-Lewensohn LR, et al. Malignant melanoma of the vulva in a nationwide, 25-year study of 219 Swedish females: predictors of survival. Cancer 1999;86:1285–93.
93. Rogo KO, Andersson R, Edbom G, et al. Conservative surgery for vulvovaginal melanoma. Eur J Gynaecol Oncol 1991;12:113–9.
94. Phillips GL, Bundy BN, Okagaki T, et al. Malignant melanoma of the vulva treated by radical hemivulvectomy. A prospective study of the Gynecologic Oncology Group. Cancer 1994;73:2626–32.
95. Rose PG, Piver MS, Tsukada Y, et al. Conservative therapy for melanoma of the vulva. Am J Obstet Gynecol 1988;159:52–5.
96. Trimble EL, Lewis JL Jr, Williams LL, et al. Management of vulvar melanoma. Gynecol Oncol 1992;45:254–8.

Sentinel Lymph Node Biopsy for Melanoma: Critical Assessment at its Twentieth Anniversary

Merrick I. Ross, MD[a],*, John F. Thompson, MD[c,d],
Jeffrey E. Gershenwald, MD[a,b,e]

KEYWORDS

- Sentinel lymph node • Biopsy • Melanoma
- Lymphadenectomy • Lymphatic mapping

The increasing incidence of cutaneous melanoma over the past few decades has created the need as well as the opportunity to establish standards of surgical care designed to achieve the following goals: (1) accurate staging and prognosis, (2) long-term locoregional disease control, and (3) optimizing the chance for cure. Establishing how best to manage the clinically negative regional lymph node basin(s) in newly diagnosed American Joint Committee on Cancer (AJCC) stage I and II patients has been identified as one of the strategies to fulfill these goals and has been the focus of intense global clinical research efforts. Significant emphasis has also been placed on accomplishing these goals while minimizing treatment-related morbidities. The technique of lymphatic mapping and sentinel lymph node (SLN) biopsy, first presented in 1990 and published in 1992 by Morton and colleagues,[1] was introduced as a minimally invasive method to accurately stage the clinically negative regional nodal basins

This work was supported in part by The University of Texas MD Anderson Cancer Center Melanoma SPORE (P50 CA93459) and the Grossman Family Foundation.
The authors have nothing to disclose.
[a] Department of Surgical Oncology, The University of Texas MD Anderson Cancer Center, 1515 Holcombe Boulevard, Unit 444, Houston, TX 77030, USA
[b] Department of Cancer Biology, The University of Texas MD Anderson Cancer Center, 1515 Holcombe Boulevard, Unit 444, Houston, TX 77030, USA
[c] Melanoma Institute Australia, North Sydney, NSW, Australia
[d] The University of Sydney, Sydney, NSW, Australia
[e] Melanoma and Skin Center, The University of Texas MD Anderson Cancer Center, 1515 Holcombe Boulevard, Houston, TX 77030, USA
* Corresponding author.
E-mail address: mross@mdanderson.org

in patients with stage I and II melanoma, and fostered adoption of a selective approach to formal lymphadenectomy in the treatment of microscopic lymph node metastases. Now recognized as a paradigm-changing landmark approach, global interest developed quickly for this rational management strategy. Several confirmatory studies, including completion of prospective randomized trials, have together generated a wealth of information regarding many issues related to the use of SLN biopsy, including accuracy, prognostic value, selection of appropriate candidates, use of enhanced histologic techniques, novel lymphatic drainage imaging studies, impact on regional disease control, and impact on morbidity and survival. While this technique has been widely regarded as one of the most important advances ever made in melanoma treatment, several controversies have nonetheless emerged.

On the eve of the twentieth anniversary since the introduction of SLN biopsy for patients with early-stage melanoma, it is appropriate and relevant to review the lessons learned and to critically evaluate the published SLN biopsy experience to assess its current role in the management of patients with stage I and II melanoma, to discuss some of the major controversies, and to outline likely future directions.

THE EVOLUTION OF SLN BIOPSY AS A RATIONAL MANAGEMENT STRATEGY IN PATIENTS WITH AJCC STAGE I AND II MELANOMA

The surgical approach in patients with stage I and II melanoma is often considered thematically by addressing 2 principles: (1) wide excision of the primary melanoma and (2) approach to regional lymph node evaluation. Whereas recommendations for the extent of excision margins are largely based on clinical trials and are therefore well established and widely accepted,[2] the approach to patients with clinically uninvolved regional lymph nodes has been the subject of extensive debate and ongoing controversy. The following clinical vignette further illustrates this clinical debate. An otherwise healthy 36-year old patient noted a changing pigmented lesion over the left scapula, and following narrow excisional biopsy of this site, was diagnosed with a 1.8-mm nonulcerated melanoma. On presentation for further evaluation and treatment planning, physical examination revealed no other suspicious cutaneous lesions and no palpable regional lymph nodes in any potential regional lymph node group. A chest radiograph was normal.

Historically, in addition to a recommendation for wide excision of the primary tumor, this patient would have likely been offered one of two approaches to the regional nodal basin: (1) nodal observation followed by formal lymph node dissection only if clinically evident (ie, palpable) nodal disease subsequently developed, a procedure termed therapeutic lymph node dissection (TLND), or (2) formal lymph node dissection as a component of the initial surgical treatment, commonly referred to as elective lymph node dissection (ELND). Although a detailed discussion is beyond the scope of this article, both approaches have theoretical and real disadvantages.[3]

A significant fraction of patients with melanoma, predicted by primary tumor and other factors, including increasing primary tumor thickness, ulceration, high mitotic rate, or other unfavorable histologic features of the primary tumor,[4] harbor clinically undetectable regional lymph node metastases at the time of presentation. Evolving data indicate that such microscopic regional disease will ultimately lead to palpable (ie, macroscopic) nodal disease.[5,6] Once clinical nodal involvement develops, however, the ability to achieve long-term survival and durable regional disease control with a TLND may be compromised as compared with surgical approaches targeted at treating microscopic nodal burden.[5,7] The clinical challenge is that following TLND, the rates of distant metastatic disease and relapse in the treated nodal basin are at least 50% and 15% to 50%, respectively.

Of importance, the practice of ELND was popularized with the intent of reducing these high rates of disease recurrence. Proponents of ELND suggested that removal of microscopically involved lymph nodes would prevent the development of clinically apparent lymph node metastasis and, at least in theory, eliminate a potential source of distant failure. Furthermore, regional lymph node surgery performed when the lymph node disease burden is microscopic and when few nodes are involved would minimize the risk of clinical recurrence in the affected basin, and potentially spare the patient from tumor burden–related sequelae including pain, skin ulceration, blood vessel and nerve involvement, and advanced lymphedema that can be associated with this pattern of recurrence.

In the majority of patients with clinically node-negative primary cutaneous melanoma, microscopic nodal disease is fortunately absent at diagnosis. It follows that such patients cannot benefit from an ELND; however, if ELND is performed, patients would be subjected to the cost and morbidity of an unnecessary operation. Because only approximately 20% of newly diagnosed stage I and II melanoma patients are considered to have an intermediate or high risk of harboring occult regional nodal disease, it is not surprising that overall survival advantages were not observed in prospective randomized trials comparing ELND to nodal observation in stage I and II patients predicted to have an intermediate or high risk for harboring microscopic regional nodal disease.[8–11] As a result, the routine practice of ELND was appropriately challenged.

Stemming in part from this controversy, and formally introduced and detailed in the next section, a rational strategy emerged when the technique of lymphatic mapping and SLN biopsy was introduced as a minimally invasive method for identifying patients who harbor occult nodal microscopic metastases.[1] Patients with proven occult regional nodal disease in the SLN could undergo an "early" TLND, and the majority of patients without nodal disease could be safely observed. This approach, termed selective lymphadenectomy, has been extensively studied worldwide and has gained widespread global use.

SCIENTIFIC SUPPORT FOR THE SENTINEL NODE CONCEPT

Lymphatic mapping relies on the hypothesis that the dermal lymphatic drainage from cutaneous sites to the regional lymph node basin(s) occurs as an orderly and definable process, and that these lymphatic drainage patterns should mimic or predict the potential routes of metastatic spread of melanoma cells via the lymphatics to regional lymph nodes (**Figs. 1**, **2A**, and **3**). Accordingly, the first lymph node(s) receiving direct afferent lymphatic drainage (ie, the SLNs) are the most likely to contain metastatic disease if any regional lymph nodes are involved. It then follows that successful identification, surgical removal, and careful histologic examination of all SLNs in a patient should provide accurate regional nodal staging.

To test this hypothesis, clinical studies were performed using intradermal injections of blue dyes (isosulfan blue or patent blue V) around the primary tumor site that are taken up and transported via the lymphatics (essentially "staining" the lymphatic fluid blue), followed by the visual identification and removal of SLNs in the regional nodal basin(s). These studies established the following: (1) SLN identification rates and (2) the accuracy of the SLN in determining the presence or absence of regional nodal metastases.

The landmark study that formally introduced this concept to the melanoma community was published by Donald Morton's group in 1992; among 237 evaluated patients,

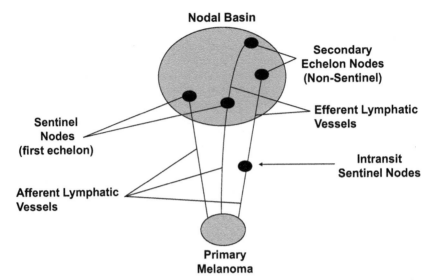

Fig. 1. Potential afferent lymphatic vessels draining from a primary cutaneous site to sentinel (first echelon) nodes in the regional nodal basin. Secondary echelon nodes may be identified by pass-through of the intradermally injected blue dye or radiolabeled colloid. Occasionally, a sentinel node is located between the injection site and the major nodal basin, and is defined as an "in-transit" sentinel node (as labeled here), but may also be referred to as an "interval" or "ectopic" sentinel node. (*Courtesy of* Merrick I. Ross, MD, copyright retained by the author and the U.T. MD Anderson Cancer Center.)

the SLN identification rate was 82%.[1] Subsequent studies from the University of Texas MD Anderson Cancer Center, the Sydney Melanoma Unit, and Moffitt Cancer Center reported similar findings.[12-14] In the early 1990s, accuracy was assessed through the use of synchronous ELND performed at the time of the SLN biopsy procedure. A false-negative event was defined as the detection of microscopic disease in non-SLNs when the SLN(s) from the same basin was histologically negative. Accordingly, the false-negative rate was then calculated as the number of false-negative events divided by the total number of patients with microscopic nodal disease. These initial studies collectively evaluated 402 patients with successful SLN localization, 86 of whom were found to have regional node metastases (81 patients with a positive SLN and 5 additional patients with disease only in a non-SLN).[3,12-14] This low false-negative rate of approximately 5% supported the SLN concept.

Additional evidence that regional node metastasis constitutes an orderly and nonrandom event was provided from an MD Anderson study that examined 105 lymphadenectomy specimens in patients with at least one positive SLN.[15] Investigators found that the SLN was the only lymph node involved in 83 (79%) of the basins, with microscopic nodal metastasis identified in an additional 21% of the lymphadenectomy specimens. Overall, among these patients with at least one positive SLN, 68% of all the SLNs harvested and only 1.8% of all non-SLNs removed contained metastatic disease.[15]

Tremendous interest was generated by these initial studies, and many centers subsequently adopted the selective lymphadenectomy approach for newly diagnosed intermediate- and high- risk stage I and II melanoma patients. Improvements in SLN localization techniques, insights into the biologic relevance of the SLN (see later discussion), and additional findings supporting the SLN concept emerged. In a report

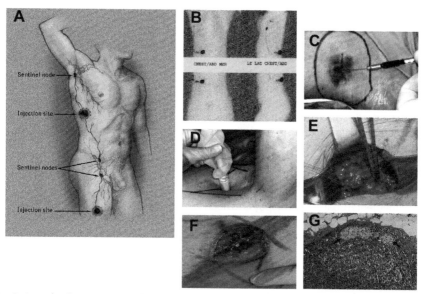

Fig. 2. Lymphatic mapping and sentinel lymph node (SLN) biopsy concept and technique. (*A*) The concept of lymphatic mapping. In this example, "melanoma" of right flank "drains" first via afferent lymphatics to both right axilla and right groin, while afferent lymphatics also "drain" to right groin from "melanoma" of right thigh. (*B*) Lymphoscintigraphy is an important component of the procedure that identifies nodal basin(s) at risk for primary melanomas arising in ambiguous lymphatic drainage sites and the number sentinel nodes in the basin. In (*B*), afferent lymphatic drainage from the low back is to the axilla rather than the anatomically more proximate inguinal basin. (*C*) Isosulfan blue is injected intradermally around melanoma biopsy site. (*D*) Transcutaneous localization of SLNs using gamma detection probe. (*E, F*) Exploration of nodal basin and visualization of SLNs. (*G*) Histologic detection of occult SLN metastasis (*arrows*) in subcapsular sinus (H&E stain, original magnification ×100). (Panels *A–F courtesy of* the authors, with copyright retained by the authors and the U.T. MD Anderson Cancer Center.) (Panel *G from* Gershenwald JE, Colome MI, Lee JE, et al. Patterns of recurrence following a negative sentinel lymph node biopsy in 243 patients with stage I or II melanoma. J Clin Oncol 1998;16(6):2257; with permission.)

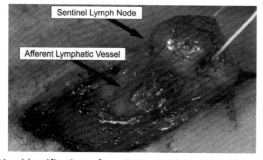

Fig. 3. Intraoperative identification of an SLN. Intradermal injection of a vital blue dye around the intact melanoma or biopsy site leads to uptake of the dye by the lymphatic system and transport of the dye to the draining regional nodal basins, thereby allowing for identification of SLNs. Note the isosulfan blue–stained afferent lymphatic vessel leading to blue-stained SLN. (*Courtesy of* Jeffrey E. Gershenwald, MD, copyright retained by the author and the U.T. MD Anderson Cancer Center.)

of nearly 250 SLN-negative patients followed for over 3 years, only 10 patients (4%) developed subsequent nodal failure within the previously mapped regional lymph node basins.[16] Such failures represent a false-negative rate similar to the 5% determined by concomitant ELND. Of note, this study represented patients who had SLN biopsy early in the global experience, when individual SLNs were subjected only to "routine" histologic analysis. More intense histologic scrutiny of the "negative" SLNs from these same 10 patients as part of this study revealed the presence of disease in 8 patients (8/10). These data not only further supported the validity of the SLN concept but also suggested that routine histologic examinations of SLNs may occasionally fail to detect clinically relevant disease.

HISTOLOGIC EXAMINATION OF SLNS

The fundamental goal of SLN biopsy is to accurately stage the regional lymph node basin, and is accomplished by the accurate identification and complete surgical removal of all the SLNs from the appropriate nodal basins at risk, followed by careful histologic examination of these SLNs. Although the definition of careful histologic examination continues to evolve, it is clear that it is logistically more feasible to apply sensitive techniques such as multiple sections or immunohistochemical analysis to a few lymph nodes (ie, the SLNs), rather than to the 20 to 30 lymph nodes submitted following a formal ELND. By carefully evaluating the nodes most likely to contain metastatic disease—the SLNs— more accurate nodal staging is possible, and with little morbidity to the patient.

Historically, the standard approach for evaluating lymph nodes, and therefore initially applied to the evaluation of SLNs as well, was to bivalve each clinically negative node and evaluate a section from each half using hematoxylin and eosin (H&E) staining. As a result, only a very small percentage of each lymph node(s) was actually sampled, and this likely explains why conventional histologic techniques underestimated the incidence of regional nodal disease in stage I and II melanoma patients. For example, the incidence of nodal failure following wide excision alone (ie, nodal observation) for primary melanomas 2 to 4 mm in thickness is approximately 35% to 50%, whereas the incidence of microscopic nodal disease as determined by ELND or SLN biopsy specimens, as determined by routine pathologic technique (ie, bivalving the nodes), is approximately 25% to 40%.[9] While subsequent nodal failure may in part result from clinically occult in-transit disease, several lines of evidence support the concept that nodal disease is more often present at diagnosis than is demonstrated by routine conventional histology: (1) step-sectioning of the SLN (ie, better sampling) increases detection of microscopic disease,[16] (2) up to 80% of patients who recur in the mapped nodal basin after a negative SLN biopsy initially assessed by routine pathology are determined to be node-positive following more careful analysis of the SLN paraffin blocks,[16,17] and (3) evaluation of SLNs using reverse transcriptase–polymerase chain reaction (RT-PCR) to detect the presence of messenger RNA encoding melanoma-related proteins (eg, tyrosinase) as potential surrogate markers for the presence of melanoma cells results in higher SLN-positive rates.[18–20] Studies demonstrate that essentially all H&E-positive SLNs and approximately 25% to 50% of H&E-negative SLNs are PCR-positive. It is intriguing that although preliminary clinical correlation studies demonstrated that recurrence rates for the PCR-positive/H&E-negative group were intermediate between the PCR-negative and H&E-positive patients,[18–21] longer-term follow-up in prospective studies from the Sunbelt Melanoma Trial and Memorial Sloan-Kettering Cancer Center each failed to demonstrate an overall decreased survival in the PCR-positive/H&E-negative patients compared with the PCR-negative/H&E-negative patients.[21,22] As histologic techniques become more sensitive, specificity may be compromised, but the more careful and complete the evaluation of SLNs, the more likely that a truly homogeneous SLN-negative subset can be defined.

Current recommendations include multiple H&E sections (ie, step-sectioning) and "routine" use of immunohistochemistry using HMB-45 and MART-1 antibodies; established standards continue to evolve[17,23–26] and are detailed elsewhere in this issue (see article on melanoma pathology by Scolyer and Prieto). Frozen section analysis at the time of SLN biopsy probably reduces the sensitivity and is therefore not recommended,[27,28] but imprint touch cytology performed on multiple sections of the SLN at the time of the SLN procedure can accurately detect microscopic disease in a significant fraction of patients with occult metastases, and may facilitate same-day completion lymphadenectomy without compromising the formal permanent histologic examination in patients who are SLN-positive and for whom concomitant completion lymphadenectomy was discussed preoperatively.[29] RT-PCR evaluation or other molecular-based studies is currently appropriate only in the context of a clinical trial.

TECHNICAL ADVANCES

Initial SLN identification rates of up to 85% using blue dye injections alone provided early promise for this technique. The use of high-resolution cutaneous lymphoscintigraphy[30–32] and an intraoperative hand-held gamma detection device to locate focal accumulation of radiotracer in SLNs following intradermal injection around the primary site have together dramatically improved SLN identification rates.[15,30,33,34] The use of an intraoperative gamma probe was first described by Krag and colleagues,[34] who reported a 95% SLN identification rate using this technique. Studies comparing combined modality techniques (ie, radiocolloid plus blue dye) to blue dye alone demonstrated a significant increase in SLN identification (to 99%) with the combined approach.[15,33] Furthermore, Gershenwald and colleagues[15] from MD Anderson observed that the number of SLNs identified was greater when both modalities were employed as compared with blue dye alone (1.74 vs 1.31, respectively). Overall, intraoperative use of the gamma probe provides an independent and complementary method of detection that is more sensitive for SLN identification than visualization of blue-stained nodes alone, and facilitates localization of SLNs that may otherwise go undetected during the SLN biopsy procedure. It follows, therefore, that more complete identification and removal of SLNs using the combined modality approach may further reduce an already low false-negative rate (see **Fig. 2**).

These techniques also facilitate localization of SLNs that may exist outside of the formal named nodal basins; such SLNs are commonly referred to as unusual, interval, in-transit, or ectopic SLNs (**Fig. 4**).[32,35–39] The incidence of SLNs in such locations is approximately 5% to 10%; interestingly, the frequency of microscopic involvement in such SLNs is similar to that observed in SLNs harvested from formal named major basins.[35] The failure to identify these SLNs risks understaging some patients and leaving behind potential sources of clinical recurrences. More recently, the use of SPECT/CT (a fusion imaging technique of nuclear [single-photon emission] and computed tomography images) provides enhanced and 3-dimensional spatial resolution of areas of increased focal radiotracer uptake activity that correspond to SLNs, and is particularly helpful in identifying the anatomic location of SLNs in the head and neck region.[40]

BIOLOGIC AND PROGNOSTIC SIGNIFICANCE OF THE SENTINEL NODE

Studies have demonstrated that the incidence of SLN metastases correlates directly with increasing tumor thickness.[15,41–44] SLN involvement is also associated with

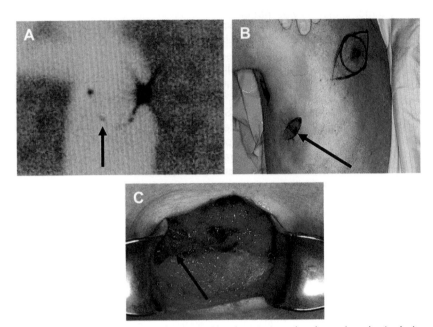

Fig. 4. In-transit sentinel node. (*A*) Planar lymphoscintigraphy shows lymphatic drainage pattern from injection site over left upper back to the ipsilateral axilla and an in-transit SLN (*arrow*) over the scapular spine. (*B*) Intraoperative photograph showing the left para-median upper back primary site and SLN biopsy sites in the ipsilateral axilla and in-transit region (*arrow*). (*C*) Close-up view of exposed in-transit SLN (*arrow*) with blue-stained afferent channel. (*Courtesy of* Merrick I. Ross, MD, copyright retained by the author and the U.T. MD Anderson Cancer Center.)

a variety of other known primary tumor factors predictive of survival, including ulceration, lymphatic invasion,[45,46] mitotic rate, Clark level, anatomic site, and host factors such as age.[42,43,47–49] In a multivariate analysis by Rousseau and colleagues[43] of 1375 patients with primary melanoma who underwent SLN biopsy, tumor thickness and the presence of ulceration both independently predicted SLN involvement (**Table 1**). Of

Table 1
Incidence of SLN metastases stratified by tumor thickness and ulceration

Tumor Thickness (mm)	Total Patients (%)	Positive SLN All (%)	Not Ulcerated (%)	Not Ulcerated AJCC Stage[b]	Ulcerated (%)	Ulcerated AJCC Stage[b]	P Value[a] Ulcerated vs Not Ulcerated
≤1.00	28	4	3	IA	16	IB	.026
1.01–2.00	38	12	11	IB	22	IIA	.007
2.01–4.00	23	28	25	IIA	34	IIB	.115
>4.00	11	44	33	IIB	53	IIC	.021
All patients	100	17	12		35		<.0001

[a] Fisher's exact test for each tumor thickness group.
[b] Stage groupings calculated using tumor thickness and ulceration data only.
   Data from Rousseau DL, Ross MI, Johnson MM, et al. Revised American Joint Committee on Cancer staging criteria accurately predict sentinel lymph node positivity in clinically node-negative melanoma patients. Ann Surg Oncol 2003;10:572.

note, the 2002 AJCC melanoma staging committee database analysis demonstrated that the same 2 factors were also the strongest predictors of survival in stage I and II patients.[4,7,47,50] This analysis uncovered a unique interaction between tumor thickness and ulceration in that the presence of ulceration within a specific tumor thickness stage worsened the prognosis of patients equivalent to those in the next higher thickness group without ulceration.[47] A similar relationship was also observed between thickness and ulceration in terms of predicting the incidence of SLN metastases.[43] These observations support the hypothesis that the prognostic value of tumor thickness and ulceration is largely dependent on the fact that these 2 same factors predict SLN metastases, and in this way provide convincing evidence that SLN involvement is a biologically important event. As noted in the article elsewhere in this issue on staging and prognosis by Dickson and Gershenwald, mitotic activity has been shown to be an important independent predictor of survival, and at a cut point of $1/mm^2$ has recently been incorporated into the new AJCC seventh edition definition of T1b primary melanoma.[50] It is interesting that preliminary data also indicate that SLN involvement correlates with mitotic activity for the subset of patients with a primary melanoma less than 1 mm in thickness.

Further support for the SLN concept stems from survival analyses of large numbers of stage I and II melanoma patients managed in prospective selective lymphadenectomy programs. These reports consistently revealed that SLN-positive patients experienced a significantly lower survival than SLN-negative patients (**Fig. 5**), and that the histologic status of the SLN was the most powerful independent predictor of survival in clinically node-negative melanoma patients when analyses included previously

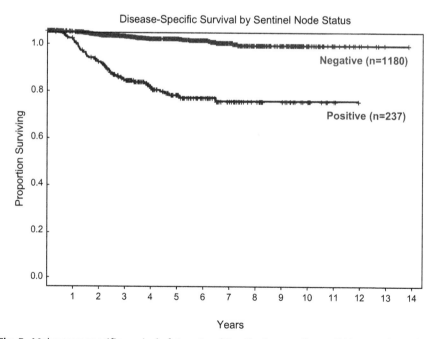

Fig. 5. Melanoma-specific survival of stage I and II patients according to SLN status. (*Data from* Gershenwald JE, Thompson W, Mansfield PF, et al. Multi-institutional melanoma lymphatic mapping experience: the prognostic value of sentinel lymph node status in 612 stage I or II melanoma patients. J Clin Oncol 1999;17:976–83. *Courtesy of* Jeffrey E. Gershenwald, MD, Houston, TX, copyright retained by the author and the U.T. MD Anderson Cancer Center.)

described primary tumor prognostic factors (**Table 2**).[51] Several published large single-institutional and multicenter experiences have corroborated these findings.[5,23,52] The prognostic significance of SLN status is underscored in **Table 3**. In **Table 3**, 5-year survival according to T-category and AJCC staging edition (sixth vs seventh) demonstrates "improved" survival estimates among patients included in the seventh edition AJCC melanoma database who had stage-appropriate use of SLN biopsy (ie, SLN biopsy performed if primary tumor was at least T1b) compared with similar T-category patients in the sixth edition AJCC melanoma database, in which only some patients with primary tumors at least T1b underwent SLN biopsy.[53]

Although patients with a negative SLN as a whole enjoy a very favorable survival profile, a negative SLN is nonetheless not an absolute predictor of survival. Five-year melanoma-specific survival rates are approximately 92% for the SLN-negative patients, with recurrence and death related to a false-negative SLN or a pure hematogenous pattern of metastases. Predictors of relapse and death in the SLN-negative group include increasing tumor thickness and primary tumor ulceration. The development of clinical nodal disease in a nodal basin previously determined to be without microscopic involvement defines a false-negative event and occurs in approximately 3% to 5% of these patients. In theory, 3 possible explanations exist for these events: (1) the actual SLN(s) was not properly identified during the SLN procedure, leaving behind a microscopically involved lymph node; (2) the original SLN procedure was accurate, but microscopic in-transit disease was present at the outset but had not yet traveled to the nodal basin; (3) the correct SLN was removed and microscopic disease was present, but was not detected by histologic examination either as a result of a very small burden of disease or because it was within a portion of the node that was not sampled.[16]

QUESTIONS AND CONTROVERSIES

The original motivation to develop the technique of SLN biopsy was to establish an effective method of early detection (and treatment) of regional lymph node involvement, thereby "preventing" the development of clinically palpable regional disease in stage I and II melanoma patients without performing unnecessary formal lymph

Table 2
Prognostic factors influencing disease-specific survival in stage I and II patients undergoing SLN biopsy

Prognostic Factor	Univariate	Multiple Covariate	
		Hazard Ratio	P value
Age	.82	1.01	.57
Sex	.35	1.11	.78
Axial location	.07	1.72	.13
Tumor thickness	<.00001	1.32	.0004
Clark level >III	.0045	2.23	.04
Ulceration	.0001	1.23	.14
SLN status	<.00001	6.32	<.00001

From Gershenwald JE, Thompson W, Mansfield PF, et al. Multi-institutional melanoma lymphatic mapping experience: the prognostic value of sentinel lymph node status in 612 stage I or II melanoma patients. J Clin Oncol 1999;17:980; with permission.

Table 3		
AJCC collaborative melanoma database stage I/II 5-year survival rate by T-classification		
T-Category	Sixth Edition	Seventh Edition SLN Subset[a]
T1a	95 ± 0.4	97 ± 1.1
T1b	91 ± 1.0	95 ± 1.5
T2a	89 ± 0.7	95 ± 0.6
T2b	77 ± 1.7	86 ± 2.0
T3a	79 ± 1.2	85 ± 1.5
T3b	63 ± 1.5	76 ± 2.5
T4a	67 ± 2.4	76 ± 3.6
T4b	45 ± 1.9	67 ± 3.6

[a] Stage-appropriate use of SLN biopsy.
From Balch, CM, Gershenwald JE, Soong SJ, et al. Melanoma staging and classification, In: Balch CM, Houghton AN, Sober AJ, et al, editors. Cutaneous melanoma. St Louis: Quality Medical Publishing, Inc; 2009. p. 67; with permission.

node dissections. The collective experience with this approach demonstrates that this goal has been achieved. Furthermore, its role as a staging tool has been well established and offers particular motivation for its use. Nonetheless, many have questioned its therapeutic value, and several other questions and controversies have emerged, which are now discussed.

Does Early Node Dissection Impart a Survival Benefit?

The potential for improved survival with early formal lymph node dissection was the goal for the routine application of ELND in the initial management of newly diagnosed stage I and II patients. The question of survival impact with the use of ELND relative to nodal observation and therapeutic dissection for those patients who develop clinically detectable nodal disease has been evaluated in 4 prospective randomized trials. The first 2 trials were performed in the 1970s (one from the World Health Organization [WHO] Melanoma Program and another from the Mayo Clinic)[10,11] during a time period before significant knowledge concerning primary tumor prognostic factors; not surprisingly, no survival advantages were noted. Accordingly, ELND was strongly contested and largely abandoned. These trials were subsequently criticized because in retrospect, the study populations were at low risk for occult regional nodal disease and therefore were unlikely to benefit from the surgical treatment being tested.

Subsequently, 2 additional ELND trials were performed targeting higher-risk, clinically node-negative melanoma patients.[8,9] Trends for improved survival following ELND were observed in both trials; however, these differences were not statistically significant. Whereas many concluded that early treatment of nodal metastases had little impact on disease progression, others suggested that these trials were underpowered because only the 20% of patients harboring nodal disease could potentially benefit from the procedure.[3] Long-term results were published in 1998 from the WHO ELND Trial, which included patients with truncal primaries larger than 1.5 mm, and demonstrated that patients with microscopic nodal disease in the ELND treatment arm had improved overall survival compared with patients who developed clinical adenopathy after randomization to wide excision of the primary tumor and nodal observation alone.[9] In 2000, results published from the Intergroup Melanoma ELND Trial, in which patients with melanomas 1 to 4 mm in thickness were included, demonstrated that prospectively stratified subgroups (patients with 1–2 mm and all nonulcerated primaries) derived a survival benefit from ELND.[8] Although overall survival rates for the entire study cohorts in both trials were not statistically different, supporting the proposal that not all patients can benefit from ELND, these studies did suggest that specific subsets of patients (most notably those with microscopic nodal disease and possibly additional patients with nodal disease undetected by routine histologic techniques) can benefit from earlier dissections. These data offer evidence-based support to the theoretical concerns of delaying the lymphadenectomy until palpable nodal disease develops, and support the selective lymphadenectomy approach.

The survival impact of the selective lymphadenectomy strategy, using SLN biopsy as an alternative to ELND, was formally studied in a prospective randomized multicenter, international trial comparing the outcomes of patients who had nodal observation after wide excision with patients who had wide excision and SLN biopsy, and had completion dissection if microscopic SLN involvement was identified.[5] The design and primary and secondary end points of the Multicenter Selective Lymphadenectomy Trial-1 (MSLT-1) are schematized in **Fig. 6**. The results of the third interim analysis (of 5 planned analyses) for this trial were published in 2006.[5] Data were available for 1269 patients. In the cohort randomized to SLN biopsy, the presence of SLN metastases was the most important prognostic factor.[54] The 5-year melanoma-specific survival rate was 72.3% ± 4.6% among patients with tumor-positive SLNs and 90.2% ± 1.3% among those with tumor-negative SLNs (P<.001), recapitulating in a prospective randomized trial the previously reported observations from several other groups. The 5-year melanoma-specific death rate was similar in the 2 groups (13.8% in the nodal observation group and 12.5% in the SLN biopsy group), as was 3-year and 5-year melanoma-specific survival (90.1% ± 1.4% and 93.2% ± 0.9%, respectively and 86.6% ± 1.6% and 87.1% ± 1.3%, respectively). Although no overall survival advantage was observed when comparing the entire cohort of patients randomized to SLN biopsy with those patients who had wide excision only and nodal observation, a small but statistically significant 5-year disease-free survival advantage was observed (78.3% ± 1.6% vs 73.1% ± 2.1%, hazard ratio [HR] 0.74, 95% confidence interval [CI] 0.59–0.93; P = .009) (**Fig. 7**). It is intriguing that the incidence of SLN

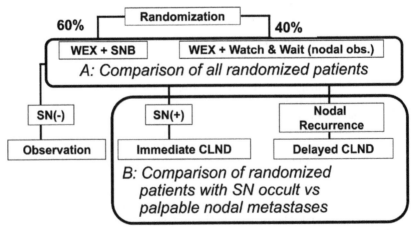

Fig. 6. Treatment algorithm for Multicenter Selective Lymphadenectomy Trial (MSLT-1). CLND, completion lymph node dissection; SN, sentinel lymph node; SNB, SLN biopsy; nodal obs., nodal observation; WEX, wide local excision of primary.

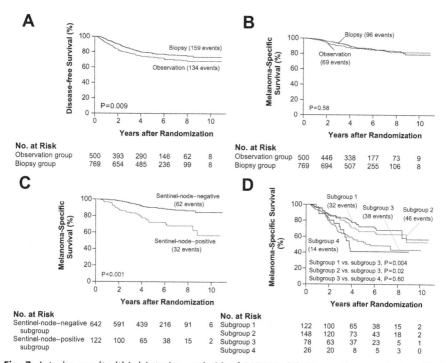

Fig. 7. Interim results (third interim analysis) of MSLT-1. (*A*) Disease-free survival and (*B*) melanoma-specific survival, respectively, according to the type of treatment. (*C*) Melanoma-specific survival according to the tumor status of the sentinel node in patients who underwent sentinel node biopsy. (*D*) Melanoma-specific survival among patients with nodal metastases: subgroup 1 comprised patients with a tumor-positive sentinel node; subgroup 2, the patients in subgroup 1 plus those in subgroup 4 with a nodal recurrence after a negative result on biopsy; subgroup 3, those with nodal recurrence during observation; and subgroup 4, those with nodal recurrence after a negative result on biopsy. (*From* Morton, DL, Thompson JF, Cochran AJ, et al. Sentinel-node biopsy or nodal observation in melanoma. N Engl J Med 2006;355(13):1307–17; with permission.)

micrometastases was 16%, and the rate of relapse in regional nodes in the observation group was nearly identical: 15.6%. The mean number of tumor-involved nodes at lymphadenectomy was 1.4 in the SLN biopsy group and 3.3 in the nodal observation group that recurred (*P*<.001). A pronounced overall survival advantage was observed when the survival analysis was limited to only the node-positive patients. Compared with the patients who underwent a therapeutic (delayed dissection) for clinical nodal failure after nodal observation, the SLN-positive patients had an improved 5-year melanoma-specific survival (72.3% ± 4.6% vs 52.4% ± 5.9%; HR for death 0.51, 95% CI 0.32–0.81; *P* = .004), as shown in **Fig. 7**.

Overall, the interim results of the MSLT-1 trial provide important insights into the value of selective lymphadenectomy as compared with delayed lymphadenectomy. The lack of an overall survival difference between the 2 treatment arms is not surprising. This trial likely suffers from the same limitation as the ELND trials: being underpowered because of the low percentage of patients (approximately 16% in this trial) who could benefit from complete lymphadenectomy. Assuming that early lymphadenectomy for SLN-positive patients is associated with an approximately

20% survival advantage, one would predict an overall survival advantage of no more than 3.2% compared with delayed lymphadenectomy.[55] Nonetheless, survival differences may emerge with longer follow-up in subsequent planned analyses, particularly because disease-free survival differences have already been reported; this may be particularly true if future events follow the patterns observed in the 2 ELND trials, whereby more recurrences in the nodal observation arm may develop over time than in the SLN biopsy arm.

The results of the secondary survival analyses comparing SLN-positive patients with those who developed clinically palpable nodes following nodal observation are particularly noteworthy. The improved survival of the SLN-positive group not only corroborates the results of the WHO trial but also supports the concept that—if left intact—microscopic nodal disease progresses clinically and is associated with a worse prognosis. In some patients, therefore, increasing nodal burden can be a source of systemic dissemination; this implies that early treatment of nodal disease can favorably alter the natural history of their disease.

Is Regional Disease Control Improved When Lymphadenectomy is Performed for Microscopic Disease?

The most common first site of recurrence in primary melanoma patients initially treated with wide excision of the primary site only is palpable regional lymph node metastasis. These patients are generally treated by TLND with curative intent and to provide regional control of disease. Post-lymphadenectomy in-basin failure rates range from 9% to 50%, and depend on a variety of factors, including basin site, number and size of involved nodes, and presence of extracapsular extension. In-basin recurrences are very difficult to treat surgically and may be the source of significant morbidity in the form of pain, severe lymphedema, venous obstruction, skin ulceration, nerve involvement, and bleeding. By contrast, in-basin failures are observed in fewer than 10% of patients who undergo ELND for microscopic disease, and are likely even less frequent after completion lymph node dissection in patients with a positive SLN. The potential for improved regional disease control when lymphadenectomy is performed for microscopic disease further supports the use of SLN biopsy.

Patient Selection for SLN Biopsy

Candidates for SLN biopsy include patients with newly diagnosed clinically node-negative primary melanoma who are predicted to be at intermediate or high risk of harboring occult regional nodal disease based on primary tumor characteristics.[42,43] Although uniform risk thresholds have not been completely resolved, a tumor thickness threshold of at least 1 mm has gained wide acceptance. Overall, the routine use of SLN biopsy in patients with thin (<1 mm) melanoma is not cost effective because of the overall low risk of nodal involvement in this group.[56] However, a selective approach to SLN biopsy for patients with thin melanoma has evolved in many melanoma centers based on the presence of adverse risk factors, such as Clark level IV invasion and/or ulceration, because these 2 factors were the most powerful predictors of recurrence in the thin melanoma patients in the 2002 AJCC analysis.[4,57] Using this approach, patients with stage IB disease and higher may be offered SLN biopsy, an approach adopted by the AJCC at that time. Other primary tumor prognostic factors that have been commonly used in the decision-making process for thin melanoma patients include vertical growth phase and a positive deep biopsy margin. An emerging important primary tumor risk factor for SLN involvement is the presence and number of mitotic figures in the vertical growth phase, which may be considered a surrogate for aggressive biology.[58-60] In a study from the University of Pennsylvania, among patients with thin melanomas of at least 0.76 mm and exhibiting 1 or more mitotic figures per mm^2, the incidence SLN metastases was 12.5%.[58] The presence of mitotic figures is increasingly being used to identify the higher risk subset of patients as candidates for SLN biopsy; its absolute role in assessing the risk of SLN involvement in patients with thin melanoma is currently an area of intense investigation. Further discussion regarding the evolving prognostic significance of primary tumor mitotic activity among patients with thin melanomas may be found elsewhere in this issue (see article on staging and prognosis by Dickson and Gershenwald).

It should be emphasized that SLN biopsy is also appropriate for patients with thick melanomas (>4 mm) even though this group is also at high risk for distant disease, as recently published experiences from more than one center demonstrates that SLN status is the single most important independent predictor of survival and also affords improved regional node field control.[61–65]

Other clinical scenarios for which SLN biopsy may be useful include: (1) patients who develop a true local recurrence subsequent to a relatively narrow excision as prior treatment of a primary melanoma; (2) patients in whom the exact tumor thickness cannot be ascertained because of improper placement in the biopsy specimen within the paraffin block, resulting in tangential sectioning; (3) when residual tumor is present at the base secondary to a superficial shave biopsy; (4) when a manipulation such as cryotherapy or cauterization has been performed on the same lesion before the diagnosis of melanoma; (5) when the pathologic diagnosis of an atypical melanocytic lesion is ambiguous but includes a primary melanoma greater than 1 mm in thickness in the differential diagnosis[66]; or (6) patients who have already had a formal wide excision with or without a skin graft who are otherwise candidates for SLN biopsy based on predicted risk of the primary tumor. In this latter situation, the accuracy of the technique is at least theoretically in question because the lymphatic drainage of the remaining skin may be different to the skin that existed immediately adjacent to the original primary melanoma. A few small published series compared the incidence of positive SLNs in groups of patients who had already undergone a 1-cm or wider excision with patients who had intact lesions or an excision for diagnosis. The patient groups were matched in terms of primary tumor factors and the incidence of positive SLNs was similar, suggesting that SLN biopsy may still be accurate in selected patients who have had prior wide excision.[67]

Is Completion Dissection in Patients with a Positive SLN Necessary?

The role of completion lymph node dissection in patients with a positive SLN biopsy represents a clinically important question for patients who undergo SLN biopsy. Only 10% to 25% of patients with a positive SLN will be found to have additional microscopic nodal disease within nonsentinel nodes removed by a subsequent formal TLND.[68–70] These data must be viewed carefully, however, since the routine pathologic technique used to evaluate a therapeutic lymphadenectomy specimen for additional non-SLN involvement is generally limited to bisecting lymph nodes rather than to multiple step-sectioning or immunohistochemical staining that is "routinely" employed to evaluate SLNs, and may thus underestimate micrometastatic disease.

An international randomized trial, the Multicenter Selective Lymphadenectomy Trial-2 (MSLT-2), is currently accruing patents using the basic framework design of a prospective randomized trial that compares therapeutic node dissection to nodal basin observation in patients with a positive SLN biopsy. This trial will address and hopefully answer the following: (1) the incidence of nodal failure after removal of a positive SLN in the absence of a completion dissection; (2) the incidence and predictors of additional positive non-SLNs in the same basin; and (3) the survival impact, if any, of completion lymph node dissection for these patients. In Europe, the role of omitting completion lymph node dissection among patients with "low-burden" SLN metastasis is the subject of another trial, known as the MINITUB study. MINITUB is a prospective, single-arm registration trial conducted by the European Organization for Research and Treatment of Cancer that evaluates the efficacy of not performing a CLND in patients with minimal tumor burden in the SLN biopsy. The primary end point of MINITUB is distant metastasis-free survival, and the secondary end points are the rate of TLND for palpable regional lymph node relapse and the long-term regional lymph node basin control rate. Patients are being followed for 10 years in both trials.

Some surgeons have already begun to omit completion dissection, albeit inconsistently, in SLN-positive patients, whereas other clinicians have selectively not recommended completion dissection based on published predictors of non-SLN involvement, including patients with primary tumors smaller than 2 mm and SLN tumor burden of less than 2 mm in diameter. Such practices outside of clinical trials should be discouraged until evidence becomes available supporting the efficacy and safety of such an approach; as such, completion dissection should be considered the current standard of care.

What are the Adverse Events?

Overall, the technique of SLN biopsy is associated with low morbidity, and many fewer postoperative complications are observed after SLN biopsy than occur after formal complete lymphadenectomy. Low complication rates were observed in the Sunbelt Melanoma Trial in more than 1202 patients following SLN biopsy alone compared with the 277 patients who had a complete lymphadenectomy.[71] The same observation has been made by others, including in the MSLT-1, wherein the overall complication rate of 10% after SLN biopsy increased to 32.7% after completion lymphadenectomy. The incidence of allergic reaction to blue dye, although reported, is very low.

Despite the widespread acceptance of SLN biopsy for many reasons (eg, accurate nodal staging, enhanced regional control, possible survival benefit, limited surgical morbidity compared with formal lymphadenectomy), some have argued that this approach may itself increase the risk of in-transit metastasis by disturbing lymph flow resulting from mechanical disruption.[72,73] Despite these assertions, all available data,[74–77] including data from MSLT-1,[5] strongly support that this is not a legitimate concern; instead, they indicate that the risk of in-transit melanoma depends on tumor biology and not on the surgical approach to regional lymph nodes.

FUTURE DIRECTIONS

Recent data indicate that the extent of microscopic disease in SLNs can be used to stratify survival.[52,69,78–91] Some studies also suggest that even isolated tumor cells in regional lymph nodes are clinically relevant in patients with melanoma, although others suggest that a lower threshold may exist below which metastatic deposits may not be clinically relevant.[69,79,81–83,90–96] Longer follow-up of these and other studies is required to definitively answer this question. The concept of microscopic nodal tumor burden will likely become even more important in the era of SLN biopsy as accurate microscopic staging of SLNs becomes even more widespread and patients are better stratified on the basis of microscopic tumor burden. As our understanding of the significance of microscopic nodal tumor burden is refined, clinical decisions regarding the need for and extent of further surgery or adjuvant therapy may also be based on the extent of microscopic nodal tumor burden.[70,97] As has been demonstrated over the past 2 decades, it is also likely that continued evolution in surgical technique, enhancements in nuclear imaging technology (including the development and implementation of radiotracers labeled with novel agents and new imaging techniques) and continued refinements in pathologic analysis to potentially include molecular-based assessment paradigms, as well as better systemic therapies, will continue to shape the clinical use of lymphatic mapping and SLN biopsy for patients with clinically node-negative stage I and II melanoma. Along these lines, SLN biopsy will be <u>essential</u> once effective, non-toxic, <u>adjuvant</u> therapies become available.

SUMMARY

Over the past 20 years, the technique of lymphatic mapping and SLN biopsy, pioneered by Donald Morton, has been repeatedly demonstrated to accurately stage the regional lymph node basins at risk in patients with AJCC stages I and II melanoma with little morbidity, and facilitates the selective application of formal completion lymph node dissection to only those patients who harbor microscopic regional nodal disease. In this way, SLN-positive patients are identified (and treated) when their nodal tumor burden is microscopic, optimizing the chance for long-term survival and durable regional nodal basin control. With the introduction of more sensitive histologic techniques, SLN biopsy offers the opportunity to more accurately stage patients and defines a more pure and homogeneous node-negative population. Node-positive patients can be offered standard adjuvant therapy or participation in prospective clinical trials assessing the value of novel adjuvant therapy regimens. It is important that low-risk patients can then be safely spared the morbidity of additional surgery and adjuvant therapy. Until molecular studies are developed that accurately predict the metastatic phenotype in patients with primary melanoma, SLN biopsy currently offers the opportunity to accomplish the aforementioned clinical goals in managing stage I and II patients: optimizing the chance for cure, providing durable regional control, accurate staging, and minimizing treatment morbidity.

REFERENCES

1. Morton DL, Wen DR, Wong JH, et al. Technical details of intraoperative lymphatic mapping for early stage melanoma. Arch Surg 1992;127(4):392–9.
2. Bedrosian I, Gershenwald JE. Surgical clinical trials in melanoma. Surg Clin North Am 2003;83(2):385–403.
3. Ross MI. Surgical management of stage I and II melanoma patients: approach to the regional lymph node basin. Semin Surg Oncol 1996;12(6):394–401.
4. Balch CM, Soong SJ, Gershenwald JE, et al. Prognostic factors analysis of 17,600 melanoma patients: validation of the American Joint Committee on Cancer melanoma staging system. J Clin Oncol 2001;19(16):3622–34.
5. Morton DL, Thompson JF, Cochran AJ, et al. Sentinel-node biopsy or nodal observation in melanoma. N Engl J Med 2006;355(13):1307–17.
6. Morton DL, Cochran AJ, Thompson JF. Sentinel-node biopsy in melanoma. N Engl J Med 2007;356:419–20.
7. Balch CM, Gershenwald JE, Soong SJ, et al. Multivariate analysis of prognostic factors among 2,313 patients with stage III melanoma: comparison of nodal micrometastases versus macrometastases. J Clin Oncol 2010;28(14):2452–9.
8. Balch CM, Soong S, Ross MI, et al. Long-term results of a multi-institutional randomized trial comparing prognostic factors and surgical results for

intermediate thickness melanomas (1.0 to 4.0 mm). Intergroup Melanoma Surgical Trial. Ann Surg Oncol 2000;7(2):87–97.

9. Cascinelli N, Morabito A, Santinami M, et al. Immediate or delayed dissection of regional nodes in patients with melanoma of the trunk: a randomised trial. WHO Melanoma Programme. Lancet 1998;351(9105):793–6.

10. Sim FH, Taylor WF, Pritchard DJ, et al. Lymphadenectomy in the management of stage I malignant melanoma: a prospective randomized study. Mayo Clin Proc 1986;61(9):697–705.

11. Veronesi U, Adamus J, Bandiera DC, et al. Inefficacy of immediate node dissection in stage 1 melanoma of the limbs. N Engl J Med 1977;297(12):627–30.

12. Ross MI, Reintgen D, Balch CM. Selective lymphadenectomy: emerging role for lymphatic mapping and sentinel node biopsy in the management of early stage melanoma. Semin Surg Oncol 1993;9(3):219–23.

13. Thompson JF, McCarthy WH, Bosch CM, et al. Sentinel lymph node status as an indicator of the presence of metastatic melanoma in regional lymph nodes. Melanoma Res 1995;5(4):255–60.

14. Reintgen D, Cruse CW, Wells K, et al. The orderly progression of melanoma nodal metastases. Ann Surg 1994;220(6):759–67.

15. Gershenwald JE, Tseng CH, Thompson W, et al. Improved sentinel lymph node localization in patients with primary melanoma with the use of radiolabeled colloid. Surgery 1998;124(2):203–10.

16. Gershenwald JE, Colome MI, Lee JE, et al. Patterns of recurrence following a negative sentinel lymph node biopsy in 243 patients with stage I or II melanoma. J Clin Oncol 1998;16(6):2253–60.

17. Cook MG, Green MA, Anderson B, et al. The development of optimal pathological assessment of sentinel lymph nodes for melanoma. J Pathol 2003;200(3): 314–9.

18. Reintgen D, Balch CM, Kirkwood J, et al. Recent advances in the care of the patient with malignant melanoma. Ann Surg 1997;225(1):1–14.

19. Shivers SC, Wang X, Li W, et al. Molecular staging of malignant melanoma: correlation with clinical outcome. JAMA 1998;280(16):1410–5.

20. Wang X, Heller R, VanVoorhis N, et al. Detection of submicroscopic lymph node metastases with polymerase chain reaction in patients with malignant melanoma. Ann Surg 1994;220(6):768–74.

21. Kammula US, Ghossein R, Bhattacharya S, et al. Serial follow-up and the prognostic significance of reverse transcriptase-polymerase chain reaction–staged sentinel lymph nodes from melanoma patients. J Clin Oncol 2004;22(19):3989–96.

22. Scoggins CR, Ross MI, Reintgen DS, et al. Prospective multi-institutional study of reverse transcriptase polymerase chain reaction for molecular staging of melanoma. J Clin Oncol 2006;24(18):2849–57.

23. Clary BM, Brady MS, Lewis JJ, et al. Sentinel lymph node biopsy in the management of patients with primary cutaneous melanoma: review of a large single-institutional experience with an emphasis on recurrence. Ann Surg 2001;233(2): 250–8.

24. Prieto VG, Clark SH. Processing of sentinel lymph nodes for detection of metastatic melanoma. Ann Diagn Pathol 2002;6(4):257–64.

25. Chakera AH, Hesse B, Burak Z, et al. EANM-EORTC general recommendations for sentinel node diagnostics in melanoma. Eur J Nucl Med Mol Imaging 2009; 36(10):1713–42.

26. Scolyer RA, Murali R, McCarthy SW, et al. Pathologic examination of sentinel lymph nodes from melanoma patients. Semin Diagn Pathol 2008;25(2):100–11.

27. Scolyer RA, Thompson JF, McCarthy SW, et al. Intraoperative frozen-section eval-uation can reduce accuracy of pathologic assessment of sentinel nodes in mela-noma patients. J Am Coll Surg 2005;201(5):821–3 [author reply: 823–4].

28. Stojadinovic A, Allen PJ, Clary BM, et al. Value of frozen-section analysis of sentinel lymph nodes for primary cutaneous malignant melanoma. Ann Surg 2002;235(1):92–8.

29. Soo V, Shen P, Pichardo R, et al. Intraoperative evaluation of sentinel lymph nodes for metastatic melanoma by imprint cytology. Ann Surg Oncol 2007;14(5):1612–7.

30. Albertini JJ, Cruse CW, Rapaport D, et al. Intraoperative radio-lympho-scintigraphy improves sentinel lymph node identification for patients with melanoma. Ann Surg 1996;223(2):217–24.

31. Berger DH, Feig BW, Podoloff D, et al. Lymphoscintigraphy as a predictor of lymphatic drainage from cutaneous melanoma. Ann Surg Oncol 1997;4(3):247–51.

32. Uren RF, Howman-Giles R, Thompson JF, et al. Lymphoscintigraphy to identify sentinel lymph nodes in patients with melanoma. Melanoma Res 1994;4(6): 395–9.

33. Kapteijn BA, Nieweg OE, Liem I, et al. Localizing the sentinel node in cutaneous melanoma: gamma probe detection versus blue dye. Ann Surg Oncol 1997;4(2): 156–60.

34. Krag DN, Meijer SJ, Weaver DL, et al. Minimal-access surgery for staging of malignant melanoma. Arch Surg 1995;130(6):654–8 [discussion: 659–60].

35. Sumner WE 3rd, Ross MI, Mansfield PF, et al. Implications of lymphatic drainage to unusual sentinel lymph node sites in patients with primary cutaneous mela-noma. Cancer 2002;95(2):354–60.

36. Thompson JF, Uren RF, Shaw HM, et al. Location of sentinel lymph nodes in patients with cutaneous melanoma: new insights into lymphatic anatomy. J Am Coll Surg 1999;189(2):195–204.

37. Uren RF, Howman-Giles R, Thompson JF, et al. Interval nodes: the forgotten sentinel nodes in patients with melanoma. Arch Surg 2000;135(10):1168–72.

38. Uren RF, Thompson JF, Howman-Giles R. Sentinel nodes. Interval nodes, lymphatic lakes, and accurate sentinel node identification. Clin Nucl Med 2000; 25(3):234–6.

39. Uren RF, Thompson JF, Howman-Giles R, et al. Melanoma metastases in trian-gular intermuscular space lymph nodes. Ann Surg Oncol 1999;6(8):811.

40. Uren RF. SPECT/CT Lymphoscintigraphy to locate the sentinel lymph node in patients with melanoma. Ann Surg Oncol 2009;16(6):1459–60.

41. Cascinelli N, Belli F, Santinami M, et al. Sentinel lymph node biopsy in cutaneous melanoma: the WHO Melanoma Program experience. Ann Surg Oncol 2000;7(6): 469–74.

42. McMasters KM, Wong SL, Edwards MJ, et al. Factors that predict the presence of sentinel lymph node metastasis in patients with melanoma. Surgery 2001;130(2): 151–6.

43. Rousseau DL Jr, Ross MI, Johnson MM, et al. Revised American Joint Committee on Cancer staging criteria accurately predict sentinel lymph node positivity in clinically node-negative melanoma patients. Ann Surg Oncol 2003; 10(5):569–74.

44. Thompson JF. The Sydney Melanoma Unit experience of sentinel lymphadenec-tomy for melanoma. Ann Surg Oncol 2001;8(Suppl 9):44S–7S.

45. Petersson F, Diwan AH, Ivan D, et al. Immunohistochemical detection of lympho-vascular invasion with D2-40 in melanoma correlates with sentinel lymph node status, metastasis and survival. J Cutan Pathol 2009;36(11):1157–63.

46. Doeden K, Ma Z, Narasimhan B, et al. Lymphatic invasion in cutaneous melanoma is associated with sentinel lymph node metastasis. J Cutan Pathol 2009; 36(7):772–80.

47. Sondak VK, Taylor JM, Sabel MS, et al. Mitotic rate and younger age are predictors of sentinel lymph node positivity: lessons learned from the generation of a probabilistic model. Ann Surg Oncol 2004;11(3):247–58.

48. Thompson JF, Shaw HM. Should tumor mitotic rate and patient age, as well as tumor thickness, be used to select melanoma patients for sentinel node biopsy? Ann Surg Oncol 2004;11(3):233–5.

49. Paek SC, Griffith KA, Johnson TM, et al. The impact of factors beyond Breslow depth on predicting sentinel lymph node positivity in melanoma. Cancer 2007; 109(1):100–8.

50. Balch CM, Gershenwald JE, Soong SJ, et al. Final version of 2009 AJCC melanoma staging and classification. J Clin Oncol 2009;27(36):6199–206.

51. Gershenwald JE, Thompson W, Mansfield PF, et al. Multi-institutional melanoma lymphatic mapping experience: the prognostic value of sentinel lymph node status in 612 stage I or II melanoma patients. J Clin Oncol 1999;17(3):976–83.

52. Cascinelli N, Bombardieri E, Bufalino R, et al. Sentinel and nonsentinel node status in stage IB and II melanoma patients: two-step prognostic indicators of survival. J Clin Oncol 2006;24(27):4464–71.

53. Balch CM, Gershenwald JE, Soong SJ, et al. Melanoma staging and classification. In: Balch CM, et al, editors. Cutaneous melanoma. St. Louis (MO): Quality Medical Publishing, Inc; 2009. p. 65–85.

54. Morton DL, Cochran AJ, Thompson JF, et al. Sentinel node biopsy for early-stage melanoma: accuracy and morbidity in MSLT-I, an international multicenter trial. Ann Surg 2005;242(3):302–11 [discussion: 311–3].

55. Ross MI, Gershenwald JE. How should we view the results of the Multicenter Selective Lymphadenectomy Trial-1 (MSLT-1)? Ann Surg Oncol 2008;15(3):670–3.

56. Agnese DM, Abdessalam SF, Burak WE Jr, et al. Cost-effectiveness of sentinel lymph node biopsy in thin melanomas. Surgery 2003;134(4):542–7 [discussion: 547–8].

57. Andtbacka RH, Gershenwald JE. Role of sentinel lymph node biopsy in patients with thin melanoma. J Natl Compr Canc Netw 2009;7(3):308–17.

58. Kesmodel SB, Karakousis GC, Botbyl JD, et al. Mitotic rate as a predictor of sentinel lymph node positivity in patients with thin melanomas. Ann Surg Oncol 2005;12(6):449–58.

59. Thompson JF, Shaw HM. Sentinel node metastasis from thin melanomas with vertical growth phase. Ann Surg Oncol 2000;7(4):251–2.

60. Kruper LL, Spitz FR, Czerniecki BJ, et al. Predicting sentinel node status in AJCC stage I/II primary cutaneous melanoma. Cancer 2006;107(10):2436–45.

61. Carlson GW, Murray DR, Hestley A, et al. Sentinel lymph node mapping for thick (> or =4-mm) melanoma: should we be doing it? Ann Surg Oncol 2003;10(4):408–15.

62. Gershenwald JE, Mansfield PF, Lee JE, et al. Role for lymphatic mapping and sentinel lymph node biopsy in patients with thick (> or = 4 mm) primary melanoma. Ann Surg Oncol 2000;7(2):160–5.

63. Jacobs IA, Chang CK, Salti GI. Role of sentinel lymph node biopsy in patients with thick (>4 mm) primary melanoma. Am Surg 2004;70(1):59–62.

64. Scoggins CR, Bowen AL, Martin RC 2nd, et al. Prognostic information from sentinel lymph node biopsy in patients with thick melanoma. Arch Surg 2010; 145(7):622–7.

65. Gajdos C, Griffith KA, Wong SL, et al. Is there a benefit to sentinel lymph node biopsy in patients with T4 melanoma? Cancer 2009;115(24):5752–60.

66. Lohmann CM, Coit DG, Brady MS, et al. Sentinel lymph node biopsy in patients with diagnostically controversial spitzoid melanocytic tumors. Am J Surg Pathol 2002;26(1):47–55.

67. Gannon CJ, Rousseau DL Jr, Ross MI, et al. Accuracy of lymphatic mapping and sentinel lymph node biopsy after previous wide local excision in patients with primary melanoma. Cancer 2006;107(11):2647–52.

68. Govindarajan A, Ghazarian DM, McCready DR, et al. Histological features of melanoma sentinel lymph node metastases associated with status of the completion lymphadenectomy and rate of subsequent relapse. Ann Surg Oncol 2007; 14(2):906–12.

69. Vuylsteke RJ, Borgstein PJ, van Leeuwen PA, et al. Sentinel lymph node tumor load: an independent predictor of additional lymph node involvement and survival in melanoma. Ann Surg Oncol 2005;12(6):440–8.

70. Gershenwald JE, Andtbacka RH, Prieto VG, et al. Microscopic tumor burden in sentinel lymph nodes predicts synchronous nonsentinel lymph node involvement in patients with melanoma. J Clin Oncol 2008;26(26):4296–303.

71. Wrightson WR, Wong SL, Edwards MJ, et al. Complications associated with sentinel lymph node biopsy for melanoma. Ann Surg Oncol 2003;10:676–80.

72. Estourgie SH, Nieweg OE, Kroon BB. High incidence of in-transit metastases after sentinel node biopsy in patients with melanoma. Br J Surg 2004;91(10): 1370–1.

73. Thomas JM, Clark MA. Selective lymphadenectomy in sentinel node-positive patients may increase the risk of local/in-transit recurrence in malignant melanoma. Eur J Surg Oncol 2004;30(6):686–91.

74. van Poll D, Thompson JF, Colman MH, et al. A sentinel node biopsy does not increase the incidence of in-transit metastasis in patients with primary cutaneous melanoma. Ann Surg Oncol 2005;12(8):597–608.

75. Pawlik TM, Ross MI, Thompson JF, et al. The risk of in-transit melanoma metastasis depends on tumor biology and not the surgical approach to regional lymph nodes. J Clin Oncol 2005;23(21):4588–90.

76. Pawlik TM, Ross MI, Johnson MM, et al. Predictors and natural history of in-transit melanoma after sentinel lymphadenectomy. Ann Surg Oncol 2005;12(8):587–96.

77. Kang JC, Wanek LA, Essner R, et al. Sentinel lymphadenectomy does not increase the incidence of in-transit metastases in primary melanoma. J Clin Oncol 2005;23(21):4764–70.

78. Gershenwald JE, Berman RS, Porter G, et al. Regional nodal basin control is not compromised by previous sentinel lymph node biopsy in patients with melanoma. Ann Surg Oncol 2000;7(3):226–31.

79. Carlson GW, Murray DR, Lyles RH, et al. The amount of metastatic melanoma in a sentinel lymph node: does it have prognostic significance? Ann Surg Oncol 2003;10(5):575–81.

80. Cochran AJ, Wen DR, Huang RR, et al. Prediction of metastatic melanoma in non-sentinel nodes and clinical outcome based on the primary melanoma and the sentinel node. Mod Pathol 2004;17(7):747–55.

81. Ranieri JM, Wagner JD, Azuaje R, et al. Prognostic importance of lymph node tumor burden in melanoma patients staged by sentinel node biopsy. Ann Surg Oncol 2002;9(10):975–81.

82. Spanknebel K, Coit DG, Bieligk SC, et al. Characterization of micrometastatic disease in melanoma sentinel lymph nodes by enhanced pathology: recommendations for standardizing pathologic analysis. Am J Surg Pathol 2005;29(3): 305–17.

83. Starz H, Siedlecki K, Balda BR. Sentinel lymphadenectomy and S-classification: a successful strategy for better prediction and improvement of outcome of melanoma. Ann Surg Oncol 2004;11(Suppl 3):162S–8S.

84. Andtbacka RH, Bedrosian I, Ross MI, et al. AJCC nodal factors and microscopic tumor burden predict recurrence in sentinel lymph node positive stage III melanoma patients. Ann Surg Oncol 2006;2(Suppl 13):12.

85. Gershenwald JE, Prieto VG, Colome-Grimmer MI, et al. The prognostic significance of microscopic tumor burden in 945 melanoma patients undergoing sentinel lymph node biopsy [abstract]. Proceedings of the American Society of Clinical Oncology 36th Annual Meeting. 2000;19:551a.

86. Gershenwald JE, Prieto VG, Johnson MM, et al. Heterogeneity of microscopic stage III melanoma in the SLN era: Implications for AJCC/UICC staging and future clinical trial design. in 6th World Congress on Melanoma. Vancouver (BC), Canada, 2005.

87. Debarbieux S, Duru G, Dalle S, et al. Sentinel lymph node biopsy in melanoma: a micromorphometric study relating to prognosis and completion lymph node dissection. Br J Dermatol 2007;157(1):58–67.

88. Rossi CR, De Salvo GL, Bonandini E, et al. Factors predictive of nonsentinel lymph node involvement and clinical outcome in melanoma patients with metastatic sentinel lymph node. Ann Surg Oncol 2008;15(4):1202–10.

89. Satzger I, Volker B, Meier A, et al. Criteria in sentinel lymph nodes of melanoma patients that predict involvement of nonsentinel lymph nodes. Ann Surg Oncol 2008;15(6):1723–32.

90. Scolyer RA, Li LX, McCarthy SW, et al. Micromorphometric features of positive sentinel lymph nodes predict involvement of nonsentinel nodes in patients with melanoma. Am J Clin Pathol 2004;122(4):532–9.

91. Shaw HM, Scolyer RA, Thompson JF. Prognostic significance of histopathological parameters in sentinel nodes of melanoma patients. Histopathology 2008;52(2): 242 [author reply: 242–4].

92. Scheri RP, Essner R, Turner RR, et al. Isolated tumor cells in the sentinel node affect long-term prognosis of patients with melanoma. Ann Surg Oncol 2007; 14(10):2861–6.

93. van Akkooi AC, de Wilt JH, Verhoef C, et al. Clinical relevance of melanoma micrometastases (<0.1 mm) in sentinel nodes: are these nodes to be considered negative? Ann Oncol 2006;17(10):1578–85.

94. Satzger I, Volker B, Meier A, et al. Prognostic significance of isolated HMB45 or Melan A positive cells in melanoma sentinel lymph nodes. Am J Surg Pathol 2007; 31(8):1175–80.

95. Scolyer RA, Murali R, Gershenwald JE, et al. Clinical relevance of melanoma micrometastases in sentinel nodes: too early to tell. Ann Oncol 2007;18(4):806–8.

96. Wagner JD, Davidson D, Coleman JJ 3rd, et al. Lymph node tumor volumes in patients undergoing sentinel lymph node biopsy for cutaneous melanoma. Ann Surg Oncol 1999;6(4):398–404.

97. van Akkooi AC, Nowecki ZI, Voit C, et al. Sentinel node tumor burden according to the Rotterdam criteria is the most important prognostic factor for survival in melanoma patients: a multicenter study in 388 patients with positive sentinel nodes. Ann Surg 2008;248(6):949–55.

Regional Treatment Strategies for In-Transit Melanoma Metastasis

Ryan S. Turley, MD[a],*, Amanda K. Raymond, MD[b],
Douglas S. Tyler, MD[c]

KEYWORDS

- Melanoma • In-transit • Regional chemotherapy
- Isolated limb infusion • Isolated limb perfusion

EPIDEMIOLOGY

While the incidence of several other cancers declines, the incidence of melanoma continues to increase and is now the most common fatal malignancy of young adults, and overall the sixth most common cancer amongst Americans.[1] In fact, an estimated 1 in 50 people will be diagnosed with melanoma over the course of their lifetime.[2] In 2009, there were an estimated 68,720 people newly diagnosed with invasive melanoma, and more than 8650 people died of melanoma in the United States.[2] Unfortunately, mortality rates from melanoma have remained stable because overall poor response of patients with metastatic disease to systemic therapy.[3]

In-transit metastases represent multifocal metastases that spread through the lymphatic system and occur between the site of the primary lesion and the regional draining lymph node basin (**Fig. 1**).[4] Recently, the 2009 American Joint Committee on Cancer (AJCC) Cancer Staging Manual was published, which recommended the retention of the previous (2002) edition's staging definition for the in-transit metastases.[5]

Disclosure: Dr Tyler receives grant support from Adherex Technologies. Dr Tyler is also a coinventor on a patent entitled "Cancer treatment methods using cadherin antagonists in combination with anticancer agents". The patent application number is 59,847 and this patent was filed on 9/27/06. Dr Tyler's rights to this patent have been signed over to the United States Government. Dr Tyler has material transfer agreements with Bayer, Schering, and Genta Pharmaceuticals. Adherex Technologies funded the phase 1 and 2 clinical trials of systemic ADH-1 and regional melphalan. Bayer provided drug only (sorafenib) for the phase 1 trial of systemic sorafenib and regional melphalan.
Grant Support: Duke Melanoma Research Fund and VA Merit Review Grant.

[a] Department of Surgery, Duke University, DUMC 3443, Durham, NC 27710, USA
[b] School of Medicine, Duke University, DUMC 3443, Durham, NC 27710, USA
[c] Department of Surgery, Duke University, DUMC 3118, Durham, NC 27710, USA
* Corresponding author.
E-mail address: ryan.turley@duke.edu

Surg Oncol Clin N Am 20 (2011) 79–103
doi:10.1016/j.soc.2010.09.008
1055-3207/11/$ – see front matter © 2011 Elsevier Inc. All rights reserved.

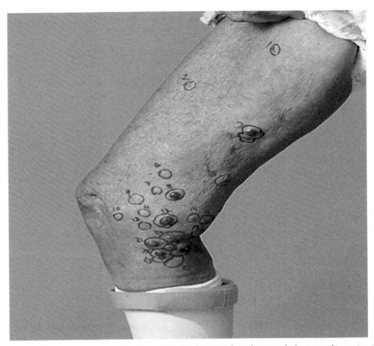

Fig. 1. In-transit melanoma metastases. Right leg with advanced, in-transit metastases of melanoma occurring between site of primary on lower leg and draining lymph node basin. (*Reproduced from* Beasley GM, Khan L, Tyler DS. Current clinical and research approaches to optimizing regional chemotherapy: novel strategies generated through a better understanding of drug pharmacokinetics, drug resistance, and the development of clinically relevant animal models. Surg Oncol Clin N Am 2008;17(4):732; with permission.)

Patients with in-transit metastases are classified as stage IIIB or IIIC, depending on their regional lymph node status (B = negative, C = positive), regardless of the number of lesions.[5,6] The number of patients that develop in-transit metastases is not insignificant, with a 30-year German study showing 21% of recurrences are in the form of in-transit or satellite metastases.[7] Another study reports that 2% to 10% of initially treated melanomas of the extremity recur in an in-transit fashion.[4] Historically, this pattern of recurrence is associated with an unfavorable prognosis, with 5-year survival rates ranging from 25% to 30%.[8–10] However, patients with IIIB in-transit disease seem to have better survival when compared with the rest of their cohort.[5,6] In the minority of patients, surgical excision of in-transit metastases can be used when the in-transit disease is limited to a few tumor deposits.[11] Unfortunately, the majority of patients have multifocal disease for which standard of care systemic chemotherapy or immunotherapy has had limited benefit.[12] However, if patients have in-transit disease confined to the extremities, regional chemotherapy delivered by isolated limb perfusion or isolated limb infusion is an effective treatment option associated with complete response rates ranging from 23% to 82% (**Table 1**).[13–27] Regional chemotherapy for in-transit disease is a rapidly progressing field and is a platform for ongoing research aimed at delineating underlying melanoma tumor biology. This review describes the current status of regional chemotherapy in treating patients with in-transit disease of the extremity, and the novel approaches being developed using targeted agents and immune modulators in an effort to improve efficacy while minimizing toxicity.

Table 1							
Response rates following melphalan-based HILP and ILI in patients with melanoma							
	Study	N	CR (%)	PR (%)	SD (%)	PD (%)	Condition
HILP	Minor et al,[13] 1985	18	82	18	0	0	Hyperthermia
	Storm and Morton,[14] 1985	26	50	31	19[a]	0	Hyperthermia
	Kroon et al,[15] 1987	18	38	44	17[a]	0	Normothermia
	Kroon et al,[16] 1993	43	77	14	9[a]	0	Normothermia
	Klaase et al,[17] 1994	120	54	25	21[a]	0	Normothermia
	Grünhagen et al,[18] 2004	100	69	26	5[a]	0	Hyperthermia
	Aloia et al,[19] 2005	59	57	31	12[a]	0	Hyperthermia
	Cornett et al,[20] 2006	58	25	39	28	11	Hyperthermia
	Sanki et al,[21] 2007	120	69	16	0	15	Hyperthermia
ILI	Mian et al,[22] 2001	9	44	56	0	0	
	Lindner et al,[23] 2002	128	41	44	12	4	
	Bonenkamp et al,[24] 2004	13	31	61	0	8	
	Brady et al,[25] 2006[b]	22	23	27	0	50	
	Beasley et al,[30] 2008	50	30	14	10	46	
	Kroon et al,[26] 2008[c]	185	38	46	10	6	
	Beasley et al,[27] 2009	128	31	33	7	29	

Abbreviations: CR, complete response; PD, progressive disease; PR, partial response; SD, stable disease.
[a] No response.
[b] Includes 1 patient with advanced sarcoma.
[c] Includes 128 patients reviewed in Lindner et al,[23] 2002.

ISOLATED LIMB PERFUSION

Regional treatment, in the form of hyperthermic isolated limb perfusion (HILP), was first performed for in-transit melanoma more than 50 years ago by Creech and colleagues.[28,29] This technique is still used today and overall remains unchanged from its original components. In brief, the femoral or subclavian vessels are surgically exposed and cannulated. When indicated, lymphadenectomy can also be performed during the vascular exposure. The artery and vein are cannulated at the root of the limb and an Esmarch tourniquet is placed proximal to the cannulated vessels. Perfusion proceeds with the use of a high-flow, melphalan-based perfusate, using a membrane oxygenator to maintain the acid-base status and oxygenation of the isolated limb in the physiologic range (**Fig. 2**). Creech and colleagues[29] used melphalan as their chemotherapeutic agent based on in vivo mouse data, and this has remained the standard agent for isolated limb perfusion (ILP). Hyperthermia of the limb is achieved due to the heated, high-flow perfusate, as well as warming blankets wrapped around the extremity for the duration of the procedure.

Retrospective studies have shown up to 82% of patients experience a complete response after ILP depending on the patient population and particular adjuncts, but larger studies seem to demonstrate complete response rates in the 50% to 70% range (see **Table 1**).[13–16,18–21] For instance, the Sydney Melanoma Unit (SMU) has reported an overall response rate of 75%, with 69% of patients experiencing a complete response when treated with ILP with regional melphalan ± actinomycin D or regional cisplatin.[21] In the authors' Duke University experience of melphalan-based ILP, 88% of patients responded and 57% were complete responders.[30] One of the larger series by Grunhagen and colleagues[18] reported an overall response rate of 95%, with 69% complete responders who received HILP with melphalan and adjunctive tumor necrosis factor-α (TNF-α). The overall 5-year survival rate for this cohort was 32%; the median survival was 25 months.

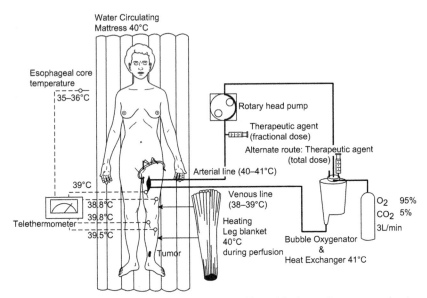

Fig. 2. Hyperthermic isolated limb perfusion. The affected limb's main artery and vein are surgically exposed and openly cannulated. Warming blankets maintain hyperthermia and temperature is monitored with temperature probes. The tourniquet is applied proximally and the melphalan chemotherapy perfusate is circulated with heated, high-flow membrane oxygenator to maintain acid-base status of the limb. (*Reproduced from* Coleman A, Augustine CK, Beasley G, et al. Optimizing regional infusion treatment strategies for melanoma of the extremities. Expert Rev Anticancer Ther 2009;9(11):1600; with permission.)

ISOLATED LIMB INFUSION

More recently, Thompson and colleagues[31] at the SMU developed an alternative to HILP, called isolated limb infusion (ILI).[32] ILI is less invasive than HILP, as it is performed via percutaneous catheterization of the involved limb. Using the Seldinger technique under fluoroscopic guidance, arterial and venous catheters are placed into the involved limb (**Fig. 3**). A pneumatic or Esmarch tourniquet is then positioned at the most proximal portion of the limb and inflated, thereby isolating the limb from systemic circulation. The extremity is wrapped with warming blankets using circulated heated water for the duration of the procedure. Next, melphalan is rapidly infused into the arterial catheter and manually circulated through a blood warmer syringe and a 3-way stopcock. After circulating for 30 minutes, a washout procedure using crystalloid fluids removes the chemotherapy from the limb via venous outflow extraction.

In contrast to ILP, ILI is a low-flow circuit with no oxygenator, resulting in the limb becoming normothermic, hypoxic, and acidotic. It is postulated that the limb acidosis and hypoxia may increase melphalan activity.[26] The simplicity of ILI has several advantages over traditional HILP. First of all, it does not require a membrane oxygenator or pump priming with blood. It is also a shorter procedure, is repeatable, and is associated with less regional toxicity when correcting for ideal body weight.[30,33] ILI is the preferred treatment for more frail patients with multiple comorbidities who may not tolerate the more involved HILP procedure. To be fair, there are also potential disadvantages of ILI. Namely, the same degree of hyperthermia as HILP cannot be

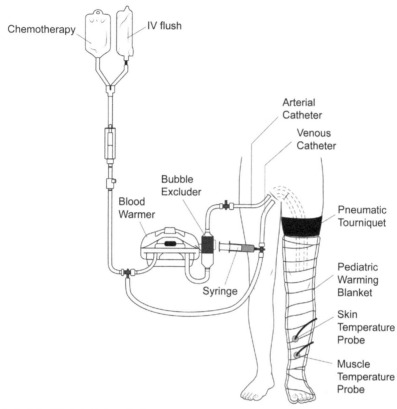

Fig. 3. Isolated limb infusion. Catheters are percutaneously inserted into the affected limb. Warming blankets are applied to the limb, but the same degree of hyperthermia in HILP cannot be achieved with ILI. The tourniquet is applied proximally and chemotherapy is circulated manually through a blood warmer using a syringe and 3-way stopcock. (*Reproduced from* Brady MS, Brown K, Patel A, et al. A phase II trial of isolated limb infusion with melphalan and dactinomycin for regional melanoma and soft tissue sarcoma of the extremity. Ann Surg Oncol 2006;13(8):1126; with permission.)

routinely achieved by ILI. Furthermore, ILI uses a lower dose of melphalan, and its duration is half as long as that with HILP.[34] These differences probably contribute to the lower overall response rates of ILI as compared with HILP in a recent multicenter combined analysis (79% in 294 patients vs 64% in 313 patients).[27] While low- to moderate-grade toxicities are similar for both ILI and HILP, HILP appears to be associated with more treatment-related limb loss.[26,27,30]

REGIONAL CHEMOTHERAPY

The major difference between systemic and regional chemotherapy treatments is the ability to deliver very high doses of chemotherapy through an isolated extremity circuit while minimizing systemic leakage and resultant systemic toxicity. Because the typical leak rate is less than 1% when performing HILP/ILI with conventional cytotoxic drugs, there are few systemic side effects and organ toxicity is rarely dose-limiting.[35] As a result, plasma melphalan can safely reach levels 10- to 100-fold times higher following regional compared with systemically delivered chemotherapy.[13,36] Drug delivery is also enhanced through its local delivery and avoidance of hepatic metabolism and renal clearance.[34] Adjuvant treatments, such as hyperthermia, may affect the pharmacokinetics of the chemotherapeutic agent, and can be applied more safely and effectively to the extremity for a regional treatment as compared with systemic chemotherapy.[37–39] HILP/ILI are also unique compared with systemic therapy in that after chemotherapy has circulated in the extremity, a washout procedure eliminates the remaining drug, reducing the risk of systemic toxicity before the tourniquet is released. Melphalan remains the most common agent used in regional chemotherapy for melanoma, and is considered the standard of care for the procedures.[34] However, alternative agents including cisplatin and temozolomide may offer significant advantages over melphalan in certain circumstances.

Melphalan

The standard chemotherapy agent used in regional chemotherapy for melanoma is melphalan (L-phenylalanine mustard [LPAM]). LPAM is a bifunctional alkylating agent, and remains the most common drug used for HILP/ILI procedures.[40] The rationale in using melphalan stems from the essential role phenylalanine plays in melanin synthesis. In theory, the phenylalanine derivative melphalan should provide selective toxicity to melanocytes and melanoma cells in which melanin is synthesized.[41] Despite its theoretical selective toxicity for metastatic melanoma, systemic melphalan is relatively ineffective because the maximally tolerated dose is much lower than the effective dose.[34] This limitation is overcome with regional delivery techniques, because much higher doses can be achieved in the extremity than would be tolerated when administered systemically.

Regional melphalan dosing is based in part on the report by Roberts and colleagues,[42] who determined that treatment responses tend to plateau at achieved melphalan levels of 25 μg/mL. Melphalan concentrations above this value are routinely achieved by HILP/ILI, so increasing the dose of melphalan to achieve levels higher than this is not likely to affect the response rate and may only increase toxicity.[35] Properties of melphalan that make it particularly effective as a regionally delivered chemotherapy include its short half-life, limited cell cycle specificity, low vascular endothelium and soft tissue toxicity, and linear dose-response relationship with respect to cytotoxicity.[13]

Melphalan has historically been dosed and administered based on body weight over a wide dose range (0.25–2.8 g/kg) without accounting for body mass distribution.[43,44] Dosing is now based on limb volume, with a target melphalan dose of 7.5 mg/L and 10 mg/L for a lower extremity ILI and HILP, respectively, and 10 mg/L and 13 mg/L for an upper extremity ILI and HILP, respectively.[23,45] Based on experience, the authors have recommended a total dose not exceeding 100 mg for the lower extremity or 50 mg for the upper extremity, although there have been reports of maximum doses as high as 120 mg for the lower extremity and 80 mg for the upper extremity.[30,46,47]

Limb volume can be estimated using volume displacement or limb circumference. Volume displacement may offer a more accurate estimation; however, it can be more cumbersome and may necessitate the position of the tourniquet be predetermined.[48] The authors' preferred method is using the limb circumference measurement by which the volume of the limb is calculated based of serial circumference measurements (eg, every 1.5 cm). Despite this being a calculated estimate rather than a direct measurement, it allows the volume to be determined in the clinic or even during the procedure once the final position of the tourniquet has been decided. The authors find this method to be more flexible by facilitating a more real-time calculation of limb volume at the time of the actual procedure. If the hand or foot of the involved extremity is free of disease, a second optional Esmarch or pneumatic tourniquet may be used to exclude these areas from the circuit. In this situation, the hand or foot volume should be subtracted from the total limb volume.[49] Some groups, including the authors' own group, now correct melphalan dosing for ideal body weight based on evidence that this dose modification is associated with lower toxicity without altering the complete response rate.[49]

Cisplatin

Cisplatin is an attractive agent, as it is commonly used systemically for the treatment of melanoma. By cross-linking DNA, cisplatin interferes with mitosis, leading to eventual apoptosis. Essential to its utility as a regional chemotherapy agent, cisplatin does not require metabolic transformation to become an active antineoplastic agent and it is cell-cycle independent.[50] Indeed, initial animal studies using cisplatin as a regional chemotherapy agent were promising and were quickly translated into clinical trials.[51] Unfortunately, these subsequent clinical studies have produced mixed results.

Early, small clinical studies reported favorable response rates after regional cisplatin perfusion without significant toxicities.[52–55] In a larger series of 58 melanoma patients reported by Hajarizadeh and colleagues,[56] 41 patients received prophylactic HILPs with cisplatin for stage I disease and 17 others were treated for stage II, III, or IV disease. In this study, HILP was followed by wide local excision of the primary tumor or reexcision of any remaining melanoma in all patients. After a median follow-up of 29 months, local recurrence rates of 12%, 33%, and 30% were observed for stage I, II, and III disease, respectively. Unfortunately, significant complications occurred in 8 patients, leaving 2 with permanent deficits. This study concluded that HILP with cisplatin was more effective than surgery alone to achieve local control and in the short-term appeared to be at least as effective as HILP with melphalan.

However, subsequent studies have shown disappointing results for HILP with cisplatin both in terms of efficacy and toxicity. Santinami and colleagues[57] discontinued a study over concerns about toxicity after only 9 patients with melanoma had been treated. In a phase 1 trial of 15 patients of HILP with cisplatin, Coit and colleagues[58] reported only 3 patients having a complete remission lasting more than 2 years as well as 3 patients developing severe limb-threatening toxicity. These investigators eventually concluded that HILP with cisplatin was not justified as a standard therapy for metastatic in-transit melanoma. Similarly, Thompson and Gianoutsos[50] suggested cisplatin was not the drug of choice for HILP treatment of melanoma confined to the limb when 5 of 6 patients receiving therapeutic HILPs with cisplatin did not achieve complete responses and 2 of 4 patients receiving prophylactic treatments developed early recurrence. Confounding these results, toxicity was very significant, resulting in an amputation in one patient and leaving another with a permanent foot drop. In the patient who had the leg amputation, melanoma remained despite extensive necrosis of normal tissue. At present, cisplatin is not used because of the incidence of complications and the lack of a significant improvement in response over melphalan.

Temozolomide

Temozolomide (TMZ) is considered to have some activity for metastatic melanoma as an oral agent. A new intravenous (IV) formulation of temozolomide has been developed, and appears to hold tremendous potential for use in regional chemotherapeutic treatments. Temozolomide is an alkylating agent that is metabolized to the active metabolite, methyldiazonium ion (MTIC), which methylates guanine residues in DNA at the O^6 and N^7 positions.[59] Cellular apoptotic pathways become activated when DNA mismatch enzymes attempt to repair the O^6-methylguanine generated by temozolomide, resulting in single- and double-stranded DNA breaks.[60] Temozolomide is suitable to the regional model because unlike dacarbazine (DTIC), temozolomide has 100% bioavailability under physiologic conditions and does not require hepatic conversion.[61] Preclinical in vivo studies in nude rats implanted with melanoma xenografts demonstrated that regional infusion with temozolomide resulted in prolonged tumor growth delay compared with rats that received systemic temozolomide or regional melphalan, especially in tumors with low O^6-alkylguanine-DNA alkyltransferase (AGT) activity, the predominant mechanism of resistance of temozolomide.[61] Analysis across a panel of xenografts suggested that approximately 20% of tumors preferentially respond to temozolomide, 20% preferentially respond to regional melphalan, and 60% respond equally to temozolomide or melphalan.[62] The Food and Drug Administration (FDA) recently approved the IV formulation of temozolomide; a phase 1 clinical trial is under way at Duke University, The University of Texas MD Anderson (MDACC), and Moffitt Cancer Center to define the toxicity profile and maximally tolerated dose to be used in regional therapy.

ALGORITHM

Despite the frequency with which HILP and ILI are performed for in-transit melanoma, no consensus exists as to which treatment is preferable or what strategies surgeons should follow should a patient progress after regional treatment. In general, the authors perform surgical excision for small volume disease, usually defined as 1 to 2 lesions that can be resected with negative surgical margins. Often, in patients who undergo surgical excision the authors will also perform a simultaneous sentinel lymph node biopsy, which reports suggest will be positive about 50% of the time.[63] Regional therapy is used in patients who have failed surgical excision, have nonresectable extremity disease, or have multifocal disease of 3 or more lesions. The authors do not recommend excision of lesions in the field of treatment if patients are undergoing regional therapy. The rationale for this twofold: (1) potential wound-healing issues related to the chemotherapy that can cause limb swelling and tissue damage, and (2) leaving the lesions in place provides an opportunity for the surgeon to monitor the effectiveness of the treatment.

The algorithm for which type of regional treatment (HILP or ILI) the authors use is as follows. Patients with local recurrence or with evidence of pelvic, femoral, or axillary nodal involvement may be candidates for HILP, as excision of the tumor-containing lymph nodes exposes the vessels used for this procedure. For patients with femoral or axillary nodal involvement,[64] a less invasive alternative is to treat these patients with an ILI, and then perform the lymphadenectomy at the end of the ILI once the heparinization is reversed and after the infusion catheters are removed. Some centers may preferentially offer ILP as the initial treatment to patients with high disease burden, as these patients may be more likely to have regional nodal disease. However, there are no strong data suggesting that patients with high disease burden are more likely to respond to HILP as compared with ILI. The authors' group has favored using ILI first, even in patients with high disease burden, leaving HILP as a potential salvage therapy for those who do not respond to ILI. In addition, there are several protocol-based ILI trials (such as temozolomide, or melphalan in combination with other targeted agents), or systemic therapy (**Fig. 4**) for patients who either fail regional treatment or progress.

STRATEGIES TO OPTIMIZE RESPONSE

As highlighted earlier, overall and complete response rates, as well as durability of response, are variable depending on the regional chemotherapy platform as well

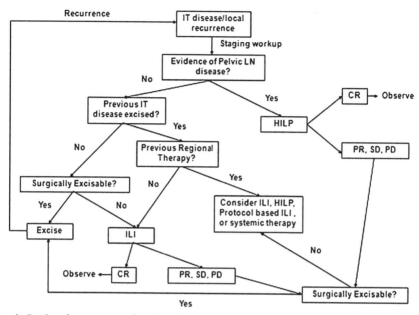

Fig. 4. Regional treatment algorithm for in-transit extremity melanoma. Patient entry is denoted at the box labeled "IT disease/local recurrence." IT, in-transit disease; LN, lymph node; HILP, hyperthermic isolated limb perfusion; ILI, isolated limb infusion; CR, complete response; PR, partial response; SD, stable disease; PD, progressive disease. (*Reproduced from* Beasley GM, Caudle A, Petersen RP, et al. A multi-institutional experience of isolated limb infusion: defining response and toxicity in the US. J Am Coll Surg 2009;208(5): 713; with permission.)

adjunctive therapies. In the context of regional chemotherapy, standard adjuncts to optimize therapy include the addition of hyperthermia and TNF-α to ILP. Newer strategies under active investigation include novel agents that overcome traditional drug resistance mechanisms, target tumor vasculature, and lower the apoptotic threshold of malignant melanoma.

Hyperthermia

Hyperthermia may augment or sensitize melanoma to cytotoxic therapy by increasing blood flow, membrane permeability, local metabolism, and drug uptake.[65–68] Indeed, hyperthermia continues to be an essential component of ILP since its introduction by Cavaliere in 1967. Based on preclinical experiments suggesting heat to be tumoricidal in a rat melanoma model, Cavaliere and colleagues[37] first explored the effects of heat alone in 22 patients with recurrent extremity tumors. The morbidity of the procedure was quite high, with 6 immediate postoperative deaths. Of the remaining 16, 12 patients were alive without evidence of disease at 3 to 28 months. Two years later, Stehlin[69] combined regional chemotherapy with heated perfusion, and established HILP in a reported experience of 37 patients. Of the 37 melanoma patients, only 12 were evaluated for measurable disease. Of these, 10 of the 12 patients (83%) had a response described as "pronounced regression" for greater than 3 months. Of note, this report used very high perfusate temperatures reaching up to 46°C. As a modern comparison, the authors initiate HILP at 38.5°C with a goal temperature of 40°C.

In 1989 the first prospective, randomized trial was conducted to evaluate the role of hyperthermia and regional extremity perfusion of in-transit melanoma.[70] In this study,

107 patients were randomized to receive either surgical excision or surgical excision followed by HILP with melphalan. With a primary end point of disease-free survival, the study was stopped prematurely (median follow-up 550 days) due to a highly significant advantage in disease-free survival in the HILP arm (89% vs 52%). In addition, there was an improvement in overall survival (98% vs 86%), with minimal local and systemic complications.

There are also strong animal model data in the context of regional therapy with the alkylating agents melphalan and temozolomide suggesting that hyperthermia augments their antitumor efficacy against both melanoma and sarcomas.[71,72] To date, no randomized controlled trial has compared hyperthermic ILP with normothermic ILP. Despite lacking level I evidence, hyperthermia remains a standard component of ILP because of the strong indirect clinical evidence and theoretical merit.

Tumor Necrosis Factor-α

The first study of TNF-α in a human trial of HILP was performed by Posner and colleagues[73] in 1995. In this study of 6 patients receiving escalating doses of TNF-α alone during HILP, only 1 patient had a complete response. A subsequent study combined TNF-α with interferon-γ (IFN-γ) and melphalan delivered via HILP.[74] Interferon was added for potential antitumor synergism. Overall, this treatment strategy was quite toxic: all patients required dopamine infusions for a severe inflammatory response, and due to limb toxicity 2 patients even required an amputation. Despite the toxicity, 89% of patients had a complete response and 11% had a partial response to the combination treatment at 11 months' follow-up.[75]

Based on this study, interest in TNF-α in addition to HILP began to increase, eventually resulting in a randomized trial of 103 patients conducted by the American College of Surgeons Oncology Group (ACOSOG).[20] This trial was stopped early after an interim analysis showed no evidence of improved patient responses, with significant increases in severe toxicities in the TNF-α plus melphalan arm. At 6 months, although there remained no significant improvement with the addition of TNF-α in the 89 patients still in the study, a difference in response rates was noted (42% complete response with combination vs 20% in single therapy; $P = .101$). Critics of this trial have cited an early time point for assessing response (3 months) as the reason for the lower response rates observed with TNF-α compared with prior trials.[76,77] However, a recent large single-institution series from the United States has also failed to demonstrate an improvement in regional in-field progression-free survival with the use of TNF-α.[64] Due to the inability to clearly demonstrate any benefit from the addition of TNF to regional therapy, it has not been FDA-approved as an adjunct for HILP in the United States.

Targeting Traditional Drug Resistance Mechanisms

Drug metabolism

One mechanism of melanoma chemoresistance is hypermetabolism of alkylating chemotherapy agents by glutathione-S-transferases (GSTs).[78] GSTs are a family of phase II detoxification enzymes that catalyze glutathione (GSH) to electrophiles including carcinogens, mutagens, and anticancer reagents. Melanoma cells as well as tumor types have been shown to express elevated GST and GSH levels,[79] which in turn have been associated with resistance to chemotherapy. Further supporting its critical role in tumor chemoresistance, melphalan exposure appears to increase tumor GSH levels by more than two-thirds.[80] Conversely, reducing GSH levels confers or restores sensitivity in vitro.[80–82] The GST enzymes, which are polymorphic and exist in both membrane-bound and cytosolic forms, are divided into 8 classes: Alpha,

Kappa, Mu, Pi, Theta, Sigma, Omega, and Zeta.[83,84] Through conjugation of GSH to intracellular melphalan, GSTs effectively neutralize melphalan by inhibiting access to DNA by the alkylating agent.[85,86] Given their great potential to augment the chemo-sensitivity of melanoma as well as other tumor types, there exists significant interest in developing novel inhibitors of GST-mediated metabolism.

One strategy in overcoming GST-mediated drug metabolism is to deplete the tumor cells of available GSH, thereby preventing conjugation of the GSH by GSTs to alkylating chemotherapy agents.[87] L-S,R-Buthionine sulfoximine (BSO) is a potent and specific inhibitor of the enzyme γ-glutamylcysteine synthetase (GCS), which is the rate-limiting step in the production of GSH.[88] BSO has been shown to decrease intra-cellular GSH levels, increase DNA cross-linking, and sensitize the cells to cytotox-icity.[89] Early, small clinical studies of continuous BSO infusion with intravenous melphalan were limited by occasional severe myelosuppression. While the addition of BSO to systemic melphalan may be associated with myelosuppression, one might predict that the combination of BSO and melphalan in regional therapy would not be limited by systemic toxicity. In a nude rat xenograft model of ILI, systemic BSO treat-ment reduced resistance to ILI melphalan.[80] Intraperitoneal administration of BSO was well tolerated and was associated with an approximately 72% reduction in tumor GSH levels. BSO treatment was associated with an increase in tumor growth delay relative to saline and melphalan-alone controls. Based on these studies, a phase 1 trial at Duke University using a 3-day infusion of BSO around the time of melphalan ILI was opened for enrollment, but was closed prematurely due to the restricted availability of the intravenous formulation of BSO.

One of the more promising targets for inhibiting the GST pathway drug metabolism is enzyme glutathione-S-transferase P1 (GSTP1). In addition to its metabolizing func-tion, GSTP1 also serves as a major regulator of cell signaling in response to stress, hypoxia, growth factors, and other stimuli. GSTP1 inhibits downstream mitogen-acti-vated protein (MAP) kinase signaling mediated by binding c-Jun N-terminal kinase (JNK), thereby preventing the phosphorylation of c-Jun.[90] The novel GSTP1 inhibitor 6-(7-nitro-2,1,3-benzoxadiazol-4-ylthio)hexanol (NBDHEX) has recently been shown to inhibit JNK pathway activation, leading to melanoma cell apoptosis in vitro as well as potent inhibition of tumor growth in vivo.[91] The exact role of GSTP1 in mela-noma tumorigenesis and its potential for augmenting currently available alkylating chemotherapy agents remains an active area of investigation.

DNA repair

Should temozolomide be shown to be an effective regional chemotherapy agent on completion of phase 1 and 2 trials, strategies to impair melanoma DNA repair induced by this compound will become important. TMZ confers its cytotoxicity by alkylating or methylating DNA at O^6-guanine, N^7-guanine, and N^3-adenine residues.[92] This methyl-ation results in DNA damage and eventual cell death. Temozolomide cytotoxicity can be overcome, however, in tumor cells through several different DNA repair mecha-nisms including the O^6-methylguanine-DNA methyltransferase (MGMT), O^6-alkylgua-nine-DNA alkyltransferase (AGT), the DNA-mismatch repair system (MMR), and the base excision repair (BER) pathways.[93–96] Two drugs, the Poly(ADP-ribose) poly-merase (PARP) inhibitor INO-1001 and the AGT inhibitor O^6-benzylguanine (O^6-BG) have been tested in a preclinical setting in an effort to delineate the importance of DNA repair inhibition in augmenting regionally delivered temozolomide.

PARP recognizes DNA damage and activates the BER pathway by recruiting the DNA repair proteins XRCC1, DNA ligase III, and DNA polymerase β. Cells without PARP activity have been to shown to be more sensitive to alkylating chemotherapy, demonstrating increased apoptosis and chromosomal instability.[97–99] Based on these data, the novel PARP inhibitor INO-1001 was tested in a melanoma model to determine whether it could augment the response to temozolomide. Toshimitsu and colleagues[92] recently tested this hypothesis using a rat xenograft model of regional chemotherapy. In this study, systemic administration of the PARP inhibitor INO-1001 followed by regional infusion of temozolomide did not significantly decrease tumor growth in melanoma xenografts with intact mismatch repair mechanisms and high MGMT activity. However, in the xenograft that exhibited deficient mismatch repair without MGMT activity, termed PRMel, systemic INO-1001 followed by regional infusion of temozolomide significantly decreased tumor growth compared with regional temozolomide alone (22.6% vs 322.8% increase in tumor volume at day 40).[92]

Inhibition of the DNA repair enzyme AGT using O^6-BG has also been tested and shown to reduce tumor AGT activity by 93.5%. Regionally administered temozolomide in conjunction with systemic O^6-BG led to significant tumor growth delay compared with either regional temozolomide alone or systemic temozolomide plus systemic O^6-BG. Two of 6 rats had tumor regression in the group treated with 750 mg/kg temozolomide alone versus 6 of 6 rats with regression in the group treated with O^6-BG for 5 days plus 750 mg/kg temozolomide.[61]

Vascular Targeting Agents

ADH-1

ADH-1 (Exherin) is a cyclic pentapeptide that disrupts N-cadherin binding interactions.[100] The cadherins are a large supergene family of proteins involved in cell-to-cell adhesion.[101] Malignant transformation in melanoma is characterized by a "switch" from E-cadherin to N-cadherin, altering intracellular signaling pathways and leading to increased proliferation, survival, and angiogenesis, as well as decreased apoptosis.[101,102] In preclinical studies, the use of systemic ADH-1 in conjunction with regional melphalan showed marked increases in tumor responses even in the most melphalan-resistant tumors.[100] Subsequent mechanistic studies suggest that the efficacy of ADH-1 in augmenting tumor responses may result from disrupting tumor cell interactions with its microenvironment. In the rat xenograft ILI model, ADH-1 significantly increased melphalan-DNA adduct formation in tumor cells, suggesting that ADH-1 may augment tumor response to melphalan by increasing delivery of the relatively small melphalan molecule into tumor cells. This finding has been further supported by in vitro and in vivo permeability assays showing increasing permeability of both normal and tumor microvasculature after treatment with ADH-1. The exact role of N-cadherin in melanoma tumor signaling remains unclear, and is an active area of investigation in the authors' laboratory.

As a direct result of the marked responses seen in preclinical experiments, a phase 1 trial was conducted. Sixteen patients were treated without dose-limiting toxicities using a single dose of ADH-1 prior to ILI and a second dose 1 week after ILI. The ADH-1 was dose-escalated while the ILI was kept at its standard dosing. In-field responses included 8 complete responders and 2 partial responders.[46] Given lack of additional toxicity from ADH-1 and a surprising 50% complete response rate, a multicenter phase 2 trial of systemic ADH-1 in combination with melphalan via ILI for patients who have AJCC Stage IIIB or IIIC extremity melanoma was performed and recently completed. This trial marks the first prospective multicenter (Duke University, MDACC, Moffit Cancer Center, and University of Florida) trial of ILI as well being the first to investigate whether a targeting agent could augment regional chemotherapy responses. In total, 45 patients were enrolled over 15 months at the 4 institutions. ADH-1 was well tolerated without significant additional toxicity.

Pretreatment using ADH-1 prior to ILI with melphalan resulted in an increase in overall and complete response rates compared with historical controls as measured at 3 months. However, many of these patients recurred 5 to 6 weeks after the 3-month time point, such that there was no significant difference in regional progression-free survival curves between the study participants and patients treated with ILI alone off this study at the same institutions.[103]

Bevacizumab

Another promising vascular targeting agent for augmenting regional chemotherapy is bevacizumab, a monoclonal antibody to vascular endothelial growth factor (VEGF). Bevacizumab has been used in combination with standard chemotherapies to treat patients with metastatic colorectal, breast, brain, kidney, and lung cancers.[104–107] The classic mechanism of bevacizumab is sequestration of VEGF and inhibition of aberrant tumor vasculature formation. Moreover, increasing evidence suggests inhibition of VEGF via bevacizumab can augment chemotherapy agents by "normalizing" tumor vasculature, leading to greater delivery of chemotherapy to tumor cells. Bevacizumab is currently being investigated in combination with other chemotherapy agents for metastatic melanoma in multiple clinical trials across the United States.[108] A recent phase 2 study examining bevacizumab in combination with the mammalian target of rapamycin (mTOR) inhibitor everolimus demonstrated moderate activity in 57 patients with metastatic melanoma.[109] When combined with dacarbazine and IFN-α2a in 26 patients, bevacizumab had moderate activity, with an overall response rate of 23% and 2 complete responders. The median overall survival for all patients in this study was 11.5 months.[110] In another phase 2 trial of 53 patients, bevacizumab in combination with paclitaxel and carboplatin was found to be moderately well tolerated, and resulted in 9 (17%) patients achieving partial regression and 30 (57%) achieving stable disease at 8 weeks.[111] Given multiple phase 2 trials suggesting improved overall response rates in combination with systemic chemotherapy as well as its inherent potential to increase drug delivery through tumor vasculature "normalization," the authors hypothesized that systemically administered bevacizumab prior to regionally delivered melphalan would significantly enhance the efficacy of regionally delivered melphalan. Indeed, preclinical evidence in a rat melanoma xenograft model suggests that a single injection of bevacizumab given 3 days before ILI with melphalan markedly improved response rates (manuscript in preparation). Tumors pretreated with bevacizumab demonstrated decreased tumor vasculature density and permeability, yet had increased melphalan-DNA adduct formation. Taken together, these studies support the concept that bevacizumab results in tumor vascular normalization, thereby enhancing drug delivery and improving overall response to regional chemotherapy (manuscript in preparation). A phase 1 trial combining bevacizumab with melphalan via ILI is currently being planned at Duke University for 2011.

Altering Apoptotic Threshold

Sorafenib

Altered cellular signaling cascades in melanoma have been shown to increase proliferation and decrease apoptosis, leading to greater chemoresistance.[112] One of the more common oncogenic pathways altered in melanoma is the BRaf serine/threonine kinase pathway. In fact, 50% to 70% of melanomas express the constitutively active mutant BRaf serine/threonine kinase.[113] Although more than 30 mutations of the BRAF gene have been identified and associated with malignancy, the most frequent mutation (~90%) is a single substitution of glutamine for valine at residue 599, which is referred to as V600E.[114] The end effect of this mutation is transformation of the BRaf kinase from the inactive to constitutively active state, resulting in continuous stimulation of MAP kinase and extracellular regulated (ERK) kinase pathways with resultant augmentation of proliferation, differentiation, angiogenesis, and apoptosis.[113] Given the high incidence of BRAF mutation in melanoma and its oncogenic effects, the BRaf kinase is a promising target for enhancing systemic as well as regional chemotherapy.

Sorafenib (Nexavar) is a commercially available drug approved for the treatment of renal cell and hepatocellular carcinomas.[115,116] This small molecule inhibits multiple tyrosine kinase pathways including the VEGF receptor-2 and -3 kinases, c-Kit, and the MAP kinases pathways, including BRaf.[117] Through its inhibition of the Raf-MEK-ERK pathway, sorafenib has been shown to inhibit cell proliferation and angiogenesis[113] as well as to induce apoptosis by downregulating the antiapoptotic protein Mcl-1 and preventing the nuclear translocation of apoptosis-inducing factor (AIF).[118–120] Although effective in preclinical in vitro and in vivo models,[121,122] clinical trials with sorafenib as a single agent in melanoma have produced disappointing results.[123] However, subsequent phase-1 to -2 trials showed greater overall tumor response rates when sorafenib was combined with cytotoxic therapies including carboplatin and paclitaxel, temozolomide, dacarbazine, or IFN-α2a.[124–127] Unfortunately, in a phase 3 randomized, controlled trial, the combination of sorafenib with carboplatin plus paclitaxel for patients with advanced melanoma failed to demonstrate improvements in any clinical end points.[128] Although sorafenib failed to synergistically enhance systemically administered cytotoxic therapy, whether it could augment regionally delivered chemotherapy whereby dose of chemotherapy can be an order of magnitude higher remained unclear.

In preclinical studies, sorafenib significantly augmented melanoma chemosensitivity to melphalan and temozolomide across a panel of 24 cell lines independent of BRaf or NRas mutational status. Using a rat xenograft model of ILI, the combination of sorafenib and either melphalan or temozolomide significantly reduced tumor growth after ILI as compared with melphalan or temozolomide alone. On immunohistochemical analysis of tumor tissue acquired 24 hours after ILI, rats pretreated with sorafenib exhibited increased apoptosis, with associated decreases in ERK activation and Mcl-1 protein levels.[129] Overall, the results of these preclinical studies suggested that sorafenib reduces tumor apoptotic threshold and thereby sensitizes melanoma tumor cells to the cytotoxic agents melphalan and temozolomide. These promising preclinical results led to an open-label, multicenter, phase 1 dose escalation study to evaluate safety, tolerability, and antitumor activity of oral sorafenib in combination with normothermic ILI with melphalan at Duke University and Memorial Sloan-Kettering Cancer Center. This study has been recently completed and involved 20 patients. From this trial, a maximally tolerated oral dose of sorafenib was defined as 200 mg twice daily. Overall response and complete response rates in this small study did not exceed historical measures of standard melphalan ILI alone, and patients pretreated with higher doses of sorafenib did seem to have an increased risk of local toxicity (ie, ulceration and myositis) without an obvious improvement in response rates. Of note, preliminary analyses have not associated response to sorafenib and melphalan with BRaf or N-ras mutational status. Final analyses of this trial are ongoing and are soon to be published.

Dasatinib

Another potential target in melanoma is the src family of kinases. Src kinase overexpression leads to increased cellular proliferation and decreased adhesion.[130] Src signals through its downstream intermediaries, called signal transducers and activators of transcription (STAT) factors. One of these factors, STAT3, has been found to be activated in the majority (85%) of melanoma cell lines.[131] STAT3 has been shown to not only promote tumor growth and survival, but also appears to upregulate VEGF and promote tumor angiogenesis.[132] Inhibition of src kinase blocked the growth of human melanoma cell lines with elevated STAT3 activity and induced apoptosis by inhibiting the expression of anti-apoptotic genes Bcl-x_L and Mcl-1.[132]

By mitigating the unchecked STAT3 activity leading to expression of prosurvival genes, Src inhibitors such as dasatinib (Sprycel) may also potentiate the effectiveness of traditional chemotherapy by lowering the apoptotic threshold. Dasatinib is manufactured by Bristol-Myers Squibb, and is a BCR-Abl and Src family tyrosine kinase inhibitor currently approved for the treatment of chronic myelogenous leukemia refractory to imatinib treatment, as well as acute lymphoblastic leukemia positive for the Philadelphia chromosome.[133] Recent in vitro studies of have shown dasatinib to synergistically enhance the effects of cisplatin, but not temozolomide or paclitaxel in melanoma.[134] In regard of the role of dasatinib in augmenting regional chemotherapy for in-transit melanoma, preclinical studies are currently ongoing and promising. Using a nude rat xenografts model of ILI, rats pretreated with orally administered dasatinib followed by regionally delivered melphalan have shown superior tumor responses compared with rats receiving regional melphalan therapy alone (unpublished data). Based on these preliminary data, the authors are planning for a phase 1 clinical trial for melanoma patients with in-transit disease.

IMMUNE MODULATION AND REGIONAL THERAPY

Immune-based therapies have demonstrated some efficacy in melanoma patients.[12,135,136] To what degree the immune system may contribute to the magnitude or durability of a tumor response to chemotherapy is currently unclear. The immune system may play a significant role in regionally treated patients, especially in light of data that response to a regional treatment, more so than lymph node status, is the strongest predictor of long-term survival.[19,26,137] Regionally treated patients do not have the immune suppression associated with systemic chemotherapy treatments and may respond differently to tumor cytotoxicity induced by the administered chemotherapeutic agent. Current studies at Duke University are trying to quantify the nature of the immune response in patients with in-transit disease, and how the immune response might contribute to regional tumor response and durability of response. The group at Memorial Sloan-Kettering Cancer Center has recently proposed an ILI trial in which patients will receive 4 doses of the CTLA-4 antibody ipilimumab after ILI. This trial is currently undergoing IRB approval, and will help determine if immune regulation can either augment a regional chemotherapy response or help generate a more robust antitumor response to it.

PERSONALIZATION

With an ever growing number of available drugs targeting specific molecular pathways, rational methods will be required to tailor individual tumor biology with appropriate molecular interventions. Although many targeting drugs have a modest effect when given alone, many can sensitize in-transit melanoma to regional chemotherapy when targeted therapies are matched correctly with the tumor's oncogenic aberration. Gene signature profiling through microarray technology is one possible method through which optimal therapy combinations for regional chemotherapy can be tailored for each patient. Gene expression profiling provides a powerful method of classifying tumors based on their underlying biology and has already been used to predict oncogenic signaling,[138] prognosis,[139] and progression.[140] In-transit melanoma is, in many ways, an ideal platform for tailored therapy because most patients will by definition have multiple lesions available for tissue sampling. In theory, tissue could be acquired relatively easily in the outpatient setting and then analyzed to guide optimal therapeutic regimen selection, verify tumor response to systemic targeted therapies prior to HILP/ILI, and even confirm response after regional chemotherapy. The practicality of this approach assumes homogeneity of gene expression across individual tumor nodules in a single patient. Recently, the authors' group tested whether gene expression differed across individual tumor nodules in a single patient, using a gene expression analysis across 55 lesions in 29 patients. Patterns of gene expression were highly similar ($P<.006$; average $r = 0.979$) across pretreatment lesions from a single patient compared with the significantly different patterns observed across patients ($P<.05$).[141]

Whether gene expression profiling can predict melphalan and temozolomide sensitivity for in-transit melanoma remains an area of active investigation. For temozolomide, the MGMT is considered by many to be the primary resistance mechanism of melanoma cells. The authors have found that quantified MGMT activity and expression across 26 melanoma cells lines correlates highly with temozolomide sensitivity.[94] However, other studies attempting to correlate MGMT activity,[142,143] expression,[144] and promoter methylation[145] to temozolomide resistance have produced mixed results. Because multiple cellular events have the potential to alter chemosensitivity of tumor cells, large-scale gene expression profiling, as opposed to single-pathway analyses, could potentially lend more insight to differential temozolomide chemosensitivity. In this regard, the authors recently tested whether a gene signature derived from larger-scale gene expression analysis could be used to create a more robust predictor of temozolomide resistance as compared with MGMT activity and expression. Using 60 cell lines from the NCI-60 panel of cancer cell lines, 45 genes were identified as predictors of temozolomide "resistance" or "sensitivity" and were used to create a gene signature of temozolomide resistance. When validated against a separate set of 26 melanoma cells lines, the temozolomide resistance gene signature did significantly correlate with measured temozolomide resistance. This correlation, however, was inferior to that derived from a single analysis of MGMT expression in the same cell lines.[94] Whether a temozolomide gene signature or MGMT expression alone best predicts response of in-transit melanoma patients to temozolomide infusion will require validation in a clinical trial.

Creating a melphalan-based ILI signature has been more challenging. Initial attempts at creating a gene signature predictor from RNA extracted from multiple melanoma cell lines have been arduous and have yet to produce a signature that can be validated. More recent attempts using RNA extracted from patient samples have been more fruitful. Using tissue samples, the authors have correlated 100 genes to response to ILI with melphalan, and are currently in the process of validating this gene signature as a predictor of response to melphalan-based regional therapy (unpublished data).

SUMMARY

Regional chemotherapy for in-transit melanoma is an effective therapy for melanoma isolated to the extremity, with response rates far exceeding those seen with current systemic therapy. ILI is a well-tolerated technique of regional chemotherapy and is considered less technically demanding to perform than HILP. Complete response rates are similar for ILI and HILP, but HILP trends to produce a higher overall response rate as well as more durable response. Novel therapeutic agents given systemically with regional ILI may augment the complete rates and improve its therapeutic index. On a grander scale, ILI is an excellent platform for conducting research aimed at improving regional as well as systemic therapy for metastatic melanoma, by gaining further insight on the underlying biology of melanoma as well as understanding the mechanisms of action of novel targeted therapies. With a proven and reproducible animal model for ILI,[100] novel targeted agents can be readily tested and quickly translated into clinical trials.[46]

In the future, the regional chemotherapy armamentarium will include agents capable of overcoming classic chemotherapy resistance pathways, normalizing abnormal tumor vasculature, modulating the immunologic response, and correcting altered cell-signaling pathways that lead to unchecked proliferation and decreased apoptosis. As the efficacy of these agents in augmenting regional chemotherapy to melanoma become more apparent, it will become essential to generate predictors to personalize appropriate therapy for each particular patient. As more trials with targeted agents are performed, patterns of gene and/or protein expression of responders and nonresponders can potentially be elucidated to give a better understanding of how targeted treatments work. The future of regional chemotherapy is not just in augmenting regional tumor responses, but also in serving as a platform to help us develop better therapeutic strategies to be used in patients with distant metastatic disease.

REFERENCES

1. Weinstock MA. Do sunscreens increase or decrease melanoma risk: an epidemiologic evaluation. J Investig Dermatol Symp Proc 1999;4(1):97–100.
2. Jemal A, Siegel R, Ward E, et al. Cancer statistics, 2009. CA Cancer J Clin 2009; 59(4):225–49.
3. de Vries E, Bray FI, Coebergh JW, et al. Changing epidemiology of malignant cutaneous melanoma in Europe 1953-1997: rising trends in incidence and mortality but recent stabilizations in western Europe and decreases in Scandinavia. Int J Cancer 2003;107(1):119–26.
4. Pawlik TM, Ross MI, Johnson MM, et al. Predictors and natural history of in-transit melanoma after sentinel lymphadenectomy. Ann Surg Oncol 2005;12(8):587–96.
5. Balch CM, Gershenwald JE, Soong SJ, et al. Final version of 2009 AJCC melanoma staging and classification. J Clin Oncol 2009;27(36):6199–206.
6. Balch CM, Buzaid AC, Soong SJ, et al. Final version of the American Joint Committee on Cancer staging system for cutaneous melanoma. J Clin Oncol 2001;19(16):3635–48.
7. Meier F, Will S, Ellwanger U, et al. Metastatic pathways and time courses in the orderly progression of cutaneous melanoma. Br J Dermatol 2002;147(1):62–70.
8. Cascinelli N, Bufalino R, Marolda R, et al. Regional nonnodal metastases of cutaneous melanoma. Eur J Surg Oncol 1986;12(2):175–80.
9. Calabro A, Singletary SE, Balch CM. Patterns of relapse in 1001 consecutive patients with melanoma nodal metastases. Arch Surg 1989;124(9):1051–5.
10. Zogakis TG, Bartlett DL, Libutti SK, et al. Factors affecting survival after complete response to isolated limb perfusion in patients with in-transit melanoma. Ann Surg Oncol 2001;8(10):771–8.
11. Dong XD, Tyler D, Johnson JL, et al. Analysis of prognosis and disease progression after local recurrence of melanoma. Cancer 2000;88(5):1063–71.
12. Bhatia S, Tykodi SS, Thompson JA. Treatment of metastatic melanoma: an overview. Oncology (Williston Park) 2009;23(6):488–96.

13. Minor DR, Allen RE, Alberts D, et al. A clinical and pharmacokinetic study of isolated limb perfusion with heat and melphalan for melanoma. Cancer 1985; 55(11):2638–44.

14. Storm FK, Morton DL. Value of therapeutic hyperthermic limb perfusion in advanced recurrent melanoma of the lower extremity. Am J Surg 1985;150(1): 32–5.

15. Kroon BB, Van Geel AN, Benckhuijsen C, et al. Normothermic isolation perfusion with melphalan for advanced melanoma of the limbs. Anticancer Res 1987;7(3 Pt B):441–2.

16. Kroon BB, Klaase JM, van Geel BN, et al. Results of a double perfusion schedule with melphalan in patients with melanoma of the lower limb. Eur J Cancer 1993;29A(3):325–8.

17. Klaase JM, Kroon BB, van Geel AN, et al. Prognostic factors for tumor response and limb recurrence-free interval in patients with advanced melanoma of the limbs treated with regional isolated perfusion with melphalan. Surgery 1994; 115(1):39–45.

18. Grünhagen DJ, Brunstein F, Graveland WJ, et al. One hundred consecutive isolated limb perfusions with TNF-alpha and melphalan in melanoma patients with multiple in-transit metastases. Ann Surg 2004;240(6):939–47 [discussion: 947–8].

19. Aloia TA, Grubbs E, Onaitis M, et al. Predictors of outcome after hyperthermic isolated limb perfusion: role of tumor response. Arch Surg 2005;140(11): 1115–20.

20. Cornett WR, McCall LM, Petersen RP, et al. Randomized multicenter trial of hyperthermic isolated limb perfusion with melphalan alone compared with melphalan plus tumor necrosis factor: American College of Surgeons Oncology Group Trial Z0020. J Clin Oncol 2006;24(25):4196–201.

21. Sanki A, Kam PC, Thompson JF. Long-term results of hyperthermic, isolated limb perfusion for melanoma: a reflection of tumor biology. Ann Surg 2007; 245(4):591–6.

22. Mian R, Henderson MA, Speakman D, et al. Isolated limb infusion for melanoma: a simple alternative to isolated limb perfusion. Can J Surg 2001;44(3):189–92.

23. Lindner P, Doubrovsky A, Kam PC, et al. Prognostic factors after isolated limb infusion with cytotoxic agents for melanoma. Ann Surg Oncol 2002;9(2):127–36.

24. Bonenkamp JJ, Thompson JF, de Wilt JH, et al. Isolated limb infusion with fotemustine after dacarbazine chemosensitisation for inoperable loco-regional melanoma recurrence. Eur J Surg Oncol 2004;30(10):1107–12.

25. Brady MS, Brown K, Patel A, et al. A phase II trial of isolated limb infusion with melphalan and dactinomycin for regional melanoma and soft tissue sarcoma of the extremity. Ann Surg Oncol 2006;13(8):1123–9.

26. Kroon HM, Moncrieff M, Kam PC, et al. Outcomes following isolated limb infusion for melanoma. A 14-year experience. Ann Surg Oncol 2008;15(11): 3003–13.

27. Beasley GM, Caudle A, Petersen RP, et al. A multi-institutional experience of isolated limb infusion: defining response and toxicity in the US. J Am Coll Surg 2009;208(5):706–15 [discussion: 715–7].

28. Creech O Jr, Ryan RF, Krementz ET. Regional chemotherapy by isolated perfusion in the treatment of melanoma of the extremities. Plast Reconstr Surg Transplant Bull 1961;28:333–46.

29. Creech O Jr, Krementz ET, Ryan RF, et al. Chemotherapy of cancer: regional perfusion utilizing an extracorporeal circuit. Ann Surg 1958;148(4):616–32.

30. Beasley GM, Petersen RP, Yoo J, et al. Isolated limb infusion for in-transit malignant melanoma of the extremity: a well-tolerated but less effective alternative to hyperthermic isolated limb perfusion. Ann Surg Oncol 2008;15(8):2195–205.
31. Thompson JF, Kam PC, Waugh RC, et al. Isolated limb infusion with cytotoxic agents: a simple alternative to isolated limb perfusion. Semin Surg Oncol 1998;14(3):238–47.
32. Thompson JF, Waugh RC, Saw RPM, et al. Isolated limb infusion with melphalan: a simple alternative to isolated limb perfusion. Reg Cancer Treat 1994;7:188–92.
33. Santillan AA, Delman KA, Beasley GM, et al. Predictive factors of regional toxicity and serum creatine phosphokinase levels after isolated limb infusion for melanoma: a multi-institutional analysis. Ann Surg Oncol 2009;16(9):2570–8.
34. Padussis JC, Steerman SN, Tyler DS, et al. Pharmacokinetics & drug resistance of melphalan in regional chemotherapy: ILP versus ILI. Int J Hyperthermia 2008;24(3):239–49.
35. Kroon HM, Moncrieff M, Kam PC, et al. Factors predictive of acute regional toxicity after isolated limb infusion with melphalan and actinomycin D in melanoma patients. Ann Surg Oncol 2009;16(5):1184–92.
36. Benckhuijsen C, Kroon BB, van Geel AN, et al. Regional perfusion treatment with melphalan for melanoma in a limb: an evaluation of drug kinetics. Eur J Surg Oncol 1988;14(2):157–63.
37. Cavaliere R, Ciocatto EC, Giovanella BC, et al. Selective heat sensitivity of cancer cells. Biochemical and clinical studies. Cancer 1967;20(9):1351–81.
38. Thompson JF, Lai DT, Ingvar C, et al. Maximizing efficacy and minimizing toxicity in isolated limb perfusion for melanoma. Melanoma Res 1994;4S:45–50.
39. Wu ZY, Smithers BM, Roberts MS. Tissue and perfusate pharmacokinetics of melphalan in isolated perfused rat hindlimb. J Pharmacol Exp Ther 1997;282(3):1131–8.
40. Eggermont AM, de Wilt JH, ten Hagen TL. Current uses of isolated limb perfusion in the clinic and a model system for new strategies. Lancet Oncol 2003;4(7):429–37.
41. Luce JK. Chemotherapy of malignant melanoma. Cancer 1972;30(6):1604–15.
42. Roberts MS, Wu ZY, Siebert GA, et al. Saturable dose-response relationships for melphalan in melanoma treatment by isolated limb infusion in the nude rat. Melanoma Res 2001;11(6):611–8.
43. Taber SW, Polk HC Jr. Mortality, major amputation rates, and leukopenia after isolated limb perfusion with phenylalanine mustard for the treatment of melanoma. Ann Surg Oncol 1997;4(5):440–5.
44. Cheng TY, Grubbs E, Abdul-Wahab O, et al. Marked variability of melphalan plasma drug levels during regional hyperthermic isolated limb perfusion. Am J Surg 2003;186(5):460–7.
45. Vrouenraets BC, Hart GA, Eggermont AM, et al. Relation between limb toxicity and treatment outcomes after isolated limb perfusion for recurrent melanoma. J Am Coll Surg 1999;188(5):522–30.
46. Beasley GM, McMahon N, Sanders G, et al. A phase 1 study of systemic ADH-1 in combination with melphalan via isolated limb infusion in patients with locally advanced in-transit malignant melanoma. Cancer 2009;115:4766–74.
47. Di Filippo F, Calabro A, Giannarelli D, et al. Prognostic variables in recurrent limb melanoma treated with hyperthermic antiblastic perfusion. Cancer 1989;63(12):2551–61.
48. Engler HS, Sweat RD. Volumetric arm measurements: technique and results. Am Surg 1962;28:465–8.

49. McMahon N, Cheng TY, Beasley GM, et al. Optimizing melphalan pharmacokinetics in regional melanoma therapy: does correcting for ideal body weight alter regional response or toxicity? Ann Surg Oncol 2009;16(4):953–61.
50. Thompson JF, Gianoutsos MP. Isolated limb perfusion for melanoma: effectiveness and toxicity of cisplatin compared with that of melphalan and other drugs. World J Surg 1992;16(2):227–33.
51. Wile AG, Guilmette E, Friedberg H, et al. A model of experimental isolation perfusion using cis-platinum. J Surg Oncol 1982;21(1):37–41.
52. Aigner K, Hild P, Henneking K, et al. Regional perfusion with cis-platinum and dacarbazine. Recent Results Cancer Res 1983;86:239–45.
53. Roseman JM. Effective management of extremity cancers using cisplatin and etoposide in isolated limb perfusions. J Surg Oncol 1987;35(3):170–2.
54. Klein ES, Ben-Ari GY. Isolation perfusion with cisplatin for malignant melanoma of the limbs. Cancer 1987;59(6):1068–71.
55. Pommier RF, Moseley HS, Cohen J, et al. Pharmacokinetics, toxicity, and short-term results of cisplatin hyperthermic isolated limb perfusion for soft-tissue sarcoma and melanoma of the extremities. Am J Surg 1988;155(5):667–71.
56. Hajarizadeh H, Mueller CR, Woltering EA, et al. Phase I-II trial of hyperthermic isolated limb perfusion with cisplatin in the treatment of high risk malignant melanoma of the extremities. Melanoma Res 1991;1(1):55–61.
57. Santinami M, Belli F, Cascinelli N, et al. Seven years experience with hyperthermic perfusions in extracorporeal circulation for melanoma of the extremities. J Surg Oncol 1989;42(3):201–8.
58. Coit DG, Bajorin DF, Menendez-Botet C. A phase I trial of hyperthermic isolation limb perfusion (HILP) using cisplatin (CDDP) for metastatic melanoma. Proceedings of ASCO. 1991;10:294.
59. Middleton MR, Grob JJ, Aaronson N, et al. Randomized phase III study of temozolomide versus dacarbazine in the treatment of patients with advanced metastatic malignant melanoma. J Clin Oncol 2000;18(1):158–66.
60. Agarwala SS, Kirkwood JM. Temozolomide, a novel alkylating agent with activity in the central nervous system, may improve the treatment of advanced metastatic melanoma. Oncologist 2000;5(2):144–51.
61. Ueno T, Ko SH, Grubbs E, et al. Modulation of chemotherapy resistance in regional therapy: a novel therapeutic approach to advanced extremity melanoma using intra-arterial temozolomide in combination with systemic O6-benzylguanine. Mol Cancer Ther 2006;5(3):732–8.
62. Yoshimoto Y, Augustine CK, Yoo JS, et al. Defining regional infusion treatment strategies for extremity melanoma: comparative analysis of melphalan and temozolomide as regional chemotherapeutic agents. Mol Cancer Ther 2007; 6(5):1492–500.
63. Yao KA, Hsueh EC, Essner R, et al. Is sentinel lymph node mapping indicated for isolated local and in-transit recurrent melanoma? Ann Surg 2003;238(5):743–7.
64. Alexander HR Jr, Fraker DL, Bartlett DL, et al. Analysis of factors influencing outcome in patients with in-transit malignant melanoma undergoing isolated limb perfusion using modern treatment parameters. J Clin Oncol 2010;28(1):114–8.
65. Dahl O, Mella O. Hyperthermia and chemotherapeutic agents. New York: Taylor and Francis; 1990.
66. Hahn GM. Potential for therapy of drugs and hyperthermia. Cancer Res 1979; 39(6 Pt 2):2264–8.
67. Wallah DFH. Basic mechanisms of tumor thermotherapy. J Mol Med 1977;17: 381–403.

68. Huang SK, Stauffer PR, Hong K, et al. Liposomes and hyperthermia in mice: increased tumor uptake and therapeutic efficacy of doxorubicin in sterically stabilized liposomes. Cancer Res 1994;54(8):2186–91.

69. Stehlin JS Jr. Hyperthermic perfusion with chemotherapy for cancers of the extremities. Surg Gynecol Obstet 1969;129(2):305–8.

70. Ghussen F, Kruger I, Smalley RV, et al. Hyperthermic perfusion with chemotherapy for melanoma of the extremities. World J Surg 1989;13(5):598–602.

71. Ko SH, Ueno T, Yoshimoto Y, et al. Optimizing a novel regional chemotherapeutic agent against melanoma: hyperthermia-induced enhancement of temozolomide cytotoxicity. Clin Cancer Res 2006;12(1):289–97.

72. Abdel-Wahab OI, Grubbs E, Viglianti BL, et al. The role of hyperthermia in regional alkylating agent chemotherapy. Clin Cancer Res 2004;10(17):5919–29.

73. Posner MC, Lienard D, Lejeune FJ, et al. Hyperthermic isolated limb perfusion with tumor necrosis factor alone for melanoma. Cancer J Sci Am 1995;1(4):274–80.

74. Brouckaert PG, Leroux-Roels GG, Guisez Y, et al. In vivo anti-tumour activity of recombinant human and murine TNF, alone and in combination with murine IFN-gamma, on a syngeneic murine melanoma. Int J Cancer 1986;38(5):763–9.

75. Lienard D, Ewalenko P, Delmotte JJ, et al. High-dose recombinant tumor necrosis factor alpha in combination with interferon gamma and melphalan in isolation perfusion of the limbs for melanoma and sarcoma. J Clin Oncol 1992;10(1):52–60.

76. Lejeune FJ, Eggermont AM. Hyperthermic isolated limb perfusion with tumor necrosis factor is a useful therapy for advanced melanoma of the limbs. J Clin Oncol 2007;25(11):1449–50 author reply 1450–1441.

77. Garrido-Laguna I, Ponz M, Espinos J. Is there any reason to delay introduction of tumor necrosis factor in the management of in-transit metastasis of unresectable melanoma? J Clin Oncol 2007;25(9):1149 author reply 1149–1151.

78. Depeille P, Cuq P, Passagne I, et al. Combined effects of GSTP1 and MRP1 in melanoma drug resistance. Br J Cancer 2005;93(2):216–23.

79. Harkey MA, Czerwinski M, Slattery J, et al. Overexpression of glutathione-S-transferase, MGSTII, confers resistance to busulfan and melphalan. Cancer Invest 2005;23(1):19–25.

80. Grubbs EG, Abdel-Wahab O, Cheng TY, et al. In-transit melanoma: the role of alkylating-agent resistance in regional therapy. J Am Coll Surg 2004;199(3):419–27.

81. Buller AL, Clapper ML, Tew KD. Glutathione S-transferases in nitrogen mustard-resistant and -sensitive cell lines. Mol Pharmacol 1987;31(6):575–8.

82. Suzukake K, Petro BJ, Vistica DT. Reduction in glutathione content of L-PAM resistant L1210 Cells confers drug sensitivity. Biochem Pharmacol 1982;31(1):121–4.

83. Townsend DM, Tew KD. The role of glutathione-S-transferase in anti-cancer drug resistance. Oncogene 2003;22(47):7369–75.

84. Okamura T, Singh S, Buolamwini J, et al. Tyrosine phosphorylation of the human glutathione S-transferase P1 by epidermal growth factor receptor. J Biol Chem 2009;284(25):16979–89.

85. McClean S, Hill BT. An overview of membrane, cytosolic and nuclear proteins associated with the expression of resistance to multiple drugs in vitro. Biochim Biophys Acta 1992;1114(2–3):107–27.

86. Suzukake K, Vistica BP, Vistica DT. Dechlorination of L-phenylalanine mustard by sensitive and resistant tumor cells and its relationship to intracellular glutathione content. Biochem Pharmacol 1983;32(1):165–7.

87. Strumeyer DH, Bloch K. Some properties of gamma-glutamylcysteine synthetase. J Biol Chem 1960;235:PC27.
88. Griffith OW, Meister A. Potent and specific inhibition of glutathione synthesis by buthionine sulfoximine (S-n-butyl homocysteine sulfoximine). J Biol Chem 1979; 254(16):7558–60.
89. Biroccio A, Benassi B, Fiorentino F, et al. Glutathione depletion induced by c-Myc downregulation triggers apoptosis on treatment with alkylating agents. Neoplasia 2004;6(3):195–206.
90. McIlwain CC, Townsend DM, Tew KD. Glutathione S-transferase polymorphisms: cancer incidence and therapy. Oncogene 2006;25(11):1639–48.
91. Pellizzari Tregno F, Sau A, Pezzola S, et al. In vitro and in vivo efficacy of 6-(7-nitro-2,1,3-benzoxadiazol-4-ylthio)hexanol (NBDHEX) on human melanoma. Eur J Cancer 2009;45(14):2606–17.
92. Toshimitsu H, Yoshimoto Y, Augustine CK, et al. Inhibition of poly(ADP-ribose) polymerase enhances the effect of chemotherapy in an animal model of regional therapy for the treatment of advanced extremity malignant melanoma. Ann Surg Oncol 2010;17:2247–54.
93. Bignami M, O'Driscoll M, Aquilina G, et al. Unmasking a killer: DNA O(6)-methylguanine and the cytotoxicity of methylating agents. Mutat Res 2000;462(2–3): 71–82.
94. Augustine CK, Yoo JS, Potti A, et al. Genomic and molecular profiling predicts response to temozolomide in melanoma. Clin Cancer Res 2009;15(2):502–10.
95. Pegg AE. Mammalian O6-alkylguanine-DNA alkyltransferase: regulation and importance in response to alkylating carcinogenic and therapeutic agents. Cancer Res 1990;50(19):6119–29.
96. Cheng CL, Johnson SP, Keir ST, et al. Poly(ADP-ribose) polymerase-1 inhibition reverses temozolomide resistance in a DNA mismatch repair-deficient malignant glioma xenograft. Mol Cancer Ther 2005;4(9):1364–8.
97. Boulton S, Pemberton LC, Porteous JK, et al. Potentiation of temozolomide-induced cytotoxicity: a comparative study of the biological effects of poly (ADP-ribose) polymerase inhibitors. Br J Cancer 1995;72(4):849–56.
98. Haince JF, Rouleau M, Hendzel MJ, et al. Targeting poly(ADP-ribosyl)ation: a promising approach in cancer therapy. Trends Mol Med 2005;11(10):456–63.
99. Tentori L, Leonetti C, Scarsella M, et al. Systemic administration of GPI 15427, a novel poly(ADP-ribose) polymerase-1 inhibitor, increases the antitumor activity of temozolomide against intracranial melanoma, glioma, lymphoma. Clin Cancer Res 2003;9(14):5370–9.
100. Augustine CK, Yoshimoto Y, Gupta M, et al. Targeting N-cadherin enhances antitumor activity of cytotoxic therapies in melanoma treatment. Cancer Res 2008; 68(10):3777–84.
101. Hsu MY, Wheelock MJ, Johnson KR, et al. Shifts in cadherin profiles between human normal melanocytes and melanomas. J Investig Dermatol Symp Proc 1996;1(2):188–94.
102. Hsu MY, Meier FE, Nesbit M, et al. E-cadherin expression in melanoma cells restores keratinocyte-mediated growth control and down-regulates expression of invasion-related adhesion receptors. Am J Pathol 2000;156(5):1515–25.
103. Beasley G, Riboh JC, Augustine CK, et al. A prospective multi-center phase II trial of systemic ADH-1 in combination with melphalan via isolated limb infusion (M-ILI) in patients with advanced extremity melanoma. In Submission.
104. Friedman HS, Prados MD, Wen PY, et al. Bevacizumab alone and in combination with irinotecan in recurrent glioblastoma. J Clin Oncol 2009;27:4733–40.

105. Hurwitz H, Fehrenbacher L, Novotny W, et al. Bevacizumab plus irinotecan, fluorouracil, and leucovorin for metastatic colorectal cancer. N Engl J Med 2004; 350(23):2335–42.
106. Miller K, Wang M, Gralow J, et al. Paclitaxel plus bevacizumab versus paclitaxel alone for metastatic breast cancer. N Engl J Med 2007;357(26):2666–76.
107. Pallis AG, Serfass L, Dziadziusko R, et al. Targeted therapies in the treatment of advanced/metastatic NSCLC. Eur J Cancer 2009;45(14):2473–87.
108. Woolam GL. Cancer statistics, 2000: a benchmark for the new century. CA Cancer J Clin 2000;50(1):6.
109. Hainsworth JD, Infante JR, Spigel DR, et al. Bevacizumab and everolimus in the treatment of patients with metastatic melanoma: a phase 2 trial of the Sarah Cannon Oncology Research Consortium. Cancer 2010;116:4122–9.
110. Vihinen PP, Hernberg M, Vuoristo MS, et al. A phase II trial of bevacizumab with dacarbazine and daily low-dose interferon-alpha2a as first line treatment in metastatic melanoma. Melanoma Res 2010;20:318–25.
111. Perez DG, Suman VJ, Fitch TR, et al. Phase 2 trial of carboplatin, weekly paclitaxel, and biweekly bevacizumab in patients with unresectable stage IV melanoma: a north central cancer treatment group study, N047A. Cancer 2009;115(1):119–27.
112. Smalley KS, Herlyn M. Targeting intracellular signaling pathways as a novel strategy in melanoma therapeutics. Ann N Y Acad Sci 2005;1059:16–25.
113. Gray-Schopfer V, Wellbrock C, Marais R. Melanoma biology and new targeted therapy. Nature 2007;445(7130):851–7.
114. Davies H, Bignell GR, Cox C, et al. Mutations of the BRAF gene in human cancer. Nature 2002;417(6892):949–54.
115. Lang L. FDA approves sorafenib for patients with inoperable liver cancer. Gastroenterology 2008;134(2):379.
116. Stein MN, Flaherty KT. CCR drug updates: sorafenib and sunitinib in renal cell carcinoma. Clin Cancer Res 2007;13(13):3765–70.
117. Wilhelm SM, Adnane L, Newell P, et al. Preclinical overview of sorafenib, a multikinase inhibitor that targets both Raf and VEGF and PDGF receptor tyrosine kinase signaling. Mol Cancer Ther 2008;7(10):3129–40.
118. Panka DJ, Wang W, Atkins MB, et al. The Raf inhibitor BAY 43-9006 (sorafenib) induces caspase-independent apoptosis in melanoma cells. Cancer Res 2006; 66(3):1611–9.
119. Rahmani M, Davis EM, Bauer C, et al. Apoptosis induced by the kinase inhibitor BAY 43-9006 in human leukemia cells involves down-regulation of Mcl-1 through inhibition of translation. J Biol Chem 2005;280(42):35217–27.
120. Yu C, Bruzek LM, Meng XW, et al. The role of Mcl-1 downregulation in the proapoptotic activity of the multikinase inhibitor BAY 43-9006. Oncogene 2005; 24(46):6861–9.
121. Gray-Schopfer VC, Karasarides M, Hayward R, et al. Tumor necrosis factor-alpha blocks apoptosis in melanoma cells when BRAF signaling is inhibited. Cancer Res 2007;67(1):122–9.
122. Sharma A, Trivedi NR, Zimmerman MA, et al. Mutant V599EB-Raf regulates growth and vascular development of malignant melanoma tumors. Cancer Res 2005;65(6):2412–21.
123. Eisen T, Ahmad T, Flaherty KT, et al. Sorafenib in advanced melanoma: a phase II randomised discontinuation trial analysis. Br J Cancer 2006;95:581–6.
124. Escudier B, Lassau N, Angevin E, et al. Phase I trial of sorafenib in combination with IFN {alpha}-2a in patients with unresectable and/or metastatic renal cell carcinoma or malignant melanoma. Clin Cancer Res 2007;13(6):1801–9.

125. Bharti AC, Donato N, Singh S, et al. Curcumin (diferuloylmethane) down-regulates the constitutive activation of nuclear factor-kappa B and IkappaBalpha kinase in human multiple myeloma cells, leading to suppression of proliferation and induction of apoptosis. Blood 2003;101(3):1053–62.

126. McDermott DF, Sosman JA, Gonzalez R, et al. Double-blind randomized phase II study of the combination of sorafenib and dacarbazine in patients With advanced melanoma: a report from the 11715 study group. J Clin Oncol 2008;26(13):2178–85.

127. Amaravadi RK, Schuchter LM, McDermott DF, et al. Phase II Trial of temozolomide and sorafenib in advanced melanoma patients with or without brain metastases. Clin Cancer Res 2009;15:7711–8.

128. Hauschild A, Agarwala SS, Trefzer U, et al. Results of a phase III, randomized, placebo-controlled study of sorafenib in combination with carboplatin and paclitaxel as second-line treatment in patients with unresectable stage III or stage IV melanoma. J Clin Oncol 2009;27(17):2823–30.

129. Augustine CK, Toshimitsu H, Jung SH, et al. Sorafenib, a multikinase inhibitor, enhances the response of melanoma to regional chemotherapy. Mol Cancer Ther 2010;9:2090–101.

130. Yeatman TJ. A renaissance for SRC. Nat Rev Cancer 2004;4(6):470–80.

131. Niu G, Bowman T, Huang M, et al. Roles of activated Src and Stat3 signaling in melanoma tumor cell growth. Oncogene 2002;21(46):7001–10.

132. Niu G, Wright KL, Huang M, et al. Constitutive Stat3 activity up-regulates VEGF expression and tumor angiogenesis. Oncogene 2002;21(13):2000–8.

133. Brave M, Goodman V, Kaminskas E, et al. Sprycel for chronic myeloid leukemia and Philadelphia chromosome-positive acute lymphoblastic leukemia resistant to or intolerant of imatinib mesylate. Clin Cancer Res 2008;14(2): 352–9.

134. Homsi J, Cubitt CL, Zhang S, et al. Src activation in melanoma and Src inhibitors as therapeutic agents in melanoma. Melanoma Res 2009;19(3):167–75.

135. Yuan J, Gnjatic S, Li H, et al. CTLA-4 blockade enhances polyfunctional NY-ESO-1 specific T cell responses in metastatic melanoma patients with clinical benefit. Proc Natl Acad Sci U S A 2008;105(51):20410–5.

136. Alexandrescu DT, Ichim TE, Riordan NH, et al. Immunotherapy for melanoma: current status and perspectives. J Immunother 2010;33(6):570–90.

137. Barbour AP, Thomas J, Suffolk J, et al. Isolated limb infusion for malignant melanoma: predictors of response and outcome. Ann Surg Oncol 2009;16(12): 3463–72.

138. Bild A, Febbo PG. Application of a priori established gene sets to discover biologically important differential expression in microarray data. Proc Natl Acad Sci U S A 2005;102(43):15278–9.

139. John T, Black MA, Toro TT, et al. Predicting clinical outcome through molecular profiling in stage III melanoma. Clin Cancer Res 2008;14(16):5173–80.

140. Winnepenninckx V, Lazar V, Michiels S, et al. Gene expression profiling of primary cutaneous melanoma and clinical outcome. J Natl Cancer Inst 2006; 98(7):472–82.

141. Augustine CK, Jung SH, Sohn I, et al. Gene expression signatures as a guide to treatment strategies for in-transit metastatic melanoma. Mol Cancer Ther 2010; 9(4):779–90.

142. Middleton MR, Lunn JM, Morris C, et al. O6-methylguanine-DNA methyltransferase in pretreatment tumour biopsies as a predictor of response to temozolomide in melanoma. Br J Cancer 1998;78(9):1199–202.

143. Middleton MR, Lee SM, Arance A, et al. O6-methylguanine formation, repair protein depletion and clinical outcome with a 4 hr schedule of temozolomide in the treatment of advanced melanoma: results of a phase II study. Int J Cancer 2000;88(3):469–73.
144. Ma S, Egyhazi S, Martenhed G, et al. Analysis of O(6)-methylguanine-DNA methyltransferase in melanoma tumours in patients treated with dacarbazine-based chemotherapy. Melanoma Res 2002;12(4):335–42.
145. Rietschel P, Wolchok JD, Krown S, et al. Phase II study of extended-dose temozolomide in patients with melanoma. J Clin Oncol 2008;26(14):2299–304.

Adjuvant Therapy for Melanoma: A Surgical Perspective

Vernon K. Sondak, MD[a,b,c],*, Ricardo J. Gonzalez, MD[a,b,d],
Ragini Kudchadkar, MD[a,b]

KEYWORDS

• Melanoma • Adjuvant therapy • Interferon • Vaccines
• GM-CSF • Ipilimumab

Adjuvant therapy is defined as treatment administered to patients who are clinically free of disease but at substantive risk of recurrence. In most tumor types, adjuvant therapy is preferentially used for patients at relatively high risk of recurrence in whom that recurrence would be difficult to treat or cure. There are 3 potential oncologic advantages a percentage of treated patients may derive from effective adjuvant therapy: (1) reduction in the risk of recurrence; (2) delay in the time to clinically evident recurrence, resulting in an increase in the time patients perceive themselves to be disease free; and (3) increase in the cure rate (overall survival) by administering therapy early in the course of disease when it is able to completely eradicate minimal residual disease that would have become incurable by the time it was clinically evident. There is one additional advantage all patients derive from adjuvant therapy, namely the sense of actively combating their disease rather than passively waiting for it to recur, often described as a feeling "I've done everything I could to beat this cancer." In exchange for these potential or real advantages, all patients accept the toxicities of adjuvant therapy— including those patients whose disease was actually cured by the initial surgery.

Recurrent melanoma, whether in a regional nodal basin, confined to a single extremity as in-transit metastases, or disseminated throughout the body, is

Statement of support: None.

Authors' financial disclosures: Dr Sondak is a paid consultant and provided expert testimony for Merck/Schering-Plough.

[a] Department of Cutaneous Oncology, H. Lee Moffitt Cancer Center and Research Institute, 12902 Magnolia Drive, Tampa, FL 33612, USA

[b] Department of Oncologic Sciences, University of South Florida College of Medicine, Tampa, FL 33612, USA

[c] Department of Surgery, University of South Florida College of Medicine, Tampa, FL 33612, USA

[d] Department of Sarcoma Oncology, H. Lee Moffitt Cancer Center and Research Institute, Tampa, FL, USA

* Corresponding author. Department of Cutaneous Oncology, H. Lee Moffitt Cancer Center and Research Institute, 12902 Magnolia Drive, Tampa, FL 33612.

E-mail address: vernon.sondak@moffitt.org

notoriously difficult to treat effectively and usually presages the patient's ultimate demise. Melanoma patients who perceive themselves at risk of recurrence, therefore, are often very motivated to pursue adjuvant therapy with even a small chance of delaying or preventing recurrence.[1] Surgeons have a profound influence on patients' decision making regarding adjuvant therapy, beginning with providing a clear understanding of the risk of specific types of recurrence (local, regional nodal, intransit, and distant). Surgeons also have an important role in explaining the morbidity of surgical treatment with and without adjuvant therapy, and of course they are instrumental in initiating the referral process to medical and radiation oncologists for consideration of specific adjuvant therapies.

RISK ASSESSMENT IN MELANOMA
Lymph Node Status as a Predictor of Distant Metastasis

In this era of "personalized medicine," it is worth emphasizing that the surgical treatment and staging of melanoma has been highly individualized for many years.[2] Sentinel node biopsy is a widely used staging procedure, intended to assess the risk of subsequent metastasis and death from melanoma.[3,4] Patients with clinically or radiographically evident nodal metastasis, whether at the time of initial diagnosis or as a recurrence after prior wide excision of the primary are more likely to relapse and die than those with a "microscopic" metastasis. (By definition in the American Joint Committee on Cancer [AJCC] staging system, any nodal metastasis discovered by sentinel node biopsy is a "micrometastasis" whereas any discovered clinically or radiographically is a "macrometastasis".) Regardless of how nodal metastases present, radical lymphadenectomy is associated with cure in up to half of patients, and so aggressive surgical therapy is an important part of the management of any stage III melanoma.[5] In addition to "tumor burden" (micrometastasis vs macrometastasis), as the number of lymph nodes involved by melanoma increases, the risk of distant metastasis and death also increases. Of note, even after nodal metastasis has occurred there is still prognostic information to be gained by knowing the thickness and ulceration status of the primary tumor.[6]

At the present time, all patients with stage III melanoma are considered appropriate candidates for radical lymphadenectomy and, if they are otherwise healthy, consideration of adjuvant therapy. There is considerable interest in trying to identify a subset of node-positive patients who may be at very low risk for regional or distant recurrence, presumably those with very small tumor deposits in the regional nodes ("micrometastases" in a different sense of the word than the AJCC employs).[7] To date, however, a threshold below which the risk of further recurrence in the regional basin and beyond is low enough to safely allow observation of the patient without either lymphadenectomy or adjuvant therapy has not been defined, but prospective trials are ongoing.[8]

Lymph Node Status as a Predictor of Regional Recurrence

While a subset of "low-risk" stage III melanoma patients who do not require lymphadenectomy may eventually be defined, currently many patients have "high-risk" stage III disease at risk of recurrence in the nodal basin despite radical node dissections. Available evidence suggests that radiation can decrease the risk of recurrence after lymphadenectomy,[9] but controversy remains regarding which patients are at sufficient risk of regional recurrence to possibly warrant radiation, as well as whether adjuvant radiation should be used in these patients following lymphadenectomy or be reserved only for the subset of patients with regional recurrence who can be re-resected to a disease-free state. To date, the presence of very large tumor-containing nodes or multiple involved lymph nodes and the finding of invasion of melanoma through the lymph node capsule into the surrounding tissue (extracapsular extension) are the most established indicators of increased risk of regional recurrence after lymphade-nectomy, and are the most commonly employed criteria used to select patients for adjuvant nodal basin irradiation.[9,10] Further discussion of adjuvant radiation in mela-noma is provided in an article by Rao and colleagues elsewhere in this issue.

Risk of Recurrence After Resection of Oligometastatic Melanoma

In recent years, patients with one or a few distant metastases have increasingly been considered for surgical management.[11] The combination of improved perioperative care combined with more effective imaging techniques has increased enthusiasm for this approach, and it is clear that some patients with resected stage IV disease have a prolonged disease-free interval after metastasectomy and a favorable overall outcome compared with patients with unresectable stage IV melanoma. At present, however, most patients recur relatively quickly after metastasectomy, and the prog-nostic factors associated with long-term recurrence-free survival for resected stage IV melanoma are not well defined. Clinical factors that appear to be most strongly associated with a short recurrence-free interval after metastasectomy are visceral metastatic disease (particularly liver metastases), multiple metastases and particularly multiple sites of metastasis, a rapid tumor doubling time as assessed radiographically, and a short disease-free interval between resection of the primary and development of stage IV disease.[11] Nonetheless, given the overall high risk of recurrence after meta-stasectomy in melanoma and the absence of defined standard adjuvant therapy for this group, the authors consider all resected stage IV melanoma patients to be appro-priate candidates for investigational trials of adjuvant therapy.

ADJUVANT SYSTEMIC THERAPY TO REDUCE DISEASE RECURRENCE AND DEATH
Lack of Efficacy of Chemotherapy and Nonspecific Immunotherapies

Over the past 40 years, more than 100 randomized clinical trials have investigated cytotoxic chemotherapeutic agents and nonspecific immunostimulants such as bacille Calmette-Guérin (BCG), *Corynebacterium parvum*, and levamisole.[12] Despite the fact that statistically one would expect 1 clinical trial in 20 using ineffective therapy to yield a false-positive result, none of these trials were positive. Interest in nonspecific immunotherapy declined as more active immunostimulatory cytokines, in particular interferon (IFN), came into clinical practice.

Adjuvant Immunotherapy with Interferon

Interferon α-2b (IFNα-2b) is the only adjuvant regimen approved by the Food and Drug Administration (FDA) for patients with stage IIB and stage III melanoma, and is consid-ered the standard of care for these patients in the United States. Here the authors review clinical trials addressing the benefit of adjuvant IFN and discuss the controver-sies of these trials.

The Eastern Cooperative Oncology Group (ECOG) trial E1684 was the first random-ized, placebo-controlled study of high-dose IFNα-2b (HDI), involving 287 patients with stage IIB (n = 31) or stage III melanoma. HDI was administered as 20 million units (MU) per m^2 intravenously 5 days per week for 1 month followed by 10 MU/m^2 subcutane-ously 3 times per week for 48 weeks. At initial publication, after a median follow-up time of 6.9 years, relapse-free survival (RFS) was increased from 1.0 to 1.7 years and overall survival (OS) was increased from 2.8 to 3.8 years, both of which were statistically significant.[13] Updated results after a median follow-up of 12.6 years showed the RFS benefit to have been maintained, but the statistical significance of the survival benefit had been lost.[14] The diminished survival benefit after longer follow-up was of uncertain cause, but led many physicians to question whether HDI was worth the significant side effects.[15]

The next cooperative group trial of IFN only increased the uncertainty about adjuvant therapy in melanoma. ECOG trial E1690 accrued 642 patients to a 3-arm study comparing HDI (n = 215) with low-dose IFN (LDI; 3 MU 3 times per week for 2 years, n = 215) and with observation (n = 212). HDI showed an improvement in RFS (44% relapse-free at 5-years) compared with LDI and observation (40% and 35%, respectively). However, unlike E1684, there was no OS benefit seen with either HDI or LDI compared with observation.[16] Because HDI was approved by the FDA during the conduct of this trial, and patients with thick melanomas were allowed to enter the trial without any nodal staging or dissection, crossover of observation-arm patients to HDI after nodal relapse was a confounding factor that may have affected the survival results. This factor emphasizes the important role that surgical staging can play in adjuvant therapy trials and clinical decisions.

A third study, trial E1694, accrued 880 patients and compared an investigational ganglioside vaccine with HDI. HDI demonstrated a statistically significant benefit compared with the vaccine in RFS and OS.[17] This result raised the question of whether HDI led to benefit or the vaccine caused harm, a question that has gained additional credence after a randomized trial of the same vaccine compared with observation in patients with stage II melanoma was stopped early because of a possible decrease in survival for vaccine-treated patients in the face of definite evidence of no impact on RFS.[18] With further follow-up, however, the results of that randomized trial now show no significant adverse impact of the vaccine on either relapse or survival.[19]

With more than 2000 patients treated on clinical trials of adjuvant HDI, several questions still remain. After reviewing these trials and combining the data into a meta-analysis, it is clear that HDI delays recurrences and improves disease-free survival.[20] The OS benefit of HDI, if any, is small; in the meta-analysis all IFN-treated patients, regardless of dose and schedule, experienced a 10% relative decrease in the risk of death, which translated into a 2.8% increase in 5-year survival rate. Therefore when counseling patients regarding treatment with adjuvant HDI, several issues must be discussed at length. (1) How important is RFS for this individual patient? Patients and physicians often have differing opinions on this matter, with patients often placing more emphasis of RFS than physicians.[1] (2) What is the toxicity of HDI? It is clear that with a relatively small overall benefit, one is less likely to give adjuvant IFN to patients with an increased risk of toxicities, such as those with already underlying severe psychiatric disorder, autoimmune disease, or poor cardiac, liver, or renal function. (3) What is the risk of relapse in any given patient?

Overall, most stage III melanoma patients should be counseled about adjuvant IFN and a lengthy discussion of its risks and benefits should be undertaken, with active patient participation. Observation alone or experimental trials are also valid choices to offer patients with stage III disease. High-risk stage II patients were included in all of the aforementioned trials, and though the benefit of adjuvant IFN in this subgroup of patients is even less clear than in stage III, some such patients will choose to pursue adjuvant treatment.

Pegylated Interferon as an Alternative to Standard Interferon

The many questions around the benefits of HDI, combined with the significant challenges patients face in undertaking this therapy (not the least of which are a month of daily visits to a hospital or clinic for intravenous infusions followed by thrice-weekly injections), has led to many clinical trials seeking alternatives. Pegylated IFN has a much longer half-life, allowing once a week injections to provide continuous drug exposure without the high peaks and long troughs (periods of time with undetectable blood IFN levels) associated with HDI. In Europe, where HDI has not been widely adopted, a large randomized trial (involving more than 1250 patients with stage III melanoma) compared pegylated IFNα-2b (Peg-IFN) administered for 5 years with observation. RFS, but not OS, was statistically significantly increased for patients randomized to Peg-IFN. Of particular interest, however, was the observation that patients with clinically occult nodal metastases diagnosed by sentinel node biopsy appeared to fare particularly well with Peg-IFN adjuvant therapy: both RFS and distant metastasis–free survival were significantly increased and there was a trend toward improved survival as well.[21] Peg-IFN in this dose and schedule shares many of the substantial toxicities of HDI, but some patients will find it more convenient and, with appropriate and aggressive dose reduction to keep toxicities to a minimum level, many patients will find it possible to stay on therapy long-term with little or no impact on daily function.[22] Recently, the Oncology Drug Advisory Committee voted to recommend that the FDA approve Peg-IFN as an alternative adjuvant approach for melanoma patients, but a final FDA decision on this point is still awaited.

Investigational Approaches with Vaccines and New Immunotherapies

Even if Peg-IFN is approved as an additional option for adjuvant therapy, it represents at best a small advance over existing approaches.[22] Numerous other approaches have been tested, particularly vaccines designed to stimulate an immune response against any remaining melanoma cells in the body, but although some have shown promise in subsets of patients,[23] none have reached the stage of FDA approval or widespread use. Indeed, the recent finding that some treated patients in several vaccine studies (including the ganglioside vaccine trial referred to previously) have fared worse than patients on observation or placebo has caused considerable consternation in the melanoma community.[18] Even if (as is likely to be the case) long-term follow-up shows no actual adverse impact of melanoma vaccines, the failure of these trials to demonstrate an advantage for vaccination requires a rethinking of our approach to immunotherapy for melanoma in general.

Another immunomodulatory cytokine besides IFN that has been evaluated as an adjuvant therapy in melanoma is granulocyte-macrophage colony-stimulating factor (GM-CSF), alone or with vaccines. Nonrandomized trial data spurred interest in this agent,[24,25] but the latest analysis of the large (800+ patients) randomized E4697 trial shows that GM-CSF alone or with a peptide vaccine failed to improve either RFS or OS.[26] The current evidence clearly does not support the adjuvant use of GM-CSF outside the setting of a clinical trial. New agents with greater immunomodulatory effects, such as ipilimumab,[27] are beginning to undergo testing in randomized adjuvant trials in patients with a high risk of relapse.

Neoadjuvant Therapy

The role of neoadjuvant (preoperative) systemic therapy in melanoma is not well studied. In many other forms of cancer, systemic treatments with high response rates in the metastatic setting are brought into the neoadjuvant setting to reduce tumor size and potentially increase resectability of borderline or unresectable tumors. In melanoma, however, the standard treatments for metastatic disease have low response rates, with the 2 approved therapies, DTIC and high-dose interleukin-2, having response rates between 10% and 20%. Combination therapies, such as biochemotherapy (cytotoxic therapy plus immunotherapy), have yielded higher response rates in the metastatic setting, on the order of 48% to 60% in some series.[28] The regimen of cisplatin, dacarbazine, and vinblastine combined with IFN and continuous infusion interleukin-2 has been studied in the neoadjuvant setting. Of the 50 patients with measurable disease in one recent study, biochemotherapy resulted in a partial or complete response in 13 patients for an overall response rate of 26%.[29] A complete pathologic response was seen in 13 patients. However, the toxicities were significant and about 20% patients did not complete all 4 cycles of treatment secondary to toxicity. However, this does show that in a small number of select cases, biochemotherapy can have a clinical and pathologic response. HDI has also been studied in a small number of patients in the neoadjuvant setting.[30] Twenty patients with stage IIIB and IIIC melanoma were given 4 weeks of intravenous IFN followed by lymph node dissection. Eleven patients had a clinical response and 3 patients had a complete pathologic response. This response rate for IFN is remarkable, but as yet it has not been validated in a confirmatory study.

Overall, neoadjuvant therapy is clearly not the standard of care in the management of stage III melanoma. However, a select group of patients may benefit from neoadjuvant systemic treatment with high response rates, such as biochemotherapy. These patients should ideally be young, healthy patients with tumors that are not or are borderline resectable, selected after careful imaging studies and with the involvement of surgical, medical, and radiation oncologists.

ADJUVANT THERAPY TO REDUCE LOCAL, REGIONAL NODAL, AND IN-TRANSIT RECURRENCE
Adjuvant Intra-arterial Infusion or Perfusion to Decrease In-Transit Recurrence

Regional intra-arterial therapy has been used for melanoma since 1950 when Klopp and colleagues[31] observed improved symptoms and decreased tumor volume after arterial infusion of nitrogen mustard. In the late 1950s, Creech and colleagues[32] developed a vascular isolation procedure that was adapted 10 years later by Stehlin[33] for the hyperthermic perfusion of melphalan for extremity melanomas. The technique was termed isolated limb perfusion (ILP), and has been used with great success for in-transit and recurrent disease with curative intent.[34] In recent years a newer percutaneous technique introduced by Thompson and Kam,[35] isolated limb infusion (ILI), has been the focus of intense study. Both approaches have their merits for in-transit and recurrent disease; however, only the more invasive ILP has been studied in the adjuvant setting.

ILP is accomplished by exposing the inguinal or iliac vessels for the lower extremity and the axillary vessels for the upper extremity. During the preliminary vascular dissection, a lymphadenectomy may also be performed to remove nodal disease. Cannulae are inserted into the respective artery and vein for vascular isolation and hyperthermic infusion of high-dose melphalan. Little to no systemic leak of melphalan should occur to minimize the risks of bone marrow suppression or hypotension. Real-time monitoring of systemic leak can be accomplished with systemic monitoring of a radiolabeled tracer incorporated into the infusate.

ILI is a minimally invasive, percutaneous method of vascular isolation and regional chemotherapy. Cannulae are inserted in the contralateral femoral vessels and then positioned under fluoroscopy in the ipsilateral femoral artery and vein. The extremity is warmed to a final limb temperature of 38°C to 39°C, a tourniquet is used to control systemic leak, and therapy is begun. Aside from the less invasive nature of this approach, ILI is performed in an acidotic and hypoxic environment, which has been demonstrated to augment the effects of melphalan cytotoxicity.[36]

Both ILI and ILP have comparable clinical results and well-established therapeutic efficacy for patients with evaluable recurrent or in-transit disease.[34,37,38] Initial studies of adjuvant ILP were retrospective and used historical controls as a comparator. Martijn and colleagues[39] reported a combined retrospective experience from Groningen and the Sydney Melanoma Unit. These investigators compared adjuvant ILP with wide excision, and concluded that in this select group of patients the combination of ILP with excision resulted in improvements in local/regional recurrence rates, disease-free survival, and OS. This report is in contrast to that of Franklin and colleagues,[40] who studied high-risk melanomas (>1.5 mm) in 227 ILP patients and compared them with 238 matched historical controls undergoing wide excision alone. Their findings demonstrated no significant differences between the groups in terms of time to limb recurrence, time to regional lymph node metastasis, time to distant metastasis, and disease-free survival or OS. Franklin and colleagues concluded that adjuvant ILP could not be recommended for this patient population. A multicenter, randomized phase III trial of 832 patients randomized to wide excision or wide excision plus ILP identified a trend toward improved disease-free survival and local disease control with wide excision and ILP. Patients who underwent excision and ILP had lower rates of in-transit (3.3% vs 6.6%) and regional node metastases (12.6% vs 16.7%) than patients undergoing excision alone. There was, however, no difference in OS and 2 patients required amputation in the ILP group. The investigators concluded that prophylactic ILP should not be recommended as an adjunct to standard therapy for high-risk melanoma.[41] Although the less invasive ILI might ultimately find a role in the adjuvant setting, there is still substantial toxicity associated with this procedure; thus, adjuvant ILI should not be undertaken outside the context of a clinical trial.[38,42]

FUTURE PROSPECTS FOR MORE EFFECTIVE ADJUVANT THERAPIES

There is clearly reason to be optimistic about the future of adjuvant therapy for melanoma. Improvements in our ability to prognosticate, fueled by the development of new genomic or other biomarkers to identify and quantitate metastatic potential and/or the presence of residual tumor cells after surgery, will allow clinicians to eliminate treatment toxicity for patients who are cured by surgery alone and focus attention on the patients who stand to gain most from therapy. Biomarkers can also help identify those patients most likely to respond (or be resistant) to therapy, allowing those who will not respond to "standard" treatment to be entered directly into clinical trials.[43] The potential value of such an approach has been shown by the recent identification of single nucleotide polymorphisms in the interleukin-28 gene that may predict IFN sensitivity or resistance in hepatitis.[44] Finally, emerging targeted therapies that can eliminate cells bearing specific mutations may find an increasingly important role in adjuvant therapy, before multiple other mutations can take place that allow resistant clones to emerge.[45,46] Regardless of which approach or combination of approaches one pursues, effective adjuvant therapy begins with complete resection of the primary tumor and any clinically evident metastases, combined with a thorough staging evaluation and assessment of the risk of subsequent recurrence or metastasis. Because of this, surgeons will have a fundamental role to play in the future of adjuvant therapy, just as they do today.

REFERENCES

1. Kilbridge KL, Weeks JC, Sober AJ, et al. Patient preferences for adjuvant interferon alfa-2b treatment. J Clin Oncol 2001;19:812–23.
2. Riker AI, Glass F, Perez I, et al. Cutaneous melanoma: methods of biopsy and definitive surgical excision. Dermatol Ther 2005;18:387–93.

3. Morton DL, Thompson JF, Cochran AJ, et al. Sentinel-node biopsy or nodal observation in melanoma. N Engl J Med 2006;355:1307–17.
4. Balch CM, Morton DL, Gershenwald JE, et al. Sentinel node biopsy and standard of care for melanoma. J Am Acad Dermatol 2009;60:872–5.
5. Sarnaik AA, Puleo CA, Zager JS, et al. Limiting the morbidity of inguinal lymphadenectomy for metastatic melanoma. Cancer Control 2009;16:240–7.
6. Balch CM, Soong S-J, Gershenwald JE, et al. Prognostic factors analysis of 17,600 melanoma patients: validation of the American Joint Committee on Cancer melanoma staging system. J Clin Oncol 2001;19:3622–34.
7. van Akkooi AC, de Wilt JH, Verhoef C, et al. Clinical relevance of melanoma micrometastases (<0.1 mm) in sentinel nodes: are these nodes to be considered negative? Ann Oncol 2006;17:1578–85.
8. Ollila DW, Ashburn JH, Amos KD, et al. Metastatic melanoma cells in the sentinel node cannot be ignored. J Am Coll Surg 2009;208:924–9.
9. Henderson MA, Burmeister B, Thompson JF. Adjuvant radiotherapy and regional lymph node field control after lymphadenectomy: results of an intergroup randomized trial (ANZMTG 01.01/TROG 02.01). J Clin Oncol 2009;27(18S,Suppl 20): LBA9084.
10. Agrawal S, Kane JM 3rd, Guadagnolo BA, et al. The benefits of adjuvant radiation therapy after therapeutic lymphadenectomy for clinically advanced, high-risk, lymph node-metastatic melanoma. Cancer 2009;115:5836–44.
11. McLoughlin JM, Zager JS, Sondak VK. Cytoreductive surgery for melanoma. Surg Oncol Clin N Am 2007;16:683–93.
12. Kirkwood JM, Sondak VK, Hersey P, et al. Adjuvant systemic therapy for high-risk melanoma patients. In: Balch CM, Houghton AN, Sober AJ, et al, editors. Cutaneous melanoma. 5th edition. St Louis (MO): Quality Medical Publishing; 2009. p. 669–92.
13. Kirkwood JM, Strawderman MH, Ernstoff MS, et al. Interferon alfa-2b adjuvant therapy of high-risk resected cutaneous melanoma: the Eastern Cooperative Group trial EST 1684. J Clin Oncol 1996;14:7–17.
14. Kirkwood JM, Manola J, Ibrahim J, et al. A pooled analysis of ECOG and intergroup trials of adjuvant high-dose interferon for melanoma. Clin Cancer Res 2004;10:1670–7.
15. Chapman PB. Counterpoint: the case against adjuvant high-dose interferon-alpha for melanoma patients. J Natl Compr Canc Netw 2004;2:69–72.
16. Kirkwood JM, Ibrahim JG, Sondak VK, et al. High- and low-dose interferon alfa-2b in high-risk melanoma: first analysis of intergroup trial E1690/S9111/C9190. J Clin Oncol 2000;18:2444–54.
17. Kirkwood JM, Ibrahim JG, Sosman JA, et al. High-dose interferon alfa-2b significantly prolongs relapse-free and overall survival compared with the GM2-KLH/QS-21 vaccine in patients with resected stage IIB-III melanoma: results of Intergroup trial E1694/S9512/C509801. J Clin Oncol 2001;19:2370–80.
18. Eggermont AM. Vaccine trials in melanoma—time for reflection. Nat Clin Pract Oncol 2009;6:256–8.
19. Eggermont AM, Suciu S, Rutkowski P, et al. Randomized phase III trial comparing postoperative adjuvant ganglioside GM2-KLH/QS-21 vaccination versus observation in stage II (T3-T4N0M0) melanoma: final results of study EORTC 18961. J Clin Oncol 2010;28(15S):612s.
20. Mocellin S, Pasquali S, Rossi CR, et al. Interferon alpha adjuvant therapy in patients with high-risk melanoma: a systematic review and meta-analysis. J Natl Cancer Inst 2010;102:493–501.

21. Eggermont AM, Suciu S, Santinami M, et al. Adjuvant therapy with pegylated interferon alfa-2b versus observation alone in resected stage III melanoma: final results of EORTC 18991, a randomised phase III trial. Lancet 2008;372: 117–26.
22. Sondak VK, Flaherty LE. Adjuvant therapy of melanoma: is pegylated interferon alfa-2b what we've been waiting for? Lancet 2008;372:89–90.
23. Sondak VK, Liu PY, Tuthill RJ, et al. Adjuvant immunotherapy of resected, intermediate-thickness node-negative melanoma with an allogeneic tumor vaccine. Overall results of a randomized trial of the Southwest Oncology Group. J Clin Oncol 2002;20:2058–66.
24. Spitler LE, Grossbard ML, Ernstoff MS, et al. Adjuvant therapy of stage III and IV malignant melanoma using granulocyte-macrophage colony-stimulating factor. J Clin Oncol 2000;18:1614–21.
25. Daud AI, Mirza N, Lenox B, et al. Phenotypic and functional analysis of dendritic cells and clinical outcome in patients with high risk melanoma treated with adjuvant GM-CSF. J Clin Oncol 2008;26:3235–41.
26. Lawson DH, Lee SJ, Tarhini AA, et al. E4697: phase III trial cooperative group study of yeast-derived granulocyte macrophage colony-stimulating factor (GM-CSF) versus placebo as adjuvant treatment of patients with completely resected stage III-IV melanoma. J Clin Oncol 2010;28(15S):612s.
27. Phan GQ, Weber JS, Sondak VK. CTLA-4 blockade with monoclonal antibodies in patients with metastatic cancer: surgical issues. Ann Surg Oncol 2008;15: 3014–21.
28. Eton O, Legha SS, Bedikian AY, et al. Sequential biochemotherapy versus chemotherapy for metastatic melanoma: results from a phase III randomized trial. J Clin Oncol 2002;20:2411–4.
29. Lewis KD, Robinson WA, McCarter M, et al. Phase II multicenter study of neoadjuvant biochemotherapy for patients with stage III malignant melanoma. J Clin Oncol 2006;24:3157–63.
30. Moschos SJ, Edington HD, Land SR, et al. Neoadjuvant treatment of regional stage IIIB melanoma with high-dose interferon alfa-2b induces objective tumor regression in association with modulation of tumor infiltrating host cellular immune responses. J Clin Oncol 2006;24:3164–71.
31. Klopp CT, Alford TC, Bateman J, et al. Fractionated intra-arterial cancer chemotherapy with methyl bis-amine hydrochloride: a preliminary report. Ann Surg 1950;132:811–32.
32. Creech O Jr, Ryan RF, Krementz ET. Treatment of melanoma by isolation-perfusion technique. J Am Med Assoc 1959;169:339–43.
33. Stehlin JS Jr. Hyperthermic perfusion with chemotherapy for cancers of the extremities. Surg Gynecol Obstet 1969;129:305–8.
34. Fraker DL. Management of in-transit melanoma of the extremity with isolated limb perfusion. Curr Treat Options Oncol 2004;5:173–84.
35. Thompson JF, Kam PC. Isolated limb infusion for melanoma: a simple but effective alternative to isolated limb perfusion. J Surg Oncol 2004;88:1–3.
36. Siemann DW, Chapman M, Beikirch A. Effects of oxygenation and pH on tumor cell response to alkylating chemotherapy. Int J Radiat Oncol Biol Phys 1991;20: 287–9.
37. Brady MS, Brown K, Patel A, et al. A phase II trial of isolated limb infusion with melphalan and dactinomycin for regional melanoma and soft tissue sarcoma of the extremity. Ann Surg Oncol 2006;13:1123–9.

38. Beasley GM, Caudle A, Petersen RP, et al. A multi-institutional experience of isolated limb infusion: defining response and toxicity in the US. J Am Coll Surg 2009; 208:706–15.

39. Martijn H, Schraffordt Koops H, Milton GW, et al. Comparison of two methods of treating primary malignant melanomas Clark IV and V, thickness 1.5 mm and greater, localized on the extremities. Wide surgical excision with and without adjuvant regional perfusion. Cancer 1986;57:1923–30.

40. Franklin HR, Schraffordt Kroops H, Oldhoff J, et al. To perfuse or not to perfuse? a retrospective comparative study to evaluate the effect of adjuvant isolated regional perfusion in patients with stage I extremity melanoma with a thickness of 1.5 mm or greater. J Clin Oncol 1988;6:701–8.

41. Koops HS, Vaglini M, Suciu S, et al. Prophylactic isolated limb perfusion for localized, high-risk limb melanoma: results of a multicenter randomized phase III trial. J Clin Oncol 1998;16:2906–12.

42. Santillan AA, Delman KA, Beasley GM, et al. Predictive factors of regional toxicity and serum creatine phosphokinase levels after isolated limb infusion for melanoma: a multi-institutional analysis. Ann Surg Oncol 2009;16:2570–8.

43. Kirkwood JM, Tarhini AA. Biomarkers of therapeutic response in melanoma and renal cell carcinoma: potential inroads to improved immunotherapy. J Clin Oncol 2009;27:2583–5.

44. Ge D, Fellay J, Thompson AJ, et al. Genetic variation in *IL28B* predicts hepatitis C treatment-induced viral clearance. Nature 2009;461:399–401.

45. Smalley KS, Nathanson KL, Flaherty KT. Genetic subgrouping of melanoma reveals new opportunities for targeted therapy. Cancer Res 2009;69:3241–4.

46. Smalley KSM, Sondak VK. Melanoma: the unlikely poster child for personalized cancer therapy? N Engl J Med 2010;363:876–8.

The Role of Radiation Therapy in the Management of Cutaneous Melanoma

Nikhil G. Rao, MD[a,b,]*, Hsiang-Hsuan M. Yu, MD[a],
Andrea Trotti III, MD[a,b], Vernon K. Sondak, MD[b]

KEYWORDS

- Melanoma • Radiation • Chemotherapy • Metastases
- Stereotactic

Surgery, systemic therapy, and radiation therapy all play an important role in the management of cutaneous melanoma. Depending on the clinical situation, radiotherapy may be used to improve local control or for palliation. This review describes the experience with radiation for a variety of clinical indications. Specifically, the roles of radiation as definitive and adjuvant therapy to the primary site, as an adjuvant after lymph node dissection, and to the lymph node basin in the absence of complete node dissection are discussed. The use of concurrent radiation therapy with interferon, chemotherapy, and hyperthermia are also described. The rationale behind radiation dose and fractionation schemes is explained. Radiation therapy as a palliative modality in stage IV melanoma is explored, including treatment of brain, subcutaneous, and other metastases. The rationale behind choosing whole brain radiation, stereotactic radiosurgery for brain metastases, and stereotactic radiation therapy for oligometastatic disease is specifically described.

DEFINITIVE AND ADJUVANT RADIOTHERAPY TO THE PRIMARY SITE

Wide resection remains the primary initial treatment of cutaneous melanoma. In rare cases, such as inoperability because of medical comorbidities or other reasons, definitive radiation may be considered to the primary site. There are limited data

Authors' disclosures: Dr Sondak is a paid consultant and has provided expert testimony for Merck/Schering-Plough. The other authors have no financial interests to disclose.
[a] Department of Radiation Oncology, H. Lee Moffitt Cancer Center, 12902 Magnolia Drive, Tampa, FL 33612, USA
[b] Department of Cutaneous Oncology, H. Lee Moffitt Cancer Center, 12902 Magnolia Drive, Tampa, FL 33612, USA
* Corresponding author. Department of Radiation Oncology, H. Lee Moffitt Cancer Center, 12902 Magnolia Drive, Tampa, FL 33612.
E-mail address: nikhil.rao@moffitt.org

Surg Oncol Clin N Am 20 (2011) 115–131
doi:10.1016/j.soc.2010.09.005
1055-3207/11/$ – see front matter © 2011 Elsevier Inc. All rights reserved.

on the role of radiation therapy alone as primary management for invasive melanoma. In one series of 95 cases of invasive melanoma, patients received high doses of radiation with superficial x-ray therapy. Five-year survival was close to 70%.[1] There is considerably more experience using radiation therapy in the treatment of lentigo maligna or lentigo maligna melanoma. In these series, superficial x-rays have generally been used, with local control rates of greater than 90% reported.[2] However, radiotherapy is generally not used in the treatment of lentigo maligna for several reasons. These include innovations in surgical techniques, the emerging use of topical therapies such as imiquimod, and difficulties in designing radiotherapy fields in cases in which margins are poorly demarcated.

Generally, the rate of local recurrence in invasive cutaneous melanoma is less than 5% after adequately wide excision of the primary site. However, in certain circumstances local recurrence at the primary site is unacceptably high after surgery alone, and adjuvant radiation therapy may be considered to improve local control.[3] Occasionally, anatomic constraints may limit the ability to obtain widely negative margins, particularly in the head and neck. Radiotherapy has been effectively used in the setting of either positive or close margins where further reexcision was not considered feasible. Key risk factors for local recurrence are thick tumors (Breslow>4 mm), ulceration, and the presence of satellitosis and/or angiolymphatic invasion. In our practice, the presence of satellitosis is a particularly high-risk feature for local recurrence, and adjuvant radiation to the primary site is often used. Once local recurrence does occur, the risk for further recurrent disease at the primary site increases greatly. In these patients, we typically recommend reresection followed by postoperative radiation therapy.

ADJUVANT RADIOTHERAPY TO THE PRIMARY SITE: DESMOPLASTIC MELANOMA

Desmoplastic melanoma is a rare subtype of melanoma accounting for approximately 1% to 4% of all melanomas. It is characterized by variably pleomorphic, spindle-shaped cells with associated collagen production.[4] Clinically, the lesions often appear to be amelanotic. This subtype is frequently associated with perineural spread, so-called neurotropism, and has been associated with increased local failure rates.

Although some investigators have shown local failure rates in desmoplastic melanoma to be in the 20% to 50% range after surgery alone, a series of 280 patients from Australia found the rate to be on the order of only 10%, with higher recurrence rates noted with the presence of neurotropism and when surgical margins were less than 1 cm.[5] Some have advocated adjuvant radiation therapy to the primary site in all cases of desmoplastic melanoma.[6] In contrast, others have reported local failure rates of less than 5% with surgery alone and advocate close monitoring for disease recurrence.[4]

Although prospective data regarding the role of radiotherapy in desmoplastic melanoma are lacking, we currently offer postoperative radiation for tumors that exhibit perineural spread and/or for lesions thicker than 4 mm, based on retrospective reports showing improvement in local control. In addition, radiotherapy should be considered in desmoplastic melanoma that has not been resected with wide margins and in locally recurrent lesions.[7] **Fig. 1** shows an electron beam setup for a patient with desmoplastic melanoma. Indications to treat were the location on the scalp and depth of invasion (>4 mm). The patient was placed in a prone position, and the outlined radiation field included the scar with a generous margin. An immobilization mask was constructed and bolus was placed to increase the skin dose. We treated the area with simple en face electron beam technique delivering 60 Gray (Gy; 1 Gy equals 100 rad) to the area in 30 fractions at 2 Gy per fraction.

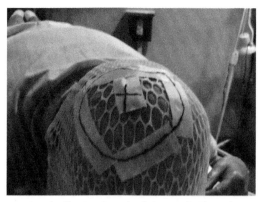

Fig. 1. Electron beam setup in the treatment of desmoplastic melanoma of the scalp: The patient is placed in the prone position with an immobilization mask. The outlined field is treated with direct electron beam radiation with appropriate lead cutout. The prescription dose is 60 Gy in 30 fractions.

RADIOTHERAPY TO THE REGIONAL LYMPH NODE BASIN
Adjuvant Radiotherapy to the Regional Node Basin After Lymph Node Dissection

Multiple retrospective series have reported apparent improvement in regional control in high-risk resected nodal basins with the use of postoperative radiotherapy.[8,9] These studies have consistently shown high-risk factors for regional failure to include multiple positive nodes (>3 nodes and especially ≥10 nodes), 1 or more nodes of large size (>3 cm), extracapsular extension of clinically palpable disease, and/or regionally recurrent disease, with combinations of these factors conferring the greatest risk.

The addition of radiotherapy after modified or radical neck dissection has consistently been reported to result in regional control rates upwards of 90% in clinically node-positive patients.[10] The morbidity of treatment is potentially significant and includes up to a 10% rate of complications at 5 years, including hearing loss, wound breakdown, bone exposure, and ear pain. In cases of bilateral nodal metastasis, as seen occasionally arising from midline head and neck and scalp primary sites, bilateral cervical radiation has been associated with higher complication rates; a 50% rate of complications at 12 months was reported in one series.[11]

In the axilla, regional recurrence rates of 50% or more have been reported after axillary node dissection in patients with extracapsular extension and/or 2 or more nodes involved.[10] **Fig. 2** shows the treatment of the axilla in a patient who had undergone axillary dissection for a large tumor-containing node with extracapsular extension. After adequate recovery from surgery, postoperative radiotherapy was delivered with intensity modulated radiation therapy (IMRT) delivering standard fractions of radiation at 2 Gy per day to a total dose of 60 Gy in 30 treatments. Care was taken to minimize hot spots greater than 60 Gy to protect the brachial plexus, and the lungs and humeral head were contoured as avoidance structures.

In the axilla treated with postoperative radiotherapy, side effects may be seen in up to 30% at 5 years, with the most significant being lymphedema. The inguinal region is the nodal basin at greatest risk for lymphedema and other complications when node dissection and radiotherapy are both used. There is also evidence that patients with body mass indices greater than 30 kg/m^2 are at even higher risk for treatment-related complications (up to 80%) after combined therapy in the groin.[10] Given the higher

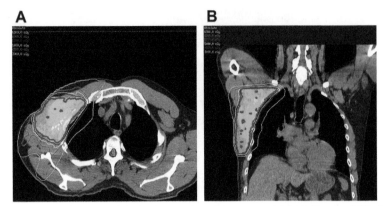

Fig. 2. Adjuvant treatment of melanoma with radiation. Axial (*A*) and coronal (*B*) distribution of radiation isodose lines in a patient treated to the right axilla after surgical resection for high-risk features (size of node 14 cm with extracapsular extension). Treatment was with intensity modulated radiation therapy (IMRT) delivering standard fractions of radiation at 2 Gy per day to a total dose of 60 Gy in 30 fractions. Care was taken to minimize hot spots and protect the lungs and humeral head.

chance for toxicity in the groin, we are cautious when recommending radiation to this nodal basin. Although the criteria used generally remain the same as in the other basins (ie, offered to those with multiple positive nodes, large nodes, extracapsular extension, or recurrent disease), a more careful risk and benefit assessment is required. Thus, we tend to be more conservative in recommending radiation to the groin, particularly in patients with significant postoperative edema, high body mass index, and those considered to be at a lower risk for recurrence.

Data from an older prospective randomized trial evaluating the role of radiation after the resection of nodal metastasis was inconclusive.[12] This study may be criticized for many reasons, including the use of low-energy x-rays, planned treatment breaks, a low total dose of radiation, and a daily fraction size less than 2 Gy per day. More recently, prospective trial data from Australia have been reported showing improved regional control with adjuvant radiation therapy in patients at high risk of regional failure.[13] In an initial phase II trial, 234 patients received 48 Gy in 20 fractions at a dose of 2.4 Gy per fraction to either the head and neck, axilla and supraclavicular basin, or the ilioinguinal basin.[14] Eligible patients had more than 1 node involved with melanoma, 1 node with extracapsular extension, regional basin recurrence, or reported intraoperative tumor spill. Regional in-field recurrences were noted in only 7% of treated patients, much less than anticipated from historical data, leading to a subsequent prospective randomized trial by the same group. Inclusion criteria for this trial included 1 or more of the following: parotid nodal involvement; at least 2 cervical or axillary or 3 inguinal nodes involved by tumor; 1 node at any site with extracapsular extension; or 1 involved node measuring at least 3 cm in greatest diameter in the head and neck or axilla or 4 cm in the groin. After lymphadenectomy, patients were randomized to receive radiation to the regional nodal field (48 Gy in 20 fractions) or observation (123 patients in the radiation arm and 127 in the observation arm). The rate of regional recurrence as the first relapse was the primary endpoint, with overall survival as a secondary endpoint. Although overall survival was not different for the 2 groups, there was a statistically significant decrease in nodal basin recurrence with the addition of radiotherapy: 20 patients (16.3%) recurred within the treatment field in the radiation arm versus 34 patients (26.8%) in the observation arm ($P = .04$, **Table 1**).

In summary, prospective randomized data have now validated criteria that identify patients with a substantial risk of regional recurrence after complete lymphadenectomy and shown a benefit in regional recurrence for the addition of radiotherapy for patients with these high-risk features. It will be important to see more detailed analysis of these study results to help refine the selection criteria for postoperative radiation (ie, to determine whether all of the criteria used were equally predictive of regional relapse), understand the long-term toxicity of therapy, and, perhaps most importantly, evaluate the success of salvage radiation therapy for those patients who failed in the regional basin after surgery alone. If overall survival is the same and ultimate regional control is also similar for patients treated with postrelapse versus routine postoperative radiation, then the risk/benefit ratio would most likely favor reserving nodal basin irradiation until the time of regional relapse. At present, a careful assessment of the risks and benefits of therapy is required to select appropriate patients for postoperative radiation to dissected nodal basins, but this approach can be used with the knowledge that there is strong evidence of improved regional control compared with surgery alone.

Radiotherapy to the Lymph Node Basin in the Absence of Complete Dissection

Some investigators have advocated the delivery of nodal basin radiotherapy instead of complete node dissection, particularly in patients with metastatic melanoma to cervical nodes from head and neck primary sites. A series of 36 patients has been reported in which patients underwent cervical nodal basin irradiation after an excisional biopsy established the presence of nodal involvement.[15] Treatment delivered 30 Gy at 6 Gy per fraction twice per week (5 treatments total). The 5-year rate of complications was reported as less than 10% and the 5-year regional control rate was greater than 90%.

Elective radiation to the clinically node-negative regional basin after wide excision of primary cutaneous melanoma of the head and neck greater than 1.5 mm in thickness or Clark level IV has been evaluated. Outcomes for 157 patients treated with this approach from 1983 to 1988 were reported in 2004.[16] Patients with desmoplastic melanoma and those who had undergone surgery for suspicion of lymph node metastasis were excluded. Ten-year locoregional control was reported as 86%.

Despite these results, the current standard of care in the treatment of melanoma includes wide excision of the primary site and sentinel lymph node biopsy for the appropriately selected patient. When the sentinel nodes are shown to contain malignancy, completion node dissection is recommended. However, circumstances may arise in which sentinel biopsy is not feasible for either medical or technical reasons. In these rare cases, we currently follow the regional basins with clinical examination and serial ultrasonography, but regional nodal irradiation is an alternative that can be considered in selected patients.

Radiotherapy with Concurrent Interferon

Although controversial, there is strong evidence that interferon α-2b improves relapse-free survival and even overall survival in stage III melanoma.[17] In addition, there may be a theoretic synergy and radiosensitization with the combination of radiation and interferon.[18] Several studies have evaluated the role of concurrent radiotherapy and interferon or radiotherapy within 1 month of the delivery of interferon in resected, high-risk, stage III melanoma.[18–21] These studies have generally reported locoregional control to be comparable with historical rates. However, despite small numbers of

Table 1
Prospective randomized trials comparing observation with adjuvant radiation therapy to dissected nodal basins

Author	Inclusion Criteria	Treatment Arms	Patients (n)	Median Survival (mo)	Regional Failure	Median Time to Recurrence (mo)
Creagan et al[12] (1978)	Any node-positive melanoma	S+RT S	27 29	33 22 ($P = .09$)	3 patients 1 patient	20 9 ($P = .07$)
Burmeister et al[13] (2009)	ECE or node size >3 cm or multiple positive nodes	S+RT S	123 127	31 47 ($P = .14$)	20 patients 34 patients ($P = .041$)	Not reported

Abbreviations: ECE, extracapsular extension; RT, radiation therapy; S, surgery (lymph node dissection).

patients in these series, most have reported greater than expected late toxicity, particularly soft tissue injury, lung injury, and myelitis.[18–21]

The use of radiotherapy with concurrent interferon has been prospectively evaluated at our center and results recently reported.[22] Inclusion criteria included stage III nodal disease involving axilla, neck, or groin, with 4 or more positive nodes or a single node of 4 cm or larger, or with microscopic or macroscopic extracapsular extension involving more than 10% of the capsule circumference. Induction interferon α-2b, 20 million U/m^2/d, was administered intravenously for 5 consecutive days every week for 4 weeks. Subsequently, radiation of 30 Gy in 5 fractions, 2 fractions per week, was given with concurrent interferon α-2b at 10 MU/m^2 subcutaneously 3 times per week on days alternating with radiation. Thereafter, maintenance interferon was continued for a total of 1 year of treatment. A total of 29 patients were enrolled between August 1997 and March 2000. The maximum (worst) grade of acute nonhematologic toxicity during concurrent treatment was grade 3 skin toxicity noted in 2 patients (9%). Late effects were limited but included 1 patient with a grade 4 brachial plexus injury. Of the evaluable patients, after a median follow-up of 80 months among surviving patients, the probability of regional control was 78% at 12 months, the median relapse-free survival was 20 months, and the median overall survival was 35 months.

Although these prospective data may be encouraging, care must be exercised when combining radiotherapy with interferon, especially when using high dose per fraction radiation. Given that a few high-grade late effects have been observed in some concurrent radiation/interferon reports, off protocol we prefer to administer the 1-month intravenous induction phase of interferon therapy, slightly delaying the subcutaneous maintenance phase until after the completion of conventionally fractionated regional basin irradiation.

Radiotherapy with Concurrent Chemotherapy

There are few data regarding the value of concurrent radiation therapy and chemotherapy in the treatment of melanoma. This is partly because of concerns about adding chemotherapy-related toxicity in a cohort for whom the treatment goal is usually palliative. In addition, the intrinsic value of cytotoxic chemotherapy when used without radiation in melanoma is limited.[23] Nonetheless, there is some evidence that chemotherapy causes sensitization of melanoma cells to treatments with radiation.[24–26] When using concurrent chemotherapy, radiation doses should be limited to no greater than 2 Gy per fraction for standard fractionated treatments. At our institution, we consider the use of radiation therapy with concurrent temozolomide in patients with unresectable melanoma, gross residual melanoma after resection, or very heavy microscopic burden. The rationale for adding temozolomide stems from evidence supporting its use in melanoma, its ease of administration (oral), and its putative radiosensitizing properties with reasonably well documented safety.[27] We deliver between 40 and 70 Gy with conventional fractionation, depending on the intent (ie, palliative vs adjuvant vs definitive), while respecting the tolerances to radiation of surrounding normal structures.

Radiotherapy with Hyperthermia

Hyperthermia in the temperature range from 40 to 45°C is cytotoxic to melanoma cells.[2] In addition, cell killing by radiation therapy is enhanced with the use of heat. In one randomized trial, patients received hyperthermia with radiation or radiation alone for metastatic or recurrent melanoma. Three fractions of 8 or 9 Gy were delivered in an 8-day period with hyperthermia (43°C for 60 minutes).[28] At 2 years, tumor control rates were 48% in the hyperthermia group compared with 28% in the radiation alone group

(P = .008). In another randomized trial, including patients with melanoma as well as other tumor types, the benefit of adding hyperthermia was only noted in lesions of less than 3 cm, and the results were less conclusive.[2] More recently a randomized trial with rigorous thermal dosimetry has been described.[29] A variety of superficial tumors less than 3 cm in depth were included with melanoma, the latter representing around 10% of the patients. Tumors were irradiated and patients were randomized to hyperthermia only if their lesions were deemed appropriate to receive hyperthermia. Local control at death or last follow-up was observed in 48% of the heated tumors versus 25% of the tumors not receiving heat (P = .02). This trial was encouraging because it showed that thermal dose could be prospectively prescribed, delivered, and correlated with outcome. However, at present, radiation therapy combined with hyperthermia is rarely used in clinical practice because of the limited availability of this technology and difficulties in controlling temperature at the treatment site.

Radiotherapy Dose and Fractionation

There are 2 distinct philosophies regarding dose and fractionation in the treatment of melanoma. Some centers have reported excellent disease control with hypofractionated radiotherapy (dose per fraction >2 Gy per treatment per day, typically, 30 Gy in 5 fractions in the adjuvant setting).[9,30] The rationale for this approach includes the ability to complete the treatment course quickly (generally <3 weeks) and in vitro and in vivo data suggesting an advantage of high dose per fraction radiation in radio-resistant melanoma cells. Those who prescribe standard fractionation in the adjuvant setting (2 Gy per day) are not convinced there is a difference in efficacy between the 2 treatment schemes, and cite the ability to increase the total dose to 60 Gy or more and the reduced risk of late side effects.[31]

The only prospective comparison of fractionation was reported by the Radiation Therapy Oncology Group in the palliative setting. This trial, with a primary endpoint of response in the treated site, randomized 137 patients with measureable metastatic melanoma to 4 fractions at 8 Gy once weekly for 21 days versus 20 fractions at 2.5 Gy, 5 days a week.[32] Response rates were nearly identical in the 2 arms (complete response rates of 24% vs 23% and partial response rates of 36% vs 34%). Survival was not reported. Grade 3 late skin morbidity was defined as marked atrophy or gross telangiectasia, and grade 4 consisted of ulceration. Three grade 4 toxicities and 3 grade 3 toxicities were noted in the 4 times 8 Gy arm compared with only 4 grade 3 toxicities in the 20 times 2.5 Gy arm. With short follow-up and with both arms receiving nonstandard treatment schemes, toxicity data from this trial are difficult to interpret. For palliation in the metastatic setting, 30 to 36 Gy at 3 Gy per fraction is usually given, as discussed later.

When using hypofractionation, it is critically important that hot spots are kept to a minimum and that the spinal cord, brain, and bowel maximum dose are kept to less than 24 Gy total. In addition, using electrons when possible may be prudent to limit the radiotherapy dose at depth and thus decrease the probability of treatment complications. Although each case is individualized, in the adjuvant setting we prefer conventionally fractionated therapy at 2 Gy per fraction, delivering a total dose between 54 Gy and 66 Gy depending on the anatomic site. We are especially wary of treating large volumes of normal tissue with large dose per fraction radiation.

PALLIATIVE RADIOTHERAPY IN MANAGEMENT OF METASTATIC MELANOMA

Radiation as a palliative intervention to reduce symptoms induced by metastasis is frequently effective. For symptomatic bone or brain metastasis, a brief course of external beam radiotherapy is commonly used; the most frequently used dose fractionation is 30 Gy given in 10 fractions over 2 weeks. When spinal cord compression is present or suspected, surgical decompression followed by postoperative radiotherapy has been shown to improve ambulatory function compared with radiotherapy alone and should be considered as the preferred approach.[33] For pathologic fracture of the extremities, we typically use 36 Gy of external beam radiotherapy in 12 fractions following internal fixation. For symptomatic subcutaneous melanoma masses or nodal metastases, palliation may be achieved with 36 Gy in 6 fractions over 3 weeks (twice a week) or comparable hypofractionation regimens. In select subsets of patients with stage IV metastasis, aggressive radiotherapy may achieve durable disease control and potentially improve survival. Palliation of pain and excellent control of the treated sites of disease may be achieved with stereotactic body radiosurgery for patients with limited vertebral metastasis and also in the treatment of a limited number of metastases at other sites.[34,35]

Multifocal, distant subcutaneous and nodal metastasis may be treated with radiation in selected cases. Overall response rates (both partial and complete response) after radiotherapy have ranged from 59% to 79%.[36,37] There is evidence that doses greater than 30 Gy may improve durable palliation for melanoma metastases.[38]

Brain Metastasis

Central nervous system (CNS) metastasis carries the worst prognosis of all visceral metastases and is a major cause of death in patients with stage IV melanoma. Melanoma is the third most common primary tumor associated with CNS metastasis, after lung and breast cancer. Approximately 10% to 40% of patients with metastatic melanoma present with cerebral metastasis; in 15% to 20% of these patients, the CNS is the first site of relapse. The overall median survival is less than 6 months, and the 1-year survival is less than 10% to 15%[39]; most patients die from complications of CNS disease. Autopsy reports have shown that up to 70% of patients who die from disseminated melanoma had brain involvement.[40]

The treatment paradigm for CNS metastasis is complex. Current management options include surgical resection, stereotactic radiosurgery, whole brain radiation therapy, and chemotherapy. Clinical decision making to select patients for 1 or more of these therapies should take into consideration such factors as performance status, number and size of intracranial lesions, extent of extracranial disease, anatomic location, neurologic deficit caused by brain metastasis, and general medical condition. **Table 2** summarizes prospective randomized studies comparing multimodality therapy with single modality therapy for management of brain metastasis in patients with limited numbers of lesions. In most of the trials evaluating treatment of brain metastasis, including the phase III randomized clinical trials that have established standard treatment paradigms, a variety of histologies were included. Therefore, the applicability of these findings to melanoma is less certain.

A recently published multi-institutional analysis of 4259 patients with newly diagnosed brain metastasis showed that prognostic factors varied by diagnosis and proposed histology-specific graded prognostic assessment.[41] For melanoma, which comprised 483 patients (11%), Karnofsky performance status and the number of brain metastases were the significant prognostic factors. The median survival of patients with performance status 90 to 100 and a single brain metastasis was 13.2 months, whereas patients with more than 3 brain metastases and performance status less than 70 had a median survival of only 3.4 months.

Table 2
Prospective randomized trials comparing multimodality therapy with single modality therapy for management of brain metastases (all histologies) in patients with limited numbers of lesions

Author	Number of Metastases	Treatment Arms	Patients (n)	Median Survival (mo)	1-y Local Control (%)	1-y Freedom from CNS Recurrence (%)
Patchell et al[46] (1990)	1	WBRT S+WBRT	23 25	3.8 10.0 (P<.01)	NR	NR
Noordijk et al[57] (1994)	1	WBRT S+WBRT	31 32	6.0 10.0 (P<.04)	NR	NR
Mintz et al[58] (1996)	1	WBRT S+WBRT	43 41	6.3 5.6	NR	NR
Patchell et al[48] (1998)	1	S S+WBRT	46 49	10.8 12.0	NR	NR
Kondziolka et al[59] (2000)	2–4	WBRT SRS+WBRT	14 13	7.5 11 (P = .22)	0 92	NR
Andrews et al[49] (2004)	1–3	WBRT SRS+WBRT	164 167	6.5 5.7	71 82 (P = .01)	NR
Aoyama et al[50] (2006)	1–4	SRS SRS+WBRT	67 65	8.0 7.5	72.5 88.7	23.6 53.2
Muacevic et al[60] (2008)	1	GKRS S+WBRT	31 33	NR	NR	NR
Chang et al[51] (2009)	1–3	SRS SRS+WBRT	30 28	15.2 5.7	67.0 100	27 73 (P = .0003)

Abbreviations: GKRS, gamma knife radiosurgery; NR, not reported; S, surgery (metastasectomy); SRS, stereotactic radiosurgery; WBRT, whole brain radiation therapy.

Whole brain radiation therapy in melanoma brain metastasis

Whole brain radiation therapy (WBRT) has been considered standard treatment of patients with brain metastases for the last 40 years. WBRT is effective in preventing new metastases, reducing symptomatic recurrences, and decreasing the need for salvage therapy. A dose of 30 Gy in 10 fractions is commonly recommended if WBRT is given alone. However, the survival of patients with melanoma after WBRT alone is dismal. Several large international studies showed that the median survival of patients with melanoma brain metastasis is 3.6 to 4.8 months after WBRT.[40] Various fractionation schemes have failed to noticeably improve overall survival for patients with brain metastasis from solid tumors including melanoma.[42] WBRT has been associated with late neurocognitive toxicity, such as progressive dementia and neurocognitive decline, presumably because of demyelination.[43] However, progression of CNS metastasis is a major competing factor in neurocognitive decline that must be weighed against the toxicity of treatment.

Combining chemotherapy with WBRT for melanoma brain metastases has been investigated by the Cytokine Working Group, which conducted 2 phase II trials of WBRT with concomitant temozolomide, a dacarbazine analogue with high CNS penetration. The first study enrolled 31 patients who underwent WBRT with concurrent temozolomide 75 mg/m^2/d for 6 out of 10 weeks followed by the same temozolomide regimen every 10 weeks. Median survival was 6 months, median progression-free survival was 2 months, and the response rate was 10% (1 complete and 2 partial responses).[44] The second trial administered temozolomide (75 mg/m^2/d for 6 weeks) plus thalidomide along with WBRT to 39 patients with melanoma brain metastasis.[45] Only 3 showed CNS response and none showed systemic response. Almost half of the patients required hospitalization for side effects and/or progression.

In patients with a single CNS metastasis or a limited number of metastases, resection in addition to WBRT conferred a survival advantage as well as improved local control rates compared with WBRT alone in a variety of primary tumor types; the median survival was 9.3 months for surgery plus radiation versus 3.5 months for WBRT alone (*P*<.01).[46] Some retrospective studies have suggested an improvement in outcomes for patients with melanoma who have limited brain metastases with resection even in the absence of postoperative whole brain radiotherapy.[40,47] Although prospective data specifically for melanoma brain metastasis are lacking, a phase III randomized study comparing surgery alone with surgery followed by WBRT for brain metastasis from various histologies showed that almost half of the patients after gross total resection of a single brain metastasis developed recurrence in the tumor bed at a median time of 27 weeks.[48] For those who received postoperative WBRT, the local recurrence was decreased to 10%. This finding supports the use of postoperative WBRT after resection for patients with single brain metastasis, particularly those with large lesions causing symptomatic mass effect in an operable location.

Stereotactic radiosurgery for brain metastases

Stereotactic radiosurgery delivers a very high dose of radiation to a stereotactically defined target in a single treatment session while sparing the adjacent normal brain tissue. Because brain metastases often displace normal brain tissue rather than infiltrating it, these lesions may be optimally treated with stereotactic radiosurgery. Both gamma knife and linear accelerator–based radiosurgery have been shown to be equally effective with similar low risks of adverse effects.

Stereotactic radiosurgery is generally used for metastases smaller than 3 to 4 cm in diameter. The maximum tolerated doses are 24 Gy for lesions up to 2 cm in maximum diameter; 18 Gy for lesions between 2 and 3 cm, and 15 Gy for lesions larger than

3 cm. **Fig. 3** shows the dose cloud or isodose distribution and a three-dimensional reconstruction of a stereotactic treatment plan for a brain lesion receiving 21 Gy in 1 fraction. Small lesions in, or immediately adjacent to, the brainstem should be treated with lower doses. Complication rates are related to the volume of the treatment target and occur in 5% to 10% of patients, most of whom recover completely with corticosteroids. Rarely, surgical decompression is required for patients who become steroid dependent because of persistent radiation-induced necrosis.

Several prospective, randomized, clinical trials investigated the benefit of combining stereotactic radiosurgery and WBRT versus either technique alone for management of a limited number of brain metastases from various histologies; these studies are summarized later.

RTOG 9508 randomized 333 patients with 1 to 3 brain metastases (patients with melanoma brain metastases constituted 5% of the study population) to either whole brain radiotherapy alone or WBRT plus stereotactic radiosurgery, and found that there was no significant improvement in survival from adding stereotactic radiosurgery after

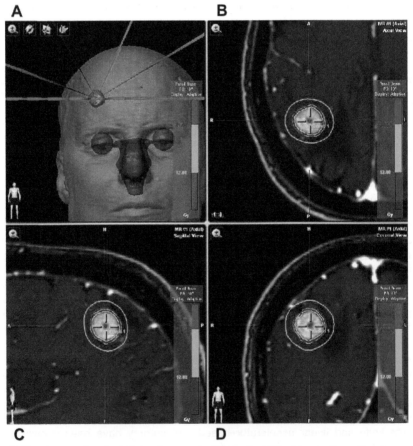

Fig. 3. Treatment of metastatic melanoma to the brain with stereotactic radiosurgery. (A) Three-dimensional reconstruction of stereotactic treatment plan. (B, C, and D) Axial, sagittal, and coronal isodose distributions for stereotactic treatment of melanoma brain metastasis receiving 21 Gy.

whole brain radiotherapy (6.5 vs 5.7 months, $P = .13$).[49] Patients who received both forms of radiation were more likely to have stable or improved performance status at 6 months (43% vs 27%, $P = .03$). In a subgroup analysis, patients with a single metastasis who underwent WBRT and radiosurgery had an improved median survival of 6.5 months versus 4.9 months in patients undergoing only WBRT ($P = .05$).

Other studies compared stereotactic radiosurgery plus WBRT with stereotactic radiosurgery alone. One trial involving 132 patients with 1 to 4 brain metastases found that adding WBRT to stereotactic radiosurgery did not improve survival but decreased the risk of intracranial relapse.[50] As a result, salvage brain therapy was required more frequently for the stereotactic radiosurgery alone group. Another trial investigated the effects of stereotactic radiosurgery with or without WBRT on neurocognitive functions.[51] The study showed that the decline in learning and memory function at 4 months after treatment was significantly higher in patients receiving both modalities compared with stereotactic radiosurgery alone. The 1-year freedom from CNS recurrence was also improved with the addition of WBRT in this study (73% vs 27%, $P = .003$). These 2 prospective trials included patients with brain metastasis from histologies not limited to melanoma.

Retrospective studies examining outcomes specifically in patients with brain metastasis from melanoma showed that the 12-month local control rate after stereotactic radiosurgery ranged from 70% to 84%, and that the risk of delayed tumoral hemorrhage was not increased.[52] Patients with 8 or fewer brain metastases, no prior WBRT, a performance status greater than 70, and controlled extracranial disease had a median survival of 54.3 months, suggesting stereotactic radiosurgery as an excellent treatment of patients with multiple brain metastasis and controlled systemic disease. Several investigators have reported experience with the use of stereotactic radiosurgery to the surgical bed following resection without WBRT; all of these reports included brain metastasis from various histologies. These reports used a median dose of 15 to 19 Gy targeting the resection bed and found the 1-year actuarial local control rate to be between 79% and 94%.[53,54]

Stereotactic Body Radiation Therapy for Extracranial Oligometastasis

Targeted radiotherapy for oligometastases is an active area of investigation. Stereotactic body radiation therapy delivers hypofractionated (high dose per fraction) treatment with high degrees of accuracy to a variety of sites, including lung, adrenal gland, liver, and spine. This treatment modality delivers 6 to 10 times the standard daily fraction dose to the tumor in 3 to 10 treatment sessions over 1 to 3 weeks, with minimum exposure to the surrounding normal tissues. Rigorous and reproducible patient immobilization is required, and organ/target motions induced by respiration should be minimized. The precision of stereotactic radiosurgery allows the spinal cord to be spared while delivering a large radiation dose to involved vertebrae or paraspinal tumors. Several institutions have published their experiences with stereotactic radiosurgery for spinal lesions in the primary and retreatment settings. A prospective cohort of 393 patients with 500 histologically verified spinal metastases, including 38 melanoma lesions (8%), were treated with a dose of 12.5 to 25 Gy in a single fraction.[55] Significant pain palliation was reported in 86% of the patients and tumor control was achieved in 90% of the patients; melanoma bone metastasis responded as well as other histologies. Another study analyzed 36 patients with melanoma spinal metastases treated with single fraction stereotactic radiosurgery and reported that 96% of patients reported improvement of axial and radicular pain and none experienced radiation-induced toxicity.[34] For those who previously received conventional external beam radiotherapy to the vertebrae, stereotactic radiosurgery may also play a role in salvage retreatment.

Early success of treating inoperable early stage non–small cell lung cancer with stereotactic radiosurgery has led to investigation of this technique for treatment of limited metastatic disease in the lung. In a multicenter phase I/II study that escalated the dose from 48 to 60 Gy in 3 fractions in increments of 6 Gy to patients with 1 to 3 pulmonary metastases from various histologies, dose-limiting toxicity was not observed and 1-year local control was 100%.[35] Another study reported local control of 87% after treating 103 lung metastases from various histologies with stereotactic radiosurgery.[56] These results suggest that stereotactic radiosurgery may be an alternative to surgery in patients with oligometastatic disease to the lung and a preferred approach for patients with significant medical comorbidities.

Experience with stereotactic radiosurgery for liver metastases is also emerging. Recent data from a multi-institutional phase I/II trial of patients with 1 to 3 hepatic lesions from various histologies treated to a dose of 60 Gy in 3 fractions showed a 2-year local control rate of 100% for lesions of 3 cm or less.[35] Further studies are underway to validate this finding and define optimal dose, schedule, and technique.

SUMMARY

Radiation therapy plays an important role in the management of melanoma. There is now level I evidence that radiation in the postoperative adjuvant setting improves regional control in the appropriately selected patient at high risk. Although hypofractionated radiation schemes are frequently used for melanoma, data to indicate that they are superior to standard fractionation schemes are lacking. Stereotactic radiosurgery is emerging as an effective treatment modality for appropriately selected patients. Treatment recommendations should be individualized and integrated into a multidisciplinary plan of care.

REFERENCES

1. Hellriegel W. Radiation therapy of primary and metastatic melanoma. Ann N Y Acad Sci 1963;100:131–41.
2. Schmidt-Ullrich RK, Johnson CR. Role of radiotherapy and hyperthermia in the management of malignant melanoma. Semin Surg Oncol 1996;12:407–15.
3. Ballo MT, Ang KK. Radiotherapy for cutaneous malignant melanoma: rationale and indications. Oncology (Williston Park) 2004;18:99–107 [discussion: 107–10, 113–4].
4. Arora A, Lowe L, Su L, et al. Wide excision without radiation for desmoplastic melanoma. Cancer 2005;104:1462–7.
5. Quinn MJ, Crotty KA, Thompson JF, et al. Desmoplastic and desmoplastic neurotropic melanoma: experience with 280 patients. Cancer 1998;83:1128–35.
6. Vongtama R, Safa A, Gallardo D, et al. Efficacy of radiation therapy in the local control of desmoplastic malignant melanoma. Head Neck 2003;25:423–8.
7. Chen JY, Hruby G, Scolyer RA, et al. Desmoplastic neurotropic melanoma: a clinicopathologic analysis of 128 cases. Cancer 2008;113:2770–8.
8. Agrawal S, Kane JM 3rd, Guadagnolo BA, et al. The benefits of adjuvant radiation therapy after therapeutic lymphadenectomy for clinically advanced, high-risk, lymph node-metastatic melanoma. Cancer 2009;115:5836–44.
9. Ballo MT, Ross MI, Cormier JN, et al. Combined-modality therapy for patients with regional nodal metastases from melanoma. Int J Radiat Oncol Biol Phys 2006;64:106–13.

10. Guadagnolo BA, Zagars GK. Adjuvant radiation therapy for high-risk nodal metastases from cutaneous melanoma. Lancet Oncol 2009;10:409–16.
11. Guadagnolo BA, Myers JN, Zagars GK. Role of postoperative irradiation for patients with bilateral cervical nodal metastases from cutaneous melanoma: a critical assessment. Head Neck 2010;32:708–13.
12. Creagan ET, Cupps RE, Ivins JC, et al. Adjuvant radiation therapy for regional nodal metastases from malignant melanoma: a randomized, prospective study. Cancer 1978;42:2206–10.
13. Burmeister B, Smithers BM, Thompson JF, et al. Adjuvant radiotherapy improves regional (lymph node field) control in melanoma patients after lymphadenectomy: results of an intergroup randomized trial (TROG 02.01/ANZMTG 01.02). Int J Radiat Oncol Biol Phys 2009;75(Suppl 3):S2.
14. Burmeister BH, Smithers BM, Davis S, et al. Radiation therapy following nodal surgery for melanoma: an analysis of late toxicity. ANZ J Surg 2002;72:344–8.
15. Ballo MT, Garden AS, Myers JN, et al. Melanoma metastatic to cervical lymph nodes: can radiotherapy replace formal dissection after local excision of nodal disease? Head Neck 2005;27:718–21.
16. Bonnen MD, Ballo MT, Myers JN, et al. Elective radiotherapy provides regional control for patients with cutaneous melanoma of the head and neck. Cancer 2004;100:383–9.
17. Mocellin S, Pasquali S, Rossi CR, et al. Interferon alpha adjuvant therapy in patients with high-risk melanoma: a systematic review and meta-analysis. J Natl Cancer Inst 2010;102:493–501.
18. Hazard LJ, Sause WT, Noyes RD. Combined adjuvant radiation and interferon-alpha 2B therapy in high-risk melanoma patients: the potential for increased radiation toxicity. Int J Radiat Oncol Biol Phys 2002;52:796–800.
19. Conill C, Jorcano S, Domingo-Domenech J, et al. Toxicity of combined treatment of adjuvant irradiation and interferon alpha2b in high-risk melanoma patients. Melanoma Res 2007;17(5):304–9.
20. Gyorki DE, Ainslie J, Joon ML, et al. Concurrent adjuvant radiotherapy and interferon-alpha2b for resected high risk stage III melanoma – a retrospective single centre study. Melanoma Res 2004;14:223–30.
21. Nguyen NP, Sallah S, Childress C, et al. Interferon-alpha combined with radiotherapy in the treatment of unresectable melanoma. Cancer Invest 2001;19:261–5.
22. Finkelstein S, Trotti A, Reintgen D, et al. The Florida Melanoma Trial I: a prospective multi-center phase I/II trial of post operative hypofractionated adjuvant radiotherapy with concurrent interferon-alfa-2b in the treatment of advanced stage III melanoma. Int J Radiat Oncol Biol Phys 2008;72(Suppl 1):S108.
23. Gogas HJ, Kirkwood JM, Sondak VK. Chemotherapy for metastatic melanoma: time for a change? Cancer 2007;109:455–64.
24. Dewit L, Bartelink H, Rumke P. Concurrent cis-diamminedichloroplatinum(II) and radiation treatment for melanoma metastases: a pilot study. Radiother Oncol 1985;3:303–9.
25. Klausner JM, Gutman M, Rozin RR, et al. Conventional fractionation radiotherapy combined with 5-fluorouracil for metastatic malignant melanoma. Am J Clin Oncol 1987;10:448–50.
26. Gill PG, Abbott RL, Ahmad A, et al. Effective palliation of melanoma with procarbazine and radiotherapy given by a low-dose fractionation schedule. Med J Aust 1986;144:126–8.
27. Quirt I, Verma S, Petrella T, et al. Temozolomide for the treatment of metastatic melanoma: a systematic review. Oncologist 2007;12:1114–23.

28. Overgaard J, Gonzalez D, Hulshof MC, et al. Randomised trial of hyperthermia as adjuvant to radiotherapy for recurrent or metastatic malignant melanoma. European Society for Hyperthermic Oncology. Lancet 1995;345:540–3.

29. Jones EL, Oleson JR, Prosnitz LR, et al. Randomized trial of hyperthermia and radiation for superficial tumors. J Clin Oncol 2005;23:3079–85.

30. Stevens G, Thompson JF, Firth I, et al. Locally advanced melanoma: results of postoperative hypofractionated radiation therapy. Cancer 2000;88:88–94.

31. Chang DT, Amdur RJ, Morris CG, et al. Adjuvant radiotherapy for cutaneous melanoma: comparing hypofractionation to conventional fractionation. Int J Radiat Oncol Biol Phys 2006;66:1051–5.

32. Sause WT, Cooper JS, Rush S, et al. Fraction size in external beam radiation therapy in the treatment of melanoma. Int J Radiat Oncol Biol Phys 1991;20: 429–32.

33. Patchell RA, Tibbs PA, Regine WF, et al. Direct decompressive surgical resection in the treatment of spinal cord compression caused by metastatic cancer: a randomised trial. Lancet 2005;366:643–8.

34. Gerszten PC, Burton SA, Quinn AE, et al. Radiosurgery for the treatment of spinal melanoma metastases. Stereotact Funct Neurosurg 2005;83:213–21.

35. Rusthoven KE, Kavanagh BD, Burri SH, et al. Multi-institutional phase I/II trial of stereotactic body radiation therapy for lung metastases. J Clin Oncol 2009;27: 1579–84.

36. Corry J, Smith JG, Bishop M, et al. Nodal radiation therapy for metastatic melanoma. Int J Radiat Oncol Biol Phys 1999;44(5):1065–9.

37. Seegenschmiedt MH, Keilholz L, Altendorf-Hofmann A, et al. Palliative radiotherapy for recurrent and metastatic malignant melanoma: prognostic factors for tumor response and long-term outcome: a 20-year experience. Int J Radiat Oncol Biol Phys 1999;44:607–18.

38. Olivier KR, Schild SE, Morris CG, et al. A higher radiotherapy dose is associated with more durable palliation and longer survival in patients with metastatic melanoma. Cancer 2007;110:1791–5.

39. Amer MH, Al-Sarraf M, Baker LH, et al. Malignant melanoma and central nervous system metastases: incidence, diagnosis, treatment and survival. Cancer 1978; 42:660–8.

40. Sampson JH, Carter JH Jr, Friedman AH, et al. Demographics, prognosis, and therapy in 702 patients with brain metastases from malignant melanoma. J Neurosurg 1998;88:11–20.

41. Sperduto PW, Chao ST, Sneed PK, et al. Diagnosis-specific prognostic factors, indexes, and treatment outcomes for patients with newly diagnosed brain metastases: a multi-institutional analysis of 4,259 patients. Int J Radiat Oncol Biol Phys 2010;77:655–61.

42. Gelber RD, Larson M, Borgelt BB, et al. Equivalence of radiation schedules for the palliative treatment of brain metastases in patients with favorable prognosis. Cancer 1981;48:1749–53.

43. Asai A, Matsutani M, Kohno T, et al. Subacute brain atrophy after radiation therapy for malignant brain tumor. Cancer 1989;63:1962–74.

44. Margolin K, Atkins B, Thompson A, et al. Temozolomide and whole brain irradiation in melanoma metastatic to the brain: a phase II trial of the Cytokine Working Group. J Cancer Res Clin Oncol 2002;128:214–8.

45. Atkins MB, Sosman JA, Agarwala S, et al. Temozolomide, thalidomide, and whole brain radiation therapy for patients with brain metastasis from metastatic melanoma: a phase II Cytokine Working Group study. Cancer 2008;113:2139–45.

46. Patchell RA, Tibbs PA, Walsh JW, et al. A randomized trial of surgery in the treatment of single metastases to the brain. N Engl J Med 1990;322:494–500.
47. Wronski M, Arbit E. Surgical treatment of brain metastases from melanoma: a retrospective study of 91 patients. J Neurosurg 2000;93:9–18.
48. Patchell RA, Tibbs PA, Regine WF, et al. Postoperative radiotherapy in the treatment of single metastases to the brain: a randomized trial. JAMA 1998;280: 1485–9.
49. Andrews DW, Scott CB, Sperduto PW, et al. Whole brain radiation therapy with or without stereotactic radiosurgery boost for patients with one to three brain metastases: phase III results of the RTOG 9508 randomised trial. Lancet 2004;363: 1665–72.
50. Aoyama H, Shirato H, Tago M, et al. Stereotactic radiosurgery plus whole-brain radiation therapy vs stereotactic radiosurgery alone for treatment of brain metastases: a randomized controlled trial. JAMA 2006;295:2483–91.
51. Chang EL, Wefel JS, Hess KR, et al. Neurocognition in patients with brain metastases treated with radiosurgery or radiosurgery plus whole-brain irradiation: a randomised controlled trial. Lancet Oncol 2009;10:1037–44.
52. Liew DN, Kano H, Kondziolka D, et al. Outcome predictors of gamma knife surgery for melanoma brain metastases. J Neurosurg 2010. [Epub ahead of print].
53. Karlovits BJ, Quigley MR, Karlovits SM, et al. Stereotactic radiosurgery boost to the resection bed for oligometastatic brain disease: challenging the tradition of adjuvant whole-brain radiotherapy. Neurosurg Focus 2009;27:E7.
54. Soltys SG, Adler JR, Lipani JD, et al. Stereotactic radiosurgery of the postoperative resection cavity for brain metastases. Int J Radiat Oncol Biol Phys 2008;70: 187–93.
55. Gerszten PC, Burton SA, Ozhasoglu C, et al. Radiosurgery for spinal metastases: clinical experience in 500 cases from a single institution. Spine (Phila Pa 1976) 2007;32:193–9.
56. Milano MT, Katz AW, Schell MC, et al. Descriptive analysis of oligometastatic lesions treated with curative-intent stereotactic body radiotherapy. Int J Radiat Oncol Biol Phys 2008;72:1516–22.
57. Noordijk EM, Vecht CJ, Haaxma-Reiche H, et al. The choice of treatment of single brain metastasis should be based on extracranial tumor activity and age. Int J Radiat Oncol Biol Phys 1994;29:711–7.
58. Mintz AH, Kestle J, Rathbone MP, et al. A randomized trial to assess the efficacy of surgery in addition to radiotherapy in patients with a single cerebral metastasis. Cancer 1996;78:1470–6.
59. Kondziolka D, Patel A, Lunsford LD, et al. Stereotactic radiosurgery plus whole brain radiotherapy versus radiotherapy alone for patients with multiple brain metastases. Int J Radiat Oncol Biol Phys 1999;45:427–34.
60. Muacevic A, Wowra B, Siefert A, et al. Microsurgery plus whole brain irradiation versus gamma knife surgery alone for treatment of single metastases to the brain: a randomized controlled multicentre phase III trial. J Neurooncol 2008;87: 299–307.

Metastasectomy for Stage IV Melanoma: For Whom and How Much?

Abigail S. Caudle, MD*, Merrick I. Ross, MD

KEYWORDS

- Stage IV melanoma • Metastasis • Surgical management
- Patient selection

Patients diagnosed with stage IV melanoma are known to have a poor prognosis, with a median survival of only 11 to 12 months, because there are no consistently effective systemic therapies available at present. The reference standard of chemotherapy, dacarbazine, is associated with response rates of only 10% to 15%, very few of which are durable.[1] Even the more aggressive approved therapy, interleukin-2, is associated with a 5-year survival rate of less than 10%.[2] Although there are several promising agents in development, such as targeted therapies and novel immunotherapy approaches, durable responses are still rare, and survival differences are measured in weeks to months instead of months to years. It seems that achieving a complete response is the only means of prolonging survival in these patients, a feat that is rarely possible with even the most aggressive systemic therapy. Because of the dismal prognosis in most patients with distant metastases, surgical referral was rarely initiated in the past. However, it is increasingly recognized that long-term survival can be achieved with surgical intervention in carefully selected patients. The rationale for surgical intervention in the management of metastatic melanoma, selection factors to be considered, published results, and future directions are discussed in this article.

RATIONALE FOR SURGICAL MANAGEMENT

Trials of systemic therapy in melanoma have consistently demonstrated that a complete response is required for a durable survival benefit.[2] However, response is accomplished in only a small percentage of treated patients, even with the administration of the most effective available therapies such as interleukin-2, which achieves a complete response in only 6% of patients.[2] Surgical metastasectomy has the unique

Department of Surgical Oncology, University of Texas MD Anderson Cancer Center, 1515 Holcombe Boulevard, Unit 444, Houston, TX 77030, USA
* Corresponding author.
E-mail address: ascaudle@mdanderson.org

Surg Oncol Clin N Am 20 (2011) 133–144
doi:10.1016/j.soc.2010.09.010
1055-3207/11/$ – see front matter © 2011 Elsevier Inc. All rights reserved.

potential to remove all tumors with a short recovery period instead of subjecting a patient to months of systemic therapy, itself associated with potential significant morbidity and occasional mortality. The importance of a complete response to systemic therapy applies to a surgical approach as well; surgery is most effective when a complete resection of all tumors is possible. However, surgery may be indicated for patients with sites of disease that are causing significant morbidity, even though a surgical approach would not render the patient disease-free. In this setting, complete resection of the symptomatic site may have the goal of palliation and improving the quality of life, while at the same time improving performance status and making the patient a better candidate for novel systemic approaches.

Although randomized prospective trials are obviously the optimal means of assessing the efficacy of surgery compared with that of other therapies, the small size and heterogeneity of this population limits true prospective analysis of survival. Some of the most convincing data supporting surgical management were obtained from an adjuvant vaccine trial, the Malignant Melanoma Active Immunotherapy Trial (MMAIT), a phase 3, randomized, double-blind trial of the polyvalent adjuvant vaccine, onamelatucel-L (Canvaxin), based on some promising retrospective matched data.[3] To be eligible, patients were required to undergo a resection of all distant metastatic disease. This resection was followed by postoperative imaging confirming no evidence of disease before being randomized to receive either Canvaxin with BCG or BCG with a placebo. Although the vaccine group had similar survival rates to the placebo group, the 5-year overall survival rate for both groups was surprisingly high (40%–45%).[4] The survival rate was much higher than previously reported, supporting that long-term survival was possible in this carefully selected stage IV population. Similar data were reported from the Southwest Oncology Group (SWOG) trial S9430, in which patients who underwent complete surgical resection for metastatic melanoma were prospectively followed up. Unlike the MMAIT trial, which included only patients who underwent a staging evaluation after complete resection and were found to still be without disease, the data from the SWOG prospective registry included all patients who underwent complete surgical resection. The SWOG registry included 62 patients from 18 institutions, with an overall median survival of 21 months and a 4-year overall survival of 29%.[5] The favorable results from these 2 trial settings support the use of surgery in a selected population.

FACTORS FOR CONSIDERATION

Surgery is not appropriate for all patients with metastatic spread of their melanoma. Patient selection is of paramount importance when discussing surgical management. In a retrospective review of 4426 patients with stage IV melanoma treated at the John Wayne Cancer Institute (JWCI), only 35% underwent surgical resection. These patients had a 5-year overall survival of 23% compared with 6% in those who were not surgical candidates ($P<.001$).[6] Surgery with the intent of providing long-term survival should be considered only when all sites of disease can be completely resected. Incomplete resection, similar to a partial response to systemic therapy, does not increase survival in these patients and should be considered only for palliation in symptomatic patients.

Radiographic Assessment

Determining the extent of disease is important. First, other primary cancers must be considered when a radiographic abnormality is seen in a patient with melanoma, particularly in the setting of an isolated lesion in the lung or the kidney. Further imaging, blood tests, and biopsy are sometimes necessary to confirm true metastatic disease. Second, the actual imaging modality is dictated by the site of known disease. For instance, an abnormality seen on chest radiograph should be further evaluated with computed tomographic (CT) imaging. Finally, a thorough evaluation must be performed to exclude or identify other sites of disease. This evaluation should include an assessment of the brain (usually with magnetic resonance imaging [MRI]), thoracic and abdominal cavities with CT or CT/positron emission tomography (PET) imaging, and a head-to-toe physical examination for the presence of skin, soft tissue, or nodal metastases. PET/CT is increasingly used in melanoma to evaluate for metastatic disease. Sensitivity rates of more than 90% and specificity rates similar to conventional CT have been reported, with the added advantage of being able to screen extremities and nodal basins for occult disease.[7] This latter information may have a significant effect on the decision to proceed with surgical intervention; the identification of unexpected widespread disease excludes patients from surgical treatment, but the identification of a few sites of additional surgically resectable disease may expand the extent of surgery and more effectively render the patient disease-free.

Patient Factors

Unlike systemic therapy, surgery theoretically provides a means of rapidly rendering the patient disease-free, with low morbidity and a short recovery period. One key is that the patient can tolerate the proposed operation. Patients should expect to recover completely from thoracotomy[8,9] or laparotomy within 4 to 8 weeks.[6] For all operations, physicians must evaluate the overall health of the patient and their ability to tolerate the stress of surgery. In addition, certain site-specific factors should also be considered, such as pulmonary function tests, if a thoracotomy is planned. In the case of skin and soft tissue resections, the surgeon should be mindful of the functional deficits inherent in the planned operation and whether the patients and their support systems will be able to adapt.

Biology of Disease

Because the disease course of melanoma is variable, many groups have tried to identify factors associated with increased survival. Certainly, there have been strides in the last several years recognizing the effect of disease biology on prognosis.

Petersen and colleagues[10] identified risk factors for poor prognosis in their study of 1720 patients with pulmonary metastases, including a nodular primary lesion, more than 1 pulmonary nodule, a disease-free interval of less than 5 years, or presence of extrathoracic metastases (synchronous or metachronous). After grouping the subjects by the number of risk factors, they found significant differences in median survival between those with no risk factors (14 months), 1 factor (12 months), and at least 3 factors (5 months). Although all the available literature is based on retrospective data of heterogenous populations, disease characteristics suggesting a more slowly growing tumor, such as a low burden of disease, solitary site of metastasis, and prolonged disease-free interval, are consistently shown to be important in outcomes despite the site of the metastases.[6,8] In an effort to quantitate this rate of growth, tumor doubling time has even been suggested as a criterion for determining whether patients should be offered pulmonary metastasectomy.[11]

Pattern of spread is another feature that may play a role in determining prognosis. In one study of 1500 patients with distant melanoma metastases, features that predicted a better survival regardless of treatment included the original site of metastasis and the stage of disease before metastasis.[12] The difference in prognosis based on the anatomic site of metastasis is well established and is even reflected in the staging system as discussed later. Other groups have also shown that patients who progress from stage I or stage II to stage IV disease fare better than those who have regional nodal spread, or stage III disease, before the discovery of distant metastases.[6] Not surprisingly, the disease-free interval between stage I or stage II disease and the development of metastases is longer (44 months) than after stage III disease (13.5 months),[6] which makes it unclear if it is truly the presence of nodal disease that portends the poor outcome or rather the shortened disease-free interval. Regardless, both are evidence of an aggressively spreading tumor.

PROGNOSIS AND OUTCOMES ACCORDING TO ANATOMIC SITE

The anatomic site of distant metastases clearly affects prognosis in melanoma. This finding is reflected in the American Joint Committee on Cancer (AJCC) staging system, which added subcategories for stage IV disease in 2001 and further corroborated this approach in the most recent AJCC dataset published in 2009.[13,14] Unlike most cancers in which patients are classified as either M0 if they have no known metastases or M1 if they have distant disease at any site, melanoma has 3 subgroups of M1 disease. M1a designates skin, soft tissue, or distant lymph node disease only; M1b represents pulmonary metastases; and M1c incorporates any visceral or brain sites or elevated lactate dehydrogenase (LDH) level (regardless of anatomic site of disease). The survival differences among these groups have been shown repeatedly, including analysis for the current seventh edition of the melanoma staging system, which was based on data from 7972 patients with stage IV melanoma from 17 institutions.[14]

Skin and Soft Tissue Metastasis

Distant skin and soft tissue metastasis represent about 40% of melanoma metastasis.[15] As reflected in the staging system, isolated skin, soft tissue, or distant nodal metastases, or M1a disease, has the most favorable prognosis of patients with stage IV melanoma, with median survival of 18 months in all patients and 1-year survival rates of 62%.[14] However, patients presenting with solitary dermal or subcutaneous metastasis that is completely resected can have survival rates of more than 80% at 8 years, although this rate represented only 11 patients of the 1800 patients with stage IV melanoma treated at that institution.[16]

There are retrospective reports describing outcomes for patients with completely resected skin, soft tissue, or nodal disease. In a report from JWCI, 260 patients with completely resected disease had a median survival of 35 months and 5-year overall survival of 25%. In this study, patients with tumors confined to the skin or soft tissue instead of nodal metastases had a better prognosis, with a median survival of 48 months.[6] This experience is similar to that at Memorial Sloan-Kettering Cancer Center (MSKCC), where 23 patients who had undergone previous lymphadenectomy for stage III disease underwent complete resections for isolated distant skin and soft tissue metastasis, with a median survival of 29 months and 5-year overall survival of 22%.[17] The differences in survival observed between these 2 groups likely reflect slightly different underlying populations. The JWCI study included all patients with distant metastases, whereas the MSKCC group focused solely on patients who had a history of nodal disease. Other factors that predict a favorable outcome include skin or soft tissue location (instead of distant nodal spread), fewer lesions, prolonged disease-free interval, and small burden of disease.[6,16,18]

The ability to aggressively resect distant skin, soft tissue, and nodal metastases has increased with the evolution of reconstructive options. In the case of bulky disease, the surgeon may need to consult with thoracic surgeons to aid with chest wall resections and/or plastic surgeons to provide tissue coverage. A variety of reconstructive options are reasonable, including skin grafts, rotational flaps, and free tissue transfer. Staged procedures are sometimes required for optimal results and definitive margin assessment (**Table 1**).

Pulmonary Metastasis

The lungs are the most common first site of distant spread (up to 40%) and represent the second most common site for distant metastasis overall.[6,8,15] Harpole and colleagues[8] estimated the probability of patients with melanoma developing pulmonary metastases at 0.13 at 5 years and up to 0.3 at 20 years, with median survival of 7 to 8 months after the development of pulmonary disease.[10,12] Patients with M1b disease have a 1-year survival rate of 53%.[14]

Resection of pulmonary metastases can be an effective therapy. With complete resection, median survival can increase to as high as 20 to 40 months.[8,9,19] One of the largest studies to explore survival after pulmonary metastasectomy is the International Registry of Lung Metastases, which collected data from 328 patients who underwent pulmonary metastasectomy for melanoma; 282 patients had a complete resection, whereas 46 had an incomplete resection. After complete resection, they reported 5- and 10-year survival rates of 22% and 16%, with no long-term survivors in the group who underwent incomplete resections.[9] These survival statistics are similar to those reported by the investigators from Duke University, who first reported survival data in 1992[8] and then updated the data 16 years later in 2007.[10] The median survival in the 2 studies remained the same (19–20 months), with similar 5-year survival rates of 20% and 21% compared with 4% among those who did not undergo resection.

Although these studies represent retrospective reviews with their inherent biases, several factors have been shown to be predictive of survival when considering resection of pulmonary metastasis, including the ability to achieve a complete resection, prolonged disease-free interval ($\geq$36 months), 2 or fewer pulmonary nodules, no history of extrathoracic metastatic disease, prior response to chemotherapy or immunotherapy, and no nodal disease.[8–10,19] Patients with a single pulmonary metastasis are particularly well served by a surgical approach.[8]

Once again, patient selection is key. Although it is estimated that almost 40% of patients with metastatic melanoma initially present with a pulmonary metastasis, a smaller group undergo thoracotomy.[15] In a review from MSKCC of patients who presented with the lungs as the first site of stage IV disease, only 21% underwent resection. However, surgery was the only treatment factor that was predictive of survival, with a median survival of 40 months compared with 13 months in those who did not undergo complete resection.[19] In addition to resectability, the patient's pulmonary condition should be weighed heavily in the decision of whether to operate. Multiple pulmonary nodules, even if bilateral, should not deter a surgical approach if all nodules

Table 1				
Survival after complete resection of distant skin or soft tissue metastases				
Author	Institution	Number of Patients	Median Survival (mo)	5-Year Overall Survival (%)
Essner et al[6]	JWCI	260	35.1	25
Gadd and Coit[17]	MSKCC	23	29	22

can be resected completely, while ensuring adequate postoperative pulmonary function (**Table 2**).

Visceral Metastasis: Gastrointestinal Tract

Although all nonpulmonary visceral metastases are grouped together as M1c in the staging system, there are differences between the different sites, such as the gastrointestinal (GI) tract and the liver. Autopsy studies have shown that melanoma metastasizes to the GI tract in 2% to 4% of patients. However, in patients who die of disseminated melanoma, up to 50% have GI tract involvement.[20] The most common sites of disease are the small bowel (75%), colon (25%), and stomach (16%).[21] Unlike patients with pulmonary metastases, which are usually asymptomatic, patients with GI tract metastases often present with symptoms such as pain (29%–59%), obstruction (27%), or bleeding/anemia (26%–60%).[22–24]

Although the overall survival of patients with nonpulmonary visceral metastasis is poor, with a median survival of 5 to 11 months depending on the specific site,[12] there are reports of long-term survival after complete surgical resection. MSKCC has reported a 5-year survival rate of 38% in patients who underwent complete resection of GI tract metastasis, similar to a rate of 41% reported by JWCI.[23,24] Once again, the importance of achieving a complete resection is evidenced by the difference in median survival between patients who underwent a complete resection (48.9 months) and those who had an incomplete or palliative resection (5.4 months). Although some of this difference is certainly attributable to the surgery itself, the extent of disease also plays a role in the disparate outcomes. For instance, patients who were not considered to be surgical candidates had a median survival of 2.9 months.[21] Features associated with favorable survival in these studies included a lower incidence of spread to contiguous organs or the retroperitoneum and low LDH level.[23,24] Disease-free interval was not associated with a survival difference, possibly because of the time involved in diagnosing GI tract metastases.

Because of the proximity of other organs in the abdominal cavity, metastases to the GI tract often involve multiple organs. Once again, this is not a contraindication to surgery as long as a complete resection can be achieved. Preoperative planning can help anticipate necessary procedures. For instance, patients may need to be counseled about the possibilities of an ileostomy or colostomy, the dietary changes after a gastrectomy, or the need for preoperative vaccinations before splenectomy. In addition, procedures such as pancreatic resections require adequate surgical experience as well as a facility with adequate postoperative support. Morbidity and mortality after surgery have been shown to be low (**Table 3**).[23,24]

Table 2				
Survival after complete resection of pulmonary metastases				
Author	Institution	Number of Patients	Median Survival (mo)	5-Year Overall Survival (%)
Leo et al[9]	International Registry of Lung Metastases	282	19	22
Petersen et al[10]	Duke (2007)	249	19	21
Harpole et al[8]	Duke (1992)	98	20	20
Essner et al[6]	JWCI		28.1	21
Andrews et al[39]	Moffitt	86	35	33
Neuman et al[19]	MSKCC	26	40	29

Table 3
Survival after complete resection of visceral metastases

Author	Institution	Number of Patients	Median Survival (mo)	5-Year Overall Survival (%)
GI Tract				
Ollila et al[23]	JWCI	46	48.9	41
Agrawal et al[24]	MSKCC	19	14.9	38
Ricaniadis et al[21]	Roswell Park	22	27.6	28
Liver				
Pawlick et al[26]	MDACC, Duke, Italy, France	24	23.6	0
Rose et al[25]	JWCI, SMU	18	18.2	23
Adrenal				
Mittendorf et al[28]	MDACC	20	20.7	NL
Collinson et al[29]	SMU	13	16	NL
Haigh et al[40]	JWCI	18	25.7	NL

Abbreviations: NL, not listed; SMU, Sydney Melanoma Unit.

Visceral Metastasis: Liver

Liver metastases occur in 15% to 20% of patients with metastatic cutaneous melanoma. Despite traditional beliefs, hepatic disease is not an absolute contraindication to surgical management, although patient selection is crucial. Patients should be considered for resection if there is evidence that the patient can be rendered surgically free of disease, a principle that dramatically limits the eligibility of most patients with liver disease. For instance, in a study combining data from JWCI and Sydney Melanoma Unit (SMU), of 1750 patients with hepatic disease, only 34 patients (2%) were considered as surgical candidates. This number decreased because only 24 patients underwent surgical resection at exploration and only 18 of those had a complete resection. Overall median survival in patients who underwent some sort of resection was 28 months compared with only 4 months for those who underwent exploration without resection and 6 months for the patients managed nonoperatively. The 5-year overall survival was 29% in patients who underwent resection (either complete or incomplete) compared with 4% in nonsurgical candidates. Although it is difficult to decide whether this prolonged survival is because of the surgical intervention or if it reflects the favorable biology of disease in these patients, the fact that a macroscopically complete resection ($P = .001$) and a histologically negative margin ($P = .3$) were associated with improved disease-free survival suggests that surgery makes a difference.[25] These results are similar to an international multi-institutional study combining patients from the MD Anderson Care Center (MDACC), Duke, Italy, and France, which reported a median survival of 23.6 months in patients with cutaneous melanoma who underwent hepatic metastasectomy. In these 24 patients, median disease-free survival was 4.7 months. Although this study included patients with ocular and cutaneous melanoma primaries, certain features seemed to be associated with a prolonged disease-free interval, including unilateral resection, metastasis less than 5 cm, and presence of a solitary metastasis, although none of these reached statistical significance in this small group.[26]

It is crucial to characterize preoperatively the location and extent of disease as much as possible when considering resection. Proximity to or involvement of major blood vessels or biliary structures and underlying liver function must be fully evaluated. In addition, intraoperative ultrasonography can improve the sensitivity of detection of small nodules and should be used at the time of laparotomy to ensure complete resection of all sites of disease. After resection, the liver is the most common site of recurrence, although select patients with low-volume disease, good hepatic function, and a prolonged interval since the first hepatectomy may be considered for repeat liver resection (see **Table 3**).[25]

Visceral Metastasis: Other Sites

Other visceral sites, such as the spleen, adrenal glands, and pancreas, can be affected by melanoma and be considered for resection. In a study of 60 patients with solid-organ metastasis, such as adrenal, pancreas, spleen, or liver metastasis, the 5-year survival rate after complete resection was 24%, whereas there were no survivors at 5 years after incomplete resection. Overall survival did not vary between patients with a single site of disease and those with multiple sites, as long as the disease was completely resected.[27] This finding is corroborated by series from MDACC and SMU showing that patients who undergo surgery for adrenal metastasis have improved survival rates compared with those that are managed nonoperatively.[28,29] Similarly, patients with completely resected isolated splenic metastases have a reported survival of 23 months (see **Table 3**).[30]

Brain Metastasis

The diagnosis of brain metastases carries a dismal prognosis and is the direct cause of death in 95% of these patients.[31] Median survival is 3 to 4 months.[31] Surgery with a curative intent has been associated with a median survival as high as 22 months,[6] although most studies report a survival of 6 to 8 months, which is not improved by adjuvant whole-brain radiotherapy.[32,33] Patients without neurologic symptoms or extracranial disease and a single focus of disease have improved results.[32,33]

Multiple Sites or Recurrent Disease

Although almost half of the patients present with a single site of disease,[6] the remaining half have multiple sites. Certainly, patients with one site of distant disease fare better than those presenting with multiple sites.[17] However, multiple sites of disease are not a contraindication to an aggressive surgical approach. In fact, in the study by Rose and colleagues,[25] 39% of the patients undergoing hepatic resection had a synchronous resection of another site. Once again, the ability to remove all sites is more important than the actual number of melanoma deposits.[34] Also, metastasectomy can be safely offered even with recurrent stage IV disease, with prolonged survival for these patients. In one study of 131 patients who developed recurrent stage IV disease after initial metastasectomy, 40 (30.5%) patients underwent repeat metastasectomy, 43 (33%) had an incomplete resection, and 48 (37%) were managed nonoperatively. Patients undergoing repeat complete resection had a median survival of 18 months, with a 5-year survival of 20%. In a multivariate analysis, time to recurrent disease and the ability to perform a complete metastasectomy were predictors of survival.[35]

SURGERY FOR PALLIATION

Because of the variable pattern of spread in melanomas, distant disease can be found anywhere and can cause unique problems that need to be addressed surgically for preservation of life or function, for patient comfort, or to facilitate the continuation of systemic therapy. For instance, skin and soft tissue disease may present with ulceration or infection, and pulmonary metastases can lead to hemoptysis or airway obstruction. Surgery for palliation is often an issue in patients with GI metastasis because patients can develop with bleeding, pain, or obstruction. Surgery is often effective at relieving symptoms of GI tract metastases in more than 90% of patients.[23,24,36,37]

Patients with intracranial disease presenting with neurologic symptoms, such as headaches, seizures, or hemorrhage, can undergo traditional surgical resection or the recently popularized approach of stereotactic radiosurgery. This type of surgery involves multiple radiation beams that converge on a single lesion, thus concentrating the dose in a small area while sparing the normal brain parenchyma. Stereotactic surgery can improve or alleviate symptoms in 78% of patients, although it has no effect on overall survival.[38]

PLANNING FOR THE FUTURE

As in the treatment of many cancers, a multidisciplinary approach is the best in melanoma. Patients presenting with resectable disease should be addressed with the entire melanoma team including medical oncologists, surgeons, radiation oncologists, and diagnostic radiologists. The initial strategy for the treatment of stage IV disease should be the result of a consensus of the entire group. Even after complete metastasectomy, melanoma usually recurs, and patients often need systemic therapy at some point. Therefore, neoadjuvant clinical trials using novel agents offer an attractive alternative for patients with potentially resectable disease. Surgery may not only render these patients disease-free but also be a means of tissue procurement for mutational analysis and basic science correlative studies to determine the mechanisms of response. Tissue procurement via surgery is also used for adoptive cell transfer, an approach with promising preliminary results, that requires the harvesting of the tumor. In this approach, tumor infiltrating lymphocytes (TILs) are identified in the patient's tumor, amplified and selected, and then reintroduced to the patient after lymphodepletion. TILs require 4 to 8 weeks between harvesting and reintroduction and can survive for prolonged periods if stored properly. Thus, in institutions that offer these modalities, surgeons should consider these future options before surgical intervention so that appropriate measures can be initiated to preserve tissue.

The recent development of novel targeted agents is one of the most promising evolutions in melanoma therapy and one that may affect the role of the surgeon in the care of these patients. Although complete tumor eradication, whether via surgery or systemic therapy, has been the only way to confer a survival advantage, these new agents may change that concept and introduce a new paradigm. Some of these agents, although not producing a complete response, may provide a durable halt to tumor progression. Other agents may induce a major response that may not be durable. The role of the surgeon may expand to encompass these patients who have a response to therapy resulting in resectable disease. Communication between surgeons and medical oncologists will become even more crucial as these agents are evaluated in clinical trials.

SUMMARY

Although the conventional paradigm for treating metastatic melanoma relies on systemic therapies, a surgical approach should be strongly considered in selected patients. A surgical approach may not be appropriate for all patients, but it can offer a rapid clearance of disease without the toxicity of systemic therapy. Patient selection is of paramount importance for surgery to be effective. Only patients with favorable biology, adequate preoperative functional state, and disease that is amenable to complete resection should be considered. Multiple sites of disease or even recurrent distant disease should not be considered as absolute contraindications for surgery as long as these principles are integrated into the decision-making process. Most importantly, surgery offers a chance of long-term survival, which is difficult to achieve in patients with melanoma by other means available at present. Thus, surgeons should be considered as vital members of the treatment team in the management of patients with stage IV melanoma. Although identifying patients who are candidates for surgery with curative intent is critical, the selective use of palliative surgery not only is important for relief of symptoms but also is a valuable strategy before the initiation or continuation of systemic therapy. In addition, the advent of new therapies that depend on the harvest of tumor specimens requires that surgeons stay abreast of all treatment options for patients with distant metastases so that they can assist in getting patients to optimal therapy as quickly as possible, regardless of the extent of disease. Also, surgical resection is central for the development of neoadjuvant programs with targeted agents.

REFERENCES

1. Middleton M, Grob J, Aaronson N, et al. Randomized phase III study of temozolomide versus dacarbazine in the treatment of patients with advanced metastatic malignant melanoma. J Clin Oncol 2000;18:158–66.
2. Atkins M, Lotze M, Dutcher J, et al. High-dose recombinant interleukin 2 therapy for patients with metastatic melanoma: analysis of 270 patients treated between 1985 and 1993. J Clin Oncol 1999;17:2105–16.
3. Hsueh E, Essner R, Foshag L, et al. Prolonged survival after complete resection of disseminated melanoma and active immunotherapy with a therapeutic cancer vaccine. J Clin Oncol 2002;20:4549–54.
4. Morton D. An international, randomized, double-blind, phase 3 study of the specific active immunotherapy agent, onamelatucel-L (Canvaxin), compared to placebo as a postsurgical adjuvant in AJCC stage IV melanoma. San Diego: Society of Surgical Oncology; 2006.
5. Sondak V, Liu P, Warneke J, et al. Surgical resection for stage IV melanoma: a Southwest Oncology Group trial (S9430). J Clin Oncol 2006;24:8019.
6. Essner R, Lee J, Wanek L, et al. Contemporary surgical treatment of advanced-stage melanoma. Arch Surg 2004;139:961–6.
7. Collins C. PET/CT in oncology: for which tumours is it the reference standard? Cancer Imaging 2007;7:S77–87.
8. Harpole D, Johnson C, Wolfe W, et al. Analysis of 945 cases of pulmonary metastatic melanoma. J Thorac Cardiovasc Surg 1992;103:743–8.
9. Leo F, Cagini L, Rocmans P, et al. Lung metastases from melanoma: when is surgical treatment warranted? Br J Cancer 2000;83:569–72.
10. Petersen R, Hanish S, Haney J, et al. Improved survival with pulmonary metastasectomy: an analysis of 1720 patients with pulmonary metastatic melanoma. J Thorac Cardiovasc Surg 2007;133:104–10.
11. Ollila D, Stern S, Morton D. Tumor doubling time: a selection factor for pulmonary resection of metastatic melanoma. J Surg Oncol 1998;69:206–11.
12. Barth A, Wanek L, Morton D. Prognostic factors in 1,521 melanoma patients with distant metastases. J Am Coll Surg 1995;181:193–201.
13. Balch C, Buzaid A, Soong S, et al. Final version of the American Joint Committee on Cancer staging system for cutaneous melanoma. J Clin Oncol 2001;19:3635–48.

14. Balch C, Gershenwald J, Soong S, et al. Final version of 2009 AJCC melanoma staging and classification. J Clin Oncol 2009;27:6199–206.
15. Balch C, Soong S, Murad T, et al. A multifactorial analysis of melanoma. IV. Prognostic factors in 200 melanoma patients with distant metastases (stage III). J Clin Oncol 1983;1:126–34.
16. Bowen G, Chang A, Lowe L, et al. Solitary melanoma confined to the dermal and/or subcutaneous tissue: evidence for revisiting the staging classification. Arch Dermatol 2000;136:1397–9.
17. Gadd M, Coit D. Recurrence patterns and outcome in 1019 patients undergoing axillary or inguinal lymphadenectomy for melanoma. Arch Surg 1992;127:1412–6.
18. Markowitz J, Cosimi L, Carey R, et al. Prognosis after initial recurrence of cutaneous melanoma. Arch Surg 1991;126:703–7.
19. Neuman H, Patel A, Hanlon C, et al. Stage-IV melanoma and pulmonary metastases: factors predictive of survival. Ann Surg Oncol 2007;14:2847–53.
20. Patel J, Didolkar M, Pickren J, et al. Metastatic pattern of malignant melanoma. A study of 216 autopsy cases. Am J Surg 1978;135:807–10.
21. Ricaniadis N, Konstadoulakis M, Walsh D, et al. Gastrointestinal metastases from malignant melanoma. Surg Oncol 1995;4:105–10.
22. Branum G, Seigler H. Role of surgical intervention in the management of intestinal metastases from malignant melanoma. Am J Surg 1991;162:428–31.
23. Ollila D, Essner R, Wanek L, et al. Surgical resection for melanoma metastatic to the gastrointestinal tract. Arch Surg 1996;131:979–80.
24. Agrawal S, Yao T, Coit D. Surgery for melanoma metastatic to the gastrointestinal tract. Ann Surg Oncol 1999;6:336–44.
25. Rose D, Essner R, Hughes T, et al. Surgical resection for metastatic melanoma to the liver: the John Wayne Cancer Institute and Sydney Melanoma Unit experience. Arch Surg 2001;136:950–5.
26. Pawlick T, Zorzi D, Abdalla E, et al. Hepatic resection for metastatic melanoma: distinct patterns of recurrence and prognosis for ocular versus cutaneous disease. Ann Surg Oncol 2006;13:712–20.
27. Wood T, DiFronzo L, Rose D, et al. Does complete resection of melanoma metastatic to solid intra-abdominal organs improve survival? Ann Surg Oncol 2001;8:658–62.
28. Mittendorf IE, Lim S, Schacherer C, et al. Melanoma adrenal metastasis: natural history and surgical management. Am J Surg 2008;195:368–9.
29. Collinson F, Lam T, Bruijn M, et al. Long-term survival and occasional regression of distant melanoma metastases after adrenal metastasectomy. Ann Surg Oncol 2008;15:1741–9.
30. de Wilt J, McCarthy W, Thompson J. Surgical treatment of splenic metastases in patients with melanoma. J Am Coll Surg 2003;197:38–43.
31. Sampson J, Carter J, Friedman A, et al. Demographics, prognosis, and therapy in 702 patients with brain metastases from malignant melanoma. J Neurosurg 1998;88:11–20.
32. Wronski M, Arbit E. Surgical treatment of brain metastases from melanoma: a retrospective study of 91 patients. J Neurosurg 2000;93:9–18.
33. Oredsson S, Ingvar C, Stromblad L, et al. Palliative surgery for brain metastases of malignant melanoma. Eur J Surg Oncol 1990;16:451–6.
34. Overett T, Shiu M. Surgical treatment of distant metastatic melanoma. Indications and results. Cancer 1985;56:1222–30.
35. Ollila D, Hsueh E, Stern S, et al. Metastasectomy for recurrent stage IV melanoma. J Surg Oncol 1999;71:209–13.

36. Reintgen D, Thompson W, Garbutt J, et al. Radiologic, endoscopic, and surgical considerations of melanoma metastatic to the gastrointestinal tract. Surgery 1984;95:635–9.

37. Gutman H, Hess K, Kokotsakis J, et al. Surgery for abdominal metastases of cutaneous melanoma. World J Surg 2001;25:750–8.

38. Lavine S, Petrovich Z, Cohen-Gadol A, et al. Gamma knife radiosurgery for metastatic melanoma: an analysis of survival, outcome, and complications. Neurosurgery 1999;44:59–64.

39. Andrews S, Robinson L, Cantor A, et al. Survival after surgical resection of isolated pulmonary metastases from malignant melanoma. Cancer Control 2006; 13:218–23.

40. Haigh PI, Essner R, Wardlaw JC, et al. Long-term survival after complete resection of melanoma metastatic to the adrenal gland. Ann Surg Oncol 1999;6(7): 633–9.

Immunotherapy of Melanoma: An Update

Jade Homsi, MD*, Joshua C. Grimm, BA, Patrick Hwu, MD

KEYWORDS

- Immunotherapy • Melanoma • Vaccine • Interleukin
- CTLA-4 • T cell

The incidence of melanoma has been steadily increasing worldwide. One in 63 Americans will develop melanoma during his/her lifetime; historically, in 1935, the risk was 1 in 1500.[1] Unlike other solid tumors, melanoma more commonly affects young people. In the 20- to 29-year-old age group, melanoma is the second most common cancer after lymphoma.[2] Local treatment strategies, such as surgery, can achieve local tumor control in the early stages of melanoma; however, the metastatic form of the disease continues to have a dismal prognosis, with a median survival rate of 6 to 9 months.[3]

An early relationship between melanoma and the immune system was established after spontaneous immune-mediated regressions of melanoma were observed. This has inspired many investigators to conduct laboratory and clinical studies to develop an effective and tolerable immunotherapeutic strategy in an attempt to transform it into a highly personalized treatment. An overview of the current status of immunotherapy in patients with melanoma and a focus on some recent success in the field are discussed in this article.

INTERFERON α-2B

Interferon (IFN) α-2b is a member of a family of cytokines with anticancer, antiviral, and immunomodulatory effects. Interferons were initially discovered as secreted glycoproteins produced by cells in response to a viral infection. Although interferon α-2b is the most widely tested interferon in melanoma, its exact mechanism of action is still unknown. The antitumor actions of IFN may be derived from its activation of signal transducer and activator of transcription (STAT) proteins and also from its direct effects on the host tissues.[4–6] The clinical manifestations of autoimmunity in patients who received IFN therapy are statistically associated with significant improvements in relapse-free survival and overall survival, which suggests a strong involvement of the immune system in its mechanism of action.[7]

Department of Melanoma Medical Oncology, University of Texas MD Anderson Cancer Center, 1515 Holcombe Boulevard, Unit 430, Houston, TX 77030, USA
* Corresponding author.
E-mail address: jhomsi@mdanderson.org

Surg Oncol Clin N Am 20 (2011) 145–163
doi:10.1016/j.soc.2010.09.004

In melanoma therapy, IFN is administered intravenously (IV) or subcutaneously (SC). Its half-life of elimination is approximately 2 hours when given IV and 3 hours when given SC.[8] The most common toxicities of IFN are neutropenia (44%), liver toxicity (29%), and fatigue (24%). During the induction phase, up to 58% of patients might require dose reductions or delays (44% due to toxicity).[9,10] High-dose IFN (HDI) is the only adjuvant therapy for stages II and III melanoma that has stood the test of time. Its role in this setting was established by the Eastern Cooperative Oncology Group (ECOG) E1684 trial and reassessed in the ECOG E1690, E1694, and E2696 trials.[9–13] HDI is administered at 20 million units/m^2/d IV for 4 weeks and 10 million units/m^2 given thrice a week SC for 48 weeks. The relapse and survival status of patients enrolled in the previous 4 studies formed the basis of a pooled analysis of nearly 2000 patients. The objective was to identify prognostic factors as well as relapse rates and survival benefits associated with adjuvant IFN in patients with stage IIB and III melanoma.[12] Relapse-free survival was significantly prolonged (2-sided log-rank P value = 0.006, hazard ratio [HR] = 1.30) with HDI treatment than with observation. Neither the univariate nor multivariate analyses demonstrated a statistically significant survival superiority with HDI treatment compared with observation. This was expected, given that the larger of the 2 trials included in this analysis (E1690) did not show a survival benefit for HDI treatment. Prognostic factors that negatively impacted relapse and survival included ulceration and age greater than 49 years.

A meta-analysis including the 4 aforementioned studies and 8 other European randomized trials using different doses of IFN has been reported.[14–21] Overall, the analysis showed a statistically significant 17% reduction in the odds of recurrence with IFN (HR = 0.83; 95% confidence interval [CI] 0.77 to 0.90; P = .000003). Similar to the previous analysis, the benefit in overall survival was not significant (0.93, 95% CI 0.85 to 1.02, P = .1). There was evidence of a dose-response relationship, with a trend for the benefit of IFN to increase with increasing doses of IFN.

Based on the available data, it is clear that IFN minimally reduces the risk of relapse after curative-intent surgery. Unfortunately, interferon toxicity is considerable and spans the entire year over which it is given. These toxicities considerably affect quality of life over the course of the treatment. Pegylated IFN (widely used in Europe) and a shorter one-month intravenous schedule of IFN have shown encouraging results but are still not considered to be the standard of care in the United States.[22,23] One thousand two hundred fifty-six patients with resected stage III melanoma were randomized to observation or pegylated IFN 6 µg/kg/wk for 8 weeks, then 3 µg/kg/wk for an intended duration of 5 years. At 3.8 years median follow-up, 328 recurrence events had occurred in the IFN group compared with 368 in the observation group (HR 0.82, 95% CI 0.71-0.96; P = .01). Patients with an ulcerated primary melanoma seemed to benefit more from pegylated IFN than patients with nonulcerated primaries.[24]

INTERLEUKIN-2

Interleukin-2 (IL-2), a natural product secreted by CD4$^+$ T lymphocytes and a T-cell growth factor, was first identified in 1976 but was not produced until 1983, when a biologically active polypeptide characteristic of human IL-2 was formulated.[25,26] Shortly thereafter, a recombinant form of IL-2 (rIL-2) was shown to have antitumor activity in murine tumor models.[27] The mechanism of this antitumor activity is not well understood. In addition to T lymphocytes, IL-2 stimulates natural killer cells,

B lymphocytes, and macrophages, as well as induces lymphokine-activated killer cells in vitro.[28]

Clinical trials conducted using patients with advanced cancer and metastatic melanoma showed antitumor effects associated with high-dose bolus intravenous IL-2 (HDIL-2) administration.[29–35] Subsequently, HDIL-2 was approved by the US Food and Drug Administration (FDA) in 1998 for the treatment of adults with advanced metastatic melanoma. The efficacy and toxicity profile of HDIL-2 were best described when the data from 270 metastatic melanoma patients treated with HDIL-2 between 1985 and 1993 were analyzed.[31,32] A bolus intravenous infusion of HDIL-2 (600,000–720,000 IU/kg every 8 hours on days 1–5 and 15–19) was used. An objective response rate of 16% (median response duration, 8.9 months; range, 4 to 106+) with a durable response rate of 4% was reported. Further analysis of the treated patients showed that patients with a good baseline performance status (ECOG of 0), no prior history of systemic therapy, a normal lactate dehydrogenase (LDH) level, and less than 3 organs involved or cutaneous and/or subcutaneous metastases had the highest probability of responding as well as achieving a durable complete response.[28,32,36,37] Autoimmune toxicity, such as treatment-related hypothyroidism, may also be associated with a favorable tumor response.[38] All reported response predictors need to be confirmed in prospective trials.

Although bolus HDIL-2 is more commonly used in the United States, continuous infusion IL-2 schedules remain common treatments in Europe. This commonly has been administered as 18×10^6 IU/d for 5 days.[39] Overall response rates have been reported to be comparable to HDIL-2, and survival rates have been documented at 4% at 5 years. Large, randomized controlled trials comparing different IL-2 schedules in melanoma have not been performed.

IL-2 toxicity can involve multiple organ systems, most significantly, the heart, lungs, kidneys, and central nervous system. Most of the toxicity is related to the capillary leak syndrome, which leads to decreased organ perfusion (oliguria and ischemia) due to the accumulation of fluid in the extravascular space.[40] The incidence of toxicities has decreased as clinicians have started to follow strict patient-eligibility criteria and have implemented standardized toxicity prevention guidelines. To minimize the toxicity, IL-2 has been administered in lower doses subcutaneously.[41] This has produced no major responses in melanoma patients.

To enhance its activity in patients with metastatic melanoma, IL-2 has been combined with vaccines. The most studied combination is IL-2 and glycoprotein 100 (gp100):209-217(210M), a peptide vaccine with a higher affinity to HLA-A2 and a better inducer of T-cell stimulation in vitro and in vivo (**Table 1**).[42–46] The HDIL-2 and gp100 vaccine is active and has been shown to be more effective in a phase III randomized trial in patients with metastatic melanoma (see **Table 1**). The combination of vaccine and low-dose IL-2 has been proven safe and tolerable but inactive against advanced melanoma.[47]

BIOCHEMOTHERAPY

To improve on the activity of immunotherapy in melanoma, combining different chemotherapy agents with IFN, IL-2, or both has been tested. Several randomized trials compared biochemotherapy to chemotherapy; all concluded that biochemotherapy is associated with increased toxicity. Inconsistent results have been reported on efficacy, with most of the variability coming from single-center studies. The overall response rate was as high as 50% in non-IL-2-based and 48% in IL-2-based biochemotherapy.

Table 1
Clinical trials evaluating gp100 vaccine and HDIL2

References	N	Design	PR	CR	Comments
[43]	31	Phase II	39%	3%	Objective regression of some brain metastases was seen.
[44]	131	Phase II	7%	9%	9% progression-free at 30+ months.
[45]	684	Retrospective	9% vs 12% (IL-2 alone vs IL2 +variety of vaccines)	4% vs 3% (IL-2 alone vs IL2 +variety of vaccines)	Patients who received the gp100:209-217 (210M) peptide plus IL-2 showed a strong trend to increased objective responses compared with HDIL-2 alone (22% vs 13%)
[46]	185	Randomized phase III of the combination vs HDIL-2 alone	7.5% vs 8%	2% vs 14% in favor of the combination	Overall response rate and PFS were significantly better with peptide vaccine and HDIL-2 compared with HDIL-2 alone. Trend for greater overall survival in the vaccine arm (18 vs 13 mo)

Abbreviations: CR, complete response; PFS, progression free survival; PR, partial response.

A doubling in median overall survival has also been reported in small studies (17 vs 8 months).[48–50]

To further investigate the benefit of biochemotherapy in metastatic melanoma, several meta-analyses have been conducted, with the most recent reported in 2007.[39,51–53] In this analysis, 11 randomized trials of chemotherapy ± IFN (1395 patients) and 7 randomized trials of chemotherapy ± IFN and IL-2 (1226 patients) were included.[48–50,54–68] Grade 3 hematologic toxicity was higher with biochemotherapy; the odds ratio for thrombocytopenia was 3.03 (95% CI, 2.16 to 4.25; $P = .00001$) and for neutropenia/leukopenia was 1.71 (95% CI, 1.25 to 2.34; $P = .0008$). Biochemotherapy was superior for partial response (odds ratio = 0.66; 95% CI, 0.53 to 0.82; $P = .0001$) and complete response (CR; odds ratio = 0.50; 95% CI, 0.35 to 0.73; $P = .0003$). There was, however, no difference between chemotherapy and biochemotherapy in duration of response (42 days), but biochemotherapy did delay the time to disease progression (odds ratio = 0.80; 95% CI, 0.71 to 0.89; $P = .0001$). There was also no advantage of biochemotherapy in terms of overall survival (OS; odds ratio = 0.99; 95% CI, 0.91 to 1.08; $P = .9$). Similar to HDIL-2, long-term survival (10 years) has been reported in 6% of patients with metastatic melanoma treated with biochemotherapy.[69] To date, biochemotherapy remains one of the treatments with the highest response rate, which makes it useful in patients with rapidly progressive melanoma by providing symptomatic relief or to render patients with locally and/or regionally advanced disease surgically resectable.

BIOTHERAPY

To improve the response rate of HDIL-2, IFN was tested in combination with high-dose and low-dose IL-2 in melanoma patients but, unfortunately, failed to show significant improvement in the response rate.[70–72] This combination was recently tested as a maintenance regimen after induction biochemotherapy and was shown to prolong progression-free survival and to improve overall survival compared with other reported multicenter trials of biochemotherapy or chemotherapy.[73] The 12-month and 24-month survival rates were 57% and 23%, respectively. Randomized controlled trials are needed to confirm the results.

CYTOTOXIC T-LYMPHOCYTE ANTIGEN-4 BLOCKADE

The activation of T cells requires the engagement of CD28 on T cells by B7 molecules expressed on the surface of antigen-presenting cells (**Fig. 1**). This CD28-B7 interaction induces T-cell proliferation, cytokine secretion, and other effector functions (Cdk-4,

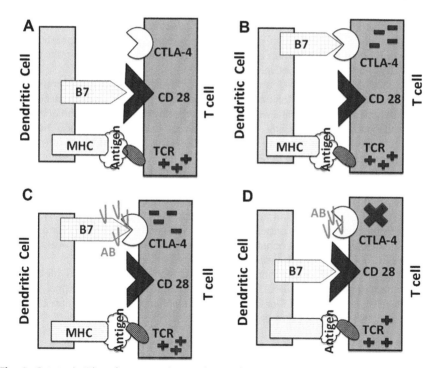

Fig. 1. Cytotoxic T-lymphocyte antigen-4 (CTLA-4) antibodies: mechanism of action. T-cell activation leads to the upregulation of CTLA-4 on the T-cell surface, which delivers a negative regulatory signal to T cells after binding to B7. CTLA-4 antibodies inhibit the interaction of B7 and CTLA-4; thus, the inhibitory signal produced by CTLA-4 is blocked and T-cell activation is prolonged. (*A*) CTLA-4 receptors are upregulated after T-cell activation. (*B*) Because of its greater affinity, CTLA-4 binds to B7 and sends and inhibitory signal within the cell. (*C*) CTLA-4 antibodies inhibit the interaction between CTLA-4 and B7. (*D*) The inhibitory signal is blocked; B7 once again binds to CD28.

Cdk-6, and cyclin D3). T-cell activation leads to the upregulation of cytotoxic T-lymphocyte antigen-4 (CTLA-4) on the T-cell surface, which delivers a negative regulatory signal to T cells after binding to B7. CTLA-4 antibodies inhibit the interaction of B7 and CTLA-4; thus, the inhibitory signal produced by CTLA-4 is blocked, and T-cell activation is prolonged.[74] Early studies in mice showed that an absence of CTLA-4 led to a lymphoproliferative disorder and to lymphocytic infiltration and destruction of major organs.[75]

Two fully human monoclonal CTLA-4 blocking antibodies, tremelimumab (IgG2; Pfizer, New York, NY, USA) and ipilimumab (IgG1; Bristol Myers Squibb, Princeton, NJ, USA), have been evaluated in clinical trials. Although it was suggested that anti-CTLA-4 antibodies deplete the T- regulatory cells, one study evaluating the changes in lymphocyte phenotype and function in melanoma patients receiving anti-CTLA-4 showed that the antitumor and autoimmune effects seen after CTLA-4 antibodies were due to direct activation of CD4+ and CD8+ effector cells, not inhibition or depletion of T regulatory cells.[76]

Both drugs have been tested as a single-agent therapy or in combination with other agents (**Tables 2** and **3**).[77–90] Most studies showed an overall response rate of 5% to 15% in patients with metastatic melanoma and reported prolonged survival in some responders. Increased response rate was associated with an increased dose of the CTLA-4 inhibitor and the presence of autoimmune toxicities in some studies. In 2010, a phase III randomized controlled trial showed ipilimumab to improve OS in comparison to gp100 vaccine in previously treated patients with metastatic melanoma.[90] In this study, ipilimumab alone (3 mg/kg) resulted in 1- and 2-year survival rates of 39% and 24%, respectively.

A unique toxicity of CTLA-4 antibody is the development of autoimmune side effects. The most common toxicities are rashes and pruritus. The most common serious adverse events are colitis with diarrhea, hypophysitis, inflammation of the pituitary gland, and hepatitis. Early administration of corticosteroids and hormone replacement are critical to the management of these toxicities. The death rate related to ipilimumab was reported to be 2%.[90]

A principal lesson learned from studies using anti-CTLA-4 antibodies was that the clinical benefit of these agents may not be well captured by the Response Evaluation Criteria In Solid Tumors (RECIST) or the World Health Organization (WHO) criteria. This led to the development of the immune-related response criteria (irRC), which focus on capturing additional response patterns observed with immune therapy.[91] According to the irRC, new lesions may not constitute progression of disease. Further evaluation of how the irRC correlate with OS improves the utility of these criteria.

Targeting of other T-cell immunoregulators is also being tested in melanoma. Programmed death ligand-1 (PDL-1), a negative regulator of T-cell signaling, and CD137(4-1BB), an inducible T-cell receptor that enhances the activation of T-cell and natural killer cells, are currently in clinical trials.[92,93]

ADOPTIVE CELL THERAPY

In adoptive cell therapy (ACT), a melanoma patient's own T lymphocytes (with antitumor activity) are expanded in vitro and are then infused into the patient along with T-cell growth factors to enhance their survival and expansion in vivo. This concept was first tested in mice, and it was shown that the intravenous injection of immune cells expanded with IL-2 could treat disseminated tumors.[94,95] The host's degree of immunosuppression (eg, levels of T-regulatory cells, such as IL7, IL15), the characteristics of the transferred cells, the immunization of the host with a vaccine expressing

Table 2
Clinical trials evaluating CTLA-4 antibodies as a single-agent therapy in melanoma

References	N	Study Design (Phase)	Drug	CTLA-4 Antibody Dose/ Schedule	RR	Survival (mo)	Grade 3 & 4 S/E	Comments
77	88	I/II	Ipi	Up to 10 mg/kg q3W	5%	13.5	14%	One complete response (21+ mo)
78	217	II	Ipi	0.3 mg/kg q3W 3 mg/kg q3W 10 mg/kg q3W	0% 4% 11%	9 9 15	0% 7% 25%	Significant increase in response with increased dose
79	29	I	Treme	0.01–15 mg/kg	14%	NR	35% in 10–15 mg/kg	Complete responses (maintained for 34+ and 25+ mo)
80	89	I/II	Treme	10 mg/kg/mo 15 mg/kg q3Mo	10% 9%	10 11.5	27% 13%	Most responses were durable (range, 3–30 + mo)
81	155	II	Ipi	10 mg/kg q3W	6%	10	22%	2-year survival rate 33%
82	246	II	Treme	15 mg/kg q90D	7%	10	11%	Durable responses ≥170 d

Abbreviations: Ipi, ipilimumab; N, number of subjects; NR, not reported; q3Mo, every 3 months; q3W, every 3 weeks; q90D, every 90 days; RR, response rate; S/E, side effects; Treme, tremelimumab.

Table 3
Clinical trials evaluating CTLA-4 antibodies in combination with other therapies in melanoma

References	N	Study Design (Phase)	Drug	CTLA-4 Antibody Dose/Schedule	RR	Survival (mo)	Grade 3 & 4 S/E	Comments
83	14	II	Ipi + gp100	3 mg/kg IV q3W	21%	NR	43%	Accrual ceased after 14 patients because of grade 3 & 4 autoimmune toxicities
84	16	I	Trem + dendritic cell vaccine	3–15 mg/kg qMo–q3Mo	25%	NR	6%	Durable response up to 4 y after study initiation
85	36	I/II	Ipi + HDIL-2	0.1–3 mg/kg q3W	22%	NR	14%	75% of responders had a response>11 mo
86	56	II	Ipi+ gp100	1–3 mg/kg q3W	13%	NR	25%	Autoimmune toxicity associated with response CR ongoing 31 mo
87	72	II	Ipi Ipi + dacarbazine (250 mg/m2/d for 5 d)	3 mg/kg q4W 3 mg/kg q4W	5% 14%	11 14	8% 17%	No statistical difference in disease control rate in 2 arms. 5 patients remain alive after 5.5+ y
88	115	II	Ipi Ipi + budesonide	10 mg/kg q3W 10 mg/kg q3W	16% 12%	19 18	47% 55%	Disease control rate was higher in patients with grade 3 & 4 S/E
89	139	II	Ipi + gp100	3–9 mg/kg q3W	17%	16	36%	Immune related adverse events were associated with a greater antitumor response
90	676	III	Gp100 Ipi Ipi+gp100	3 mg/kg q3W 3 mg/kg q3W	1.5% 11% 6%	6 10 10	11% 23% 17%	Ipi with or without gp100 vaccine improved overall survival in patients with previously treated metastatic melanoma

Abbreviations: CR, complete response; Ipi, ipilimumab; N, number of subjects; NR, not reported; qMo, every month; q3Mo, every 3 months; q3W, every 3 weeks; q4W, every 4 weeks; RR, response rate; S/E, side effects; Treme, tremelimumab.

a tumor antigen recognized by the transferred cells, the stimulation of antigen presenting cells, and the genetic modification of lymphocytes using retroviruses have all been shown to be major factors associated with treatment outcome.[96–99] Early studies evaluating ACT in melanoma patients showed a significant correlation between clinical response and the following: extranodal source of the tumor-infiltrating lymphocytes (TIL), shorter culture duration, shorter TIL doubling time, greater autologous tumor lysis by TIL, and secretion of granulocyte-macrophage colony-stimulating factor (GM-CSF) by TIL.[100] Several clinical studies have evaluated ACT in melanoma (**Table 4**).[101–109] Some of the lessons learned from the available studies are

1. ACT represents a highly personalized treatment with a new reagent created for each patient.
2. Expansion of TIL for therapy requires a significant investment in infrastructure and a high degree of clinical and laboratory expertise.
3. ACT in patients with melanoma is reported to have the highest response rate compared with other non-ACT treatments in melanoma patients.
4. Lymphodepletion before ACT is an important component of the treatment and the lymphodepletion regimen might have an effect on the response rate.
5. An approximately 50% expansion success-rate has been reported for TIL-based ACT.
6. Significant treatment-related toxicities have been reported in patients receiving total body irradiation as a component of ACT.
7. Although ACT using autologous tumor-infiltrating lymphocytes is currently the most effective strategy, the use of tumor-specific T cells derived from the peripheral blood of patients shows promise.

Current studies are focused on improving the yield of TIL cultures, using vaccines to stimulate the transferred T cells and creating more specific antigens.

VACCINES

Melanoma is an immunogenic tumor, triggering a predominately Th1-directed immune response in the host. As a result of their interaction with the tumor antigens displayed on tumor cells, antigen-presenting cells stimulate CD8+ T-lymphocytes. Consequently, vaccine therapy, because of its ability to invoke an immunologic response, provides a potentially innovative therapeutic avenue in the treatment of melanoma. The following sections provide a review of the various vaccines used thus far in the treatment of melanoma.

DNA Vaccines

The use of DNA vaccines, most commonly in the form of a plasmid vector, has recently garnered more aggressive investigation. The plasmid vector is constructed using tumor DNA sequences that code for tumor-specific antigens.[110] The precise mechanism by which these antigens induce an immune response has been debated, but 2 probable mechanisms have emerged—direct transfection of dendritic cells and cross-priming.[111] In the process of cross-priming, non-antigen-presenting cells take up the tumor DNA, and host cellular machinery transcribes and translates the tumor DNA into specific antigens.[111] These antigens are then presented in the typical fashion to T-lymphocytes by dendritic cells, triggering a cascade that results in the provocation of an immune response.[111,112] One clear advantage of DNA vaccines is their ability to activate the cellular and humoral immune systems.[113] A preclinical animal model illustrated the significant tumor protection of a gp100 DNA vaccine in the treatment of

Table 4
Clinical trials evaluating ACT in melanoma

References	N	Lymphodepletion	T Cells Source	Postinfusion	RR	Comments
101	11	None	Melan-A/MART-1-specific T-cell clones from peripheral blood	HDIL-2	27%	Responders only with cutaneous or LN metastases
102	12	None	PBMC-derived T-cells specific for gp100 or TIL	Low-dose subcutaneous IL-2 or HDIL-2	17%	Transferred cells declined to undetectable levels by 2 wk
103	13	Cy for 2 d; Flu for next 5	TIL	HDIL-2	46%	Responses in visceral metastases
105	13	Cy for 2 d; Flu for next 5	TIL genetically engineered to produce IL-2	Only 5 had HDIL-2	15%	Persistence of IL-2-transduced TIL in 3 patients (one partial responder)
105	14	None	Melan-A/MART-1-specific T-cell clones from peripheral blood	Low-dose IL-2 and IFN	43%	1 CR for 5 y and 1 CR for 28 mo; mostly cutaneous and LN
106	15	Cy for 2 d Flu for next 5 d	PBMC-derived T cells specific for gp100 or TIL	Low-dose IL-2 or HDIL-2	0%	5 patients demonstrated mixed responses
107	25	Cy and Flu for 5 d followed by a single fraction of 2 Gy of TBI	TIL	Hematopoietic stem cells and HDIL-2	52%	The 2-y survival rate: 30%
107	25	Cy and Flu for 5 d and 12 Gy of TBI for 3 d:	TIL	Hematopoietic stem cells and HDIL-2	72%	The 2-y survival rates: 42%
107,108	43	Cy for 2 d; Flu for next 5 d	TIL	HDIL-2	49%	CR up to 63 mo
109	86	67% received Cy 36 h before TIL	TIL	HDIL-2 in 2	34%	Response similar in patients treated with or without Cy

Abbreviations: CR, complete response; Cy, cyclophosphamide; Flu, fludarabine; HDIL-2, 720,000 U/kg intravenously every 8 hours to tolerance up to 15 doses; INF, interferon α; LN, lymph node; RR, response rate; TBI, total body irradiation; TIL, tumor-infiltrating lymphocytes.

melanoma.[114] A Phase I clinical trial of the gp100 DNA vaccine has been completed in melanoma patients (stage IIB, III, and IV disease); immune responses (increase in CD8+ T-cell interactions with the tumor antigens coded by the DNA vaccine) were documented in 5 of 18 patients.[115] The vaccine showed minimal toxicity, with the most common complication being an injection site reaction.[115] It is apparent that further evaluation is necessary to determine the actual clinical benefit of a DNA vaccine for patients with advanced disease.

Dendritic Cell Vaccines

Several factors make dendritic cells an exciting vaccine target for patients with melanoma. Dendritic cells are antigen-presenting cells with the unique ability to interact with major histocompatibility complex (MHC)-I and MHC-II, thus upregulating innate and acquired immunity.[116] Additionally, the affinity with which dendritic cells bind MHC-I and II receptors allows a small number of these antigen-presenting cells to elicit a considerably greater immune response.[117] It is crucial, however, that the antigens selected for presentation to dendritic cells be specific for a given tumor and able to affect the growth potential of that tumor.[118] Recent investigations have demonstrated clinical and tumor-specific T lymphocyte responses in patients who had already failed prior therapeutic interventions.[119,120] In one study, CD8+ T cells were upregulated via a Th1 immune response after administration of a dendritic cell vaccine, with concomitant clinical results.[120] A recent phase III trial investigating a standard therapy of dacarbazine chemotherapy versus a novel treatment with a peptide-pulsed dendritic vaccine showed no difference in overall survival or progression-free survival, and therefore, the trial was terminated.[121]

Peptide-Based Vaccines

Peptide vaccines use tumor-associated antigens to stimulate the immune system to incite a CD8+ T-cell predominant response against tumor cells harboring those same antigens. Initial efforts at using peptide-based vaccines for melanoma proved minimally beneficial.[122] A clinical trial of 185 patients treated with IL-2 alone or IL-2 and gp100 demonstrated better response rates and improved progression-free survival in patients who received the combination therapy (see **Table 1**).[46] Another heavily investigated antigen-rich vaccine was Canvaxin. After phase II clinical trials involving patients with stage III melanoma showed improvement in survival with Canvaxin, phase III trials in stage III and IV were initiated.[123] The trials were discontinued early, because interim analyses showed that it was unlikely that the trials would ever provide significant evidence of a survival benefit for Canvaxin-treated patients.[124]

Viral Vaccines

Viruses have long been used as a vector for inducing a host response against a specific antigen. Recent studies have attempted to use the same mechanism in the treatment of various types of cancer.[125] In a recent Phase II clinical trial, 50 patients with unresectable stage III or IV disease were treated with a granulocyte-macrophage CSF-encoding, second-generation oncolytic herpesvirus.[126] The overall response rate was 26% (CR = 6%), and regression of injected and distant (including visceral) lesions occurred. Some responses were maintained up to 31 months. Overall survival was 58% at 1 year and 52% at 24 months. This effectiveness combined with a limited toxicity profile led to a phase III trial that is currently under way.

SUMMARY

Treatment of patients with melanoma in the adjuvant and metastatic settings remains the focus of many preclinical and clinical studies. In recent years, newer strategies to modulate the immune system in melanoma (vaccines, antibodies, and adoptive T-cell therapy) have shown very promising results. Improvements in overall survival have been obtained in metastatic melanoma by inhibiting immune check points. The most unique aspect of immunotherapy is the prolonged tumor response achieved in patients with metastatic disease. Predictive biomarkers to help select patients or to evaluate tumor response are needed. There is also a need to improve the response rate and decrease the toxicity of these agents. Studies combining multiple agents with different mechanisms of action in modulating the immune system are under way. Also, targeted therapies are showing effectiveness in melanoma. The best combination of immuno-therapies and target therapies to achieve the most optimal results must be found.

REFERENCES

1. Ries LA, Wingo PA, Miller DS, et al. The annual report to the nation on the status of cancer, 1973–1997, with a special section on colorectal cancer. Cancer 2000; 88:2398–424.
2. National Cancer Institute, U.S. National Institutes of Health. Surveillance, epidemiology, and end results (SEER) Program. Available at: www.seer cancer.gov. Accessed March 1, 2010.
3. Bedikian AY, Millward M, Pehamberger H, et al. Bcl-2 antisense (oblimersensodium) plus dacarbazine in patients with advanced melanoma: the Oblimersen Melanoma Study Group. J Clin Oncol 2006;24:4738–45.
4. Qureshi SA, Salditt-Georgieff M, Darnell MA. Tyrosine-phosphorylated Stat1 and Stat2 plus a 48-kDa protein all contact DNA in forming interferon-stimulated-gene factor 3. Proc Natl Acad Sci U S A 1995;92(9):3829–33.
5. Qureshi SA, Leung S, Kerr IM, et al. Function of Stat2 protein in transcriptional activation by alpha interferon. Mol Cell Biol 1996;16(1):288–93.
6. Badgwell B, Lesinski GB, Magro C, et al. The antitumor effects of interferon-alpha are maintained in mice challenged with a STAT1-deficient murine melanoma cell line. J Surg Res 2004;116(1):129–36.
7. Gogas H, Ioannovich J, Dafni U. Prognostic significance of autoimmunity during treatment of melanoma with interferon. N Engl J Med 2006;354(7):709–18.
8. Kirkwood JM, Bender C, Agarwala S, et al. Mechanisms and management of toxicities associated with high-dose interferon alfa-2b therapy. J Clin Oncol 2002;20(17):3703–18.
9. Kirkwood JM, Strawderman MH, Ernstoff MS, et al. Interferon alfa-2b adjuvant therapy of high-risk resected cutaneous melanoma: the Eastern Cooperative Oncology Group Trial EST 1684. J Clin Oncol 1996;14(1):7–17.
10. Kirkwood JM, Ibrahim JG, Sondak VK, et al. High- and low-dose interferon alfa-2b in high-risk melanoma: first analysis of intergroup trial E1690/S9111/C9190. J Clin Oncol 2000;18(12):2444–58.
11. Kirkwood JM, Ibrahim JG, Sosman JA, et al. High-dose interferon alfa-2b significantly prolongs relapse-free and overall survival compared with the GM2-KLH/QS-21 vaccine in patients with resected stage IIB-III melanoma: results of intergroup trial E1694/S9512/C509801. J Clin Oncol 2001;19(9):2370–80.
12. Kirkwood JM, Manola J, Ibrahim J, et al. A pooled analysis of eastern cooperative oncology group and intergroup trials of adjuvant high-dose interferon for melanoma. Clin Cancer Res 2004;10(5):1670–7.

13. Kirkwood JM, Ibrahim J, Lawson DH, et al. High-dose interferon alfa-2b does not diminish antibody response to GM2 vaccination in patients with resected melanoma: results of the Multicenter Eastern Cooperative Oncology Group Phase II Trial E2696. J Clin Oncol 2001;19(5):1430–6.

14. Wheatley K, Ives N, Hancock B, et al. Does adjuvant interferon-alpha for high-risk melanoma provide a worthwhile benefit? A meta-analysis of the randomised trials. Cancer Treat Rev 2003;29(4):241–52.

15. Creagan ET, Dalton RJ, Ahmann DL, et al. Randomized, surgical adjuvant clinical trial of recombinant interferon alfa-2a in selected patients with malignant melanoma. J Clin Oncol 1995;13(11):2776–83.

16. Kleeberg UR, Sucio S, Brocker EB, et al. Final results of the EORTC 18871/DKG 80-1 randomised phase III trial. rIFN-alpha 2b versus rIFN-gamma versus ISCADOR M versus observation after surgery in melanoma patients with either high-risk primary (thickness >3 mm) or regional lymph node metastasis. Eur J Cancer 2004;40(3):390–402.

17. Grob JJ, Dreno B, de la Salmoniere P, et al. Randomised trial of interferon alpha-2a as adjuvant therapy in resected primary melanoma thicker than 1.5 mm without clinically detectable node metastases. French Cooperative Group on Melanoma. Lancet 1998;351(9120):1905–10.

18. Pehamberger H, Soyer HP, Steiner A, et al. Adjuvant interferon alfa-2a treatment in resected primary stage II cutaneous melanoma. Austrian Malignant Melanoma Cooperative Group. J Clin Oncol 1998;16(4):1425–9.

19. Cameron DA, Cornbleet MC, Mackie RM, et al. Adjuvant interferon alpha 2b in high risk melanoma - the Scottish study. Br J Cancer 2001;84(9):1146–9.

20. Cascinelli N, Belli F, MacKie RM, et al. Effect of long-term adjuvant therapy with interferon alpha-2a in patients with regional node metastases from cutaneous melanoma: a randomised trial. Lancet 2001;358(9285):866–9.

21. Hancock BW, Wheatley K, Harris S, et al. Adjuvant interferon in high-risk melanoma: the AIM HIGH Study–United Kingdom Coordinating Committee on Cancer Research randomized study of adjuvant low-dose extended-duration interferon Alfa-2a in high-risk resected malignant melanoma. J Clin Oncol 2004;22(1):53–61.

22. Eggermont AM, Suciu S, Santinami M, et al. Adjuvant therapy with pegylated interferon alfa-2b versus observation alone in resected stage III melanoma: final results of EORTC 18991, a randomised phase III trial. Lancet 2008;372(9633): 117–26.

23. Pectasides D, Dafni U, Bafaloukos D, et al. Randomized phase III study of 1 month versus 1 year of adjuvant high-dose interferon alfa-2b in patients with resected high-risk melanoma. J Clin Oncol 2009;27(6):939–44.

24. Eggermont AM, Suciu S, Testori A, et al. Ulceration of primary melanoma and responsiveness to adjuvant interferon therapy: analysis of the adjuvant trials EORTC18952 and EORTC18991 in 2,644 patients. J Clin Oncol 2009;27:15s [Suppl; abstract 9007].

25. Morgan DA, Ruscetti FW, Gallo R. Selective in vitro growth of T lymphocytes for normal human bone marrows. Science 1976;193:1007–8.

26. Taniguchi T, Matsui H, Fujita T, et al. Structure and expression of cloned cDNA for human interleukin-2. Nature 1983;302:305–10.

27. Rosenberg SA, Mule JJ, Speiss PJ, et al. Regression of established pulmonary metastases and subcutaneous tumor mediated by the systemic administration of high-dose recombinant interleukin 2. J Exp Med 1985;161: 1169–88.

28. Atkins MB, Mier JW, Parkinson DR, et al. Hypothyroidism after treatment with interleukin-2 and lymphokine-activated killer cells. N Engl J Med 1988;318: 1557–63.

29. Rosenberg SA, Lotze MT, Muul LM, et al. Observations on the systemic administration of autologous lymphokine-activated killer cells and recombinant interleukin-2 to patients with metastatic cancer. N Engl J Med 1985;313:1485–92.

30. Rosenberg SA, Lotze MT, Muul LM, et al. A progress report on the treatment of 157 patients with advanced cancer using lymphokine-activated killer cells and interleukin-2 or high-dose interleukin-2 alone. N Engl J Med 1987;316:889–97.

31. Atkins MB, Kunkel L, Sznol M, et al. High-dose recombinant interleukin-2 therapy in patients with metastatic melanoma: long-term survival update. Cancer J Sci Am 2000;6:S11–4.

32. Atkins MB, Lotze MT, Dutcher JP, et al. High-dose recombinant interleukin 2 therapy for patients with metastatic melanoma: analysis of 270 patients treated between 1985 and 1993. J Clin Oncol 1999;17:2105–16.

33. Dutcher JP, Creekmore S, Weiss GR, et al. A phase II study of interleukin-2 and lymphokine-activated killer cells in patients with metastatic malignant melanoma. J Clin Oncol 1989;7:477–85.

34. Parkinson DR, Abrams JS, Wiernik PH, et al. Interleukin-2 therapy in patients with metastatic malignant melanoma: a phase II study. J Clin Oncol 1990;8: 1650–6.

35. Rosenberg SA, Yang JC, Topalian SL, et al. Treatment of 283 consecutive patients with metastatic melanoma or renal cell cancer using high-dose bolus interleukin 2. JAMA 1999;271:907–13.

36. Petrella T, Quirt I, Verma S, et al. Single-agent interleukin-2 in the treatment of metastatic melanoma: a systematic review. Cancer Treat Rev 2007;33:484–96.

37. Chang E, Rosenberg SA. Patients with melanoma metastases at cutaneous and subcutaneous sites are highly susceptible to interleukin-2-based therapy. J Immunother 2001;24:88–90.

38. Mouawad R, Sebert M, Michels J, et al. Treatment for metastatic malignant melanoma: old drugs and new strategies. Crit Rev Oncol Hematol 2010;74(1):27–39.

39. Keilholz U, Conradt C, Legha SS, et al. Results of interleukin-2-based treatment in advanced melanoma: a case record-based analysis of 631 patients. J Clin Oncol 1998;16(9):2921–9.

40. Schwartz RN, Stover L, Dutcher J, et al. Managing toxicities of high-dose interleukin-2. Oncology (Williston Park) 2002;16(11 Suppl 13):11–20.

41. Tagliaferri P, Barile C, Caraglia M, et al. Daily low-dose subcutaneous recombinant interleukin-2 by alternate weekly administration: antitumor activity and immunomodulatory effects. Am J Clin Oncol 1998;21(1):48–53.

42. Parkhurst MR, Salgaller ML, Southwood S, et al. Improved induction of melanoma-reactive CTL with peptides from the melanoma antigen gp100 modified at HLA-A*0201-binding residues. J Immunol 1996;157:2539–48.

43. Rosenberg SA, Yang JC, Schwartzentruber DJ, et al. Immunologic and therapeutic evaluation of a synthetic peptide vaccine for the treatment of patients with metastatic melanoma. Nat Med 1998;4:321–7.

44. Sosman JA, Carrillo C, Urba WJ, et al. Three phase II cytokine working group trials of gp100 (210M) peptide plus high-dose interleukin-2 in patients with HLA-A2-positive advanced melanoma. J Clin Oncol 2008;26(14):2292–8.

45. Smith FO, Downey SG, Klapper JA, et al. Treatment of metastatic melanoma using interleukin-2 alone or in conjunction with vaccines. Clin Cancer Res 2008;14(17):5610–8.

46. Schwartzentruber DJ, Lawson D, Richards J, et al. A phase III multi-institutional randomized study of immunization with the gp100: 209–217(210M) peptide followed by high-dose IL-2 compared with high-dose IL-2 alone in patients with metastatic melanoma [abstract CRA9011]. J Clin Oncol 2009. In 2009 ASCO Annual Meeting. Orlando, Florida, 2009. 27.

47. Roberts JD, Niedzwiecki D, Carson WE, et al. Cancer and Leukemia Group B. Phase 2 study of the g209-2M melanoma peptide vaccine and low-dose interleukin-2 in advanced melanoma: Cancer and Leukemia Group B 509901. J Immunother 2006;29(1):95–101.

48. Vorobiof DA, Bezwoda WR. A randomised trial of vindesine plus interferon-2b compared with interferon-2b or vindesine alone in the treatment of advanced malignant melanoma. Eur J Cancer 1994;30A:797–800.

49. Falkson CI. Experience with interferon alpha 2b combined with dacarbazine in the treatment of metastatic malignant melanoma. Med Oncol 1995;12:35–40.

50. Eton O, Legha SS, Bedikian AY, et al. Sequential biochemotherapy versus chemotherapy for metastatic melanoma: results from a phase III randomized trial. J Clin Oncol 2002;20:2045–52.

51. Huncharek M, Caubet JF, McGarry R. Single-agent DTIC versus combination chemotherapy with or without immunotherapy in metastatic melanoma: a meta-analysis of 3273 patients from 20 randomized trials. Melanoma Res 2001;11:75–81.

52. Allen I, Kupelnick B, Kumashiro M. Efficacy of interleukin-2 in the treatment of metastatic melanoma – systemic review and metastasis analysis. Cancer Ther 1998;1:168–73.

53. Ives NJ, Stowe RL, Lorigan P, et al. Chemotherapy compared with biochemotherapy for the treatment of metastatic melanoma: a meta-analysis of 18 trials involving 2,621 patients. J Clin Oncol 2007;25(34):5426–34.

54. Kirkwood JM, Ernstoff MS, Giuliano A, et al. Interferon -2a and dacarbazine in melanoma. J Natl Cancer Inst 1990;82:1062–3.

55. Galvez CA, Bonamassa M. Advanced malignant melanoma: DTIC plus rIFN-alfa-2b vs DTIC alone [abstract 932]. Eur J Cancer 1991;27(Suppl 2):s155.

56. Thomson DB, Adena M, McLeod RC, et al. Interferon-2a does not improve response or survival when combined with dacarbazine in metastatic malignant melanoma: Results of a multi-institutional Australian randomized trial. Melanoma Res 1993;3:133–8.

57. Bajetta E, Di Leo A, Zampino MG, et al. Multicenter randomized trial of dacarbazine alone or in combination with two different doses and schedules of interferon alpha-2a in the treatment of advanced melanoma. J Clin Oncol 1994;12:806–11.

58. Falkson CI, Ibrahim J, Kirkwood JM, et al. cPhase III trial of dacarbazine versus dacarbazine with interferon alpha-2b versus dacarbazine with tamoxifen versus dacarbazine with interferon alpha-2b and tamoxifen in patients with metastatic malignant melanoma: an Eastern Cooperative Oncology Group study. J Clin Oncol 1998;16:1743–51.

59. Gorbonova VA, Egorov GN, Perevodchikova NI, et al. [Combined chemotherapy with or without interferon alpha N_1 (IFN) for advanced malignant melanoma: a randomized pilot phase III study]. Gan To Kagaku Ryoho 2000;27(Suppl 2):310–4.

60. Young AM, Marsden J, Goodman A, et al. Prospective randomized comparison of dacarbazine (DTIC) versus DTIC plus interferon-alpha (IFN-alpha) in metastatic melanoma. Clin Oncol (R Coll Radiol) 2001;13:458–65.

61. Danson S, Lorigan P, Arance A, et al. Randomised phase II study of temozolomide given every 8 hours or daily with either interferon alpha-2b or thalidomide in metastatic malignant melanoma. J Clin Oncol 2003;21:2551–7.

62. Kaufmann R, Spieth K, Leiter U, et al. Temozolomide in combination with interferon-alpha versus temozolomide alone in patients with advanced metastatic melanoma: a randomized, phase III, multicenter study from the Dermatologic Cooperative Oncology Group. J Clin Oncol 2005;23:9001–7.

63. Johnston SR, Constenla DO, Moore J, et al. Randomized phase II trial of BCDT [carmustine (BCNU), cisplatin, dacarbazine (DTIC) and tamoxifen] with or without interferon alpha (IFN-) and interleukin (IL-2) in patients with metastatic melanoma. Br J Cancer 1998;77:1280–6.

64. Rosenberg SA, Yang JC, Schwartzentruber DJ, et al. Prospective randomized trial of the treatment of patients with metastatic melanoma using chemotherapy with cisplatin, dacarbazine, and tamoxifen alone or in combination with interleukin-2 and interferon alpha-2b. J Clin Oncol 1999;17:968–75.

65. Atzpodien J, Neuber K, Kamanabrou D, et al. Combination chemotherapy with or without sc IL-2 and IFN-alpha: results of a prospectively randomized trial of the Cooperative Advanced Malignant Melanoma Chemoimmunotherapy group (ACIMM). Br J Cancer 2002;86:179–84.

66. Ridolfi R, Chiarion-Sileni V, Guida M, et al. Cisplatin, dacarbazine with or without subcutaneous interleukin-2, and interferon alfa-2b in advanced melanoma outpatients: Results from an Italian multicenter phase III randomized clinical trial. J Clin Oncol 2002;20:1600–7.

67. Atkins MB, Hsu J, Lee S, et al. Phase III trial comparing concurrent biochemotherapy with cisplatin, vinblastine, dacarbazine, interleukin-2, and interferon alfa-2b with cisplatin, vinblastine, and dacarbazine alone in patients with metastatic malignant melanoma (E3695): a trial coordinated by the Eastern Cooperative Oncology Group. J Clin Oncol 2008;26(35):5748–54.

68. Bajetta E, Del Vecchio M, Nova P, et al. Multicenter phase III randomized trial of polychemotherapy (CVD regimen) versus the same chemotherapy (CT) plus subcutaneous interleukin-2 and interferon-alpha2b in metastatic melanoma. Ann Oncol 2006;17(4):571–7.

69. Bedikian AY, Papadopoulos NE, Kim KB, et al. Does complete response (CR) with systemic therapy (SRx) translate into long term survival in stage IV melanoma (MM)? [abstract 9043]. J Clin Oncol 2008;26(Suppl).

70. Rosenberg SA, Lotze MT, Yang JC, et al. Combination therapy with interleukin-2 and alpha-interferon for the treatment of patients with advanced cancer. J Clin Oncol 1989;7:1863–74.

71. Sparano JA, Fisher RI, Sunderland M, et al. Randomized phase III trial of treatment with high-dose interleukin-2 either alone or in combination with interferon alfa-2a in patients with advanced melanoma. J Clin Oncol 1993;11:1969–77.

72. Whitehead RP, Figlin R, Citron ML, et al. A phase II trial of concomitant human interleukin-2 and interferon-alpha-2a in patients with disseminated malignant melanoma. J Immunother Emphasis Tumor Immunol 1993;13:117–21.

73. O'Day SJ, Atkins MB, Boasberg P, et al. Phase II multicenter trial of maintenance biotherapy after induction concurrent Biochemotherapy for patients with metastatic melanoma. J Clin Oncol 2009;27(36):6207–12.

74. Kirkwood JM, Tarhini AA, Panelli MC, et al. Next generation of immunotherapy for melanoma. J Clin Oncol 2008;26(20):3445–55.

75. Waterhouse P, Penninger JM, Timms E, et al. Lymphoproliferative disorders with early lethality in mice deficient in Ctla-4. Science 1995;270:985–8.

76. Maker AV, Attia P, Rosenberg SA. Analysis of the cellular mechanism of antitumor responses and autoimmunity in patients treated with CTLA-4 blockade. J Immunol 2006;176(9):5136.

77. Weber JS, O'Day S, Urba W, et al. Phase I/II study of ipilimumab for patients with metastatic melanoma. J Clin Oncol 2008;26(36):5950–6.
78. Wolchok JD, Neyns B, Linette G, et al. Ipilimumab monotherapy in patients with pretreated advanced melanoma: a randomised, double-blind, multicentre, phase 2, dose-ranging study. Lancet Oncol 2010;11(2):155–64.
79. Ribas A, Camacho LH, Lopez-Berestein G, et al. Antitumor activity in melanoma and anti-self responses in a phase I trial with the anti-cytotoxic T lymphocyte-associated antigen 4 monoclonal antibody CP-675,206. J Clin Oncol 2005; 23(35):8968–77.
80. Camacho LH, Antonia S, Sosman J, et al. Phase I/II trial of tremelimumab in patients with metastatic melanoma. J Clin Oncol 2009;27(7):1075–81.
81. O'Day SJ, Maio M, Chiarion-Sileni V, et al. Efficacy and safety of ipilimumab monotherapy in patients with pretreated advanced melanoma: a multicenter single-arm phase II study. Ann Oncol 2010;21(8):1712–7.
82. Kirkwood JM, Lorigan P, Hersey P, et al. Phase II trial of tremelimumab (CP-675,206) in patients with advanced refractory or relapsed melanoma. Clin Cancer Res 2010;16(3):1042–8.
83. Phan GQ, Yang JC, Sherry RM, et al. Cancer regression and autoimmunity induced by cytotoxic T lymphocyteassociated antigen 4 blockade in patients with metastatic melanoma. Proc Natl Acad Sci U S A 2003;100:8372–7.
84. Ribas A, Comin-Anduix B, Chmielowski B, et al. Dendritic cell vaccination combined with CTLA4 blockade in patients with metastatic melanoma. Clin Cancer Res 2009;15(19):6267–76.
85. Maker AV, Phan GQ, Attia P, et al. Tumor regression and autoimmunity in patients treated with cytotoxic T lymphocyte- associated antigen 4 blockade and inter-leukin-2: a phase I/II study. Ann Surg Oncol 2005;12:1005–16.
86. Attia P, Phan GQ, Maker AV, et al. Autoimmunity correlates with tumor regression in patients with metastatic melanoma treated with anti-cytotoxic T-lymphocyte antigen-4. J Clin Oncol 2005;23(25):6043–53.
87. Hersh EM, O'Day SJ, Powderly J, et al. A phase II multicenter study of ipilimumab with or without dacarbazine in chemotherapy-naïve patients with advanced melanoma. Invest New Drugs 2010. [Epub ahead of print].
88. Weber J, Thompson JA, Hamid O, et al. A randomized, double-blind, placebo-controlled, phase II study comparing the tolerability and efficacy of ipilimumab administered with or without prophylactic budesonide in patients with unresectable stage III or IV melanoma. Clin Cancer Res 2009;15(17):5591–8.
89. Downey SG, Klapper JA, Smith FO, et al. Prognostic factors related to clinical response in patients with metastatic melanoma treated by CTL-associated antigen-4 blockade. Clin Cancer Res 2007;13(22 Pt 1):6681–8.
90. Hodi FS, O'Day SJ, McDermott DF, et al. Improved survival with ipilimumab in patients with metastatic melanoma. N Engl J Med 2010;363:711–23.
91. Wolchok JD, Hoos A, O'Day S, et al. Guidelines for the evaluation of immune therapy activity in solid tumors: immune-related response criteria. Clin Cancer Res 2009;15(23):7412–20.
92. Blank C, Gajewski TF, Mackensen A. Interaction of PD-L1 on tumor cells with PD-1 on tumor-specific T cells as a mechanism of immune evasion: implications for tumor immunotherapy. Cancer Immunol Immunother 2005;54:307–14.
93. Mittler RS, Foell J, McCausland M, et al. Anti-CD137 antibodies in the treatment of autoimmune disease and cancer. Immunol Res 2004;29:197–208.

94. Eberlein TJ, Rosenstein M, Rosenberg SA. Regression of a disseminated syngeneic solid tumor by systemic transfer of lymphoid cells expanded in IL-2. J Exp Med 1982;156:385–97.

95. Donohue JH, Rosenstein M, Chang AE, et al. The systemic administration of purified interleukin-2 enhances the ability of sensitized murine lymphocyte to cure a disseminated syngeneic lymphoma. J Immunol 1984;132:2123–8.

96. Rosenberg SA, Aebersold P, Cornetta K, et al. Gene transfer into humans–immunotherapy of patients with advanced melanoma, using tumor-infiltrating lymphocytes modified by retroviral gene transduction. N Engl J Med 1990; 323(9):570–8.

97. Gattinoni L, Finkelstein SE, Klebanoff CA, et al. Removal of homeostatic cytokine sinks by lymphodepletion enhances the efficacy of adoptively transferred tumor-specific CD8+ T cells. J Exp Med 2005;202:907–12.

98. Abad JD, Wrzensinski C, Overwijk W, et al. T- cell receptor gene therapy of established tumors in a murine melanoma model. J Immunother 2008;31:1–6.

99. Rosenberg SA, Restifo NP, Yang JC, et al. Adoptive cell transfer: a clinical path to effective cancer immunotherapy. Nat Rev Cancer 2008;8(4):299–308.

100. Schwartzentruber DJ, Homm SS, Dadmarz R, et al. In vitro predictors of therapeutic response in melanoma patients receiving tumor infiltrating lymphocytes and interleukin-2. J Clin Oncol 1994;12:1475–83.

101. Mackensen A, Meidenbauer N, Vogl S, et al. Phase I study of adoptive T-cell therapy using antigen-specific CD8+ T cells for the treatment of patients with metastatic melanoma. J Clin Oncol 2006;24(31):5060–9.

102. Dudley ME, Wunderlich J, Nishimura MI, et al. Adoptive transfer of cloned melanoma-reactive T lymphocytes for the treatment of patients with metastatic melanoma. J Immunother 2001;24(4):363–73.

103. Dudley ME, Wunderlich JR, Robbins PF, et al. Cancer regression and autoimmunity in patients after clonal repopulation with antitumor lymphocytes. Science 2002;298:850–4.

104. Heemskerk B, Liu K, Dudley ME, et al. Adoptive cell therapy for patients with melanoma, using tumor-infiltrating lymphocytes genetically engineered to secrete interleukin-2. Hum Gene Ther 2008;19(5):496–510.

105. Khammari A, Labarrière N, Vignard V, et al. Treatment of metastatic melanoma with autologous Melan-A/MART-1-specific cytotoxic T lymphocyte clones. J Invest Dermatol 2009;129(12):2835–42.

106. Dudley ME, Wunderlich JR, Yang JC, et al. A phase I study of nonmyeloablative chemotherapy and adoptive transfer of autologous tumor antigen-specific T lymphocytes in patients with metastatic melanoma. J Immunother 2002;25(3): 243–51.

107. Dudley ME, Yang JC, Sherry R, et al. Adoptive cell therapy for patients with metastatic melanoma: evaluation of intensive myeloablative chemoradiation preparative regimens 2008;26(32):5233–9.

108. Dudley ME, Wunderlich JR, Yang JC, et al. Adoptive cell transfer therapy following nonmyeloablative but lymphodepleting chemotherapy for the treatment of patients with refractory metastatic melanoma. J Clin Oncol 2005;23: 2346–57. J Clin Oncol 2008; 26(32):5233–39.

109. Rosenberg SA, Yannelli JR, Yang JC, et al. Treatment of patients with metastatic melanoma with autologous tumor-infiltrating lymphocytes and interleukin 2. J Natl Cancer Inst 1994;86(15):1159–66.

110. Tang D, Devit M, Johnston SA. Genetic immunization is a simple method for eliciting an immune response. Nature 1992;356(6365):152–4.

111. Porgador A, Irvine KR, Iwasaki A, et al. Predominant role for directlytransfected dendritic cells in antigen presentation to CD8+ T cells after gene gun immunization. J Exp Med 1998;188:1075–82.

112. Akbari O, Panjwani N, Garcia S, et al. DNA vaccination: transfection and activation of dendritic cells as key events for immunity. J Exp Med 1999;189:169–78.

113. Wolchok JD, Livingston PO. Vaccines for melanoma: translating basic immunology into new therapies. Lancet Oncol 2001;2(4):205–11.

114. Hawkins WG, Gold JS, Dyall R. Immunisation with DNA coding for gp100 results in CD4+ T-cell independent antitumor immunity. Surgery 2000;128:273–80.

115. Yuan J, Ku GY, Gllardo HF, et al. Safety and immunogenicity of a human and mouse gp100 DNA vaccine in a phase I trial of patients with melanoma. Cancer Immun 2009;9:5.

116. Fernandez NC, Lozier A, Flament C, et al. Dendritic cells directly trigger NK cell function: cross talk relevant in innate ant-tumor immune responses in vivo. Nat Med 1999;5(4):405–11.

117. Inaba K, Pack M, Inaba M, et al. High levels of a major histocompatibility complex II-self peptide complex on dendritic cells from the T cells areas of lymph nodes. J Exp Med 1997;186(5):665–72.

118. Gilboa E, Vieweg J. Cancer immunotherapy with mRNA-transfected dendritic cells. Immunol Rev 2004;199:251–63.

119. Zhang S, Wang Q, Miao B. Review: dendritic cell-based vaccine in the treatment of patients with advanced melanoma. Cancer Biother Radiopharm 2007;22(4): 501–7.

120. Palucka AK, Ueno H, Connolly J, et al. Dendritic cells loaded with killed allogeneic melanoma cells can induce objective clinical responses and MART-1 specific CD8+ T-cell immunity. J Immunother 2006;29(5):545–57.

121. Schadendorf D, Ugurel S, Schuler-Thurner B, et al. Dacarbazine (DTIC) versus vaccination with autologous peptide-pulsed dendritic cells (DC) in first-line treatment of patients with metastatic melanoma: a randomized phase III trial of the DC study group of the DeCOG. Ann Oncol 2006;17(4):563–70.

122. Lienard D, Rimoldi D, Marchand M, et al. Ex vivo detectable activation of Melan-A-specific T cells correlating with inflammatory skin reactions in melanoma patients vaccinated with peptides in IFA. Cancer Immunol 2004;4:4.

123. Morton DL, Hsueh EC, Essner R, et al. Prolonged survival of patients receiving active immunotherapy with Canvaxin therapeutic polyvalent vaccine after complete resection of melanoma metastatic to regional lymph nodes. Ann Surg 2002;236(4):438–48.

124. Kelland L. Discontinued drugs in 2005: oncology drugs. Expert Opin Investig Drugs 2006;15(11):1309–18.

125. Jager E, Karbach J, Gnjatic S, et al. Recombinant vaccinia/fowlpox NY-ESO-1 vaccines induce both humoral and cellular NY-ESO-1-specific immune responses in cancer patient. Proc Natl Acad Sci U S A 2006;103(9):14453–8.

126. Senzer NN, Kaufman HL, Amatruda T, et al. Phase II clinical trial of granulocyte-macrophage colony-stimulating factor-encoding, second-generation oncolytic herpesvirus in patients with unresectable metastatic melanoma. J Clin Oncol 2009;27(34):5763–71.

Targeted Therapy for Melanoma: A Primer

Michael A. Davies, MD, PhD[a,b,*], Jeffrey E. Gershenwald, MD[c,d]

KEYWORDS

• Targeted therapy • BRAF • NRAS • c-KIT • PTEN • GNαQ

Melanoma is the most aggressive form of skin cancer. Unfortunately, despite recent improvements for some solid tumors, the prevalence and mortality of melanoma continue to increase. For patients with distant metastases, treatment with single-agent or combination chemotherapy regimens have generally resulted in very low response rates, with no significant impact on patient survival.[1] Immunotherapies (eg, interleukin-2, ipilimumab) have also yielded overall low response rates, although a small subset of patients have achieved durable responses and long-term survival.[2–5] These modest achievements are further limited by noting that immunotherapies may also result in significant toxicities, including treatment-related deaths. Thus, a critical need exists for new therapeutic approaches for this aggressive disease.

The treatment of many cancers is entering a new era based on an improved understanding of the molecular pathogenesis of these diseases. Although some cancers seem to be primarily driven by viral infection, most are caused by genetic events that alter the expression or function of normal genes and proteins. These events, which include gene amplifications, deletions, and mutations, disrupt the regulatory processes that normally control the growth and survival of cells. Multiple analyses have shown that although a spectrum of genetic abnormalities is present in cancer

This work was supported in part by The University of Texas MD Anderson Cancer Center Melanoma SPORE (P50 CA93459); the American Society of Clinical Oncology Career Development Award (Dr Davies); MD Anderson Physician-Scientist Award (Dr Davies); Melanoma Research Alliance Young Investigator Award (Dr Davies); and the Grossman Family Foundation (Dr Gershenwald).

Disclosures: Dr Davies receives research support from GlaxoSmithKline, Merck, and AstraZeneca.

[a] Department of Melanoma Medical Oncology, The University of Texas MD Anderson Cancer Center, 7455 Fannin, 1SCRB2.3019, Unit 0904, Houston, TX 77054, USA
[b] Department of Systems Biology, The University of Texas MD Anderson Cancer Center, 7455 Fannin, 1SCRB2.3019, Unit 0904, Houston, TX 77054, USA
[c] Department of Surgical Oncology, The University of Texas MD Anderson Cancer Center, 1515 Holcombe Boulevard, Unit 0444, Houston, TX 77030, USA
[d] Department of Cancer Biology, The University of Texas MD Anderson Cancer Center, 1515 Holcombe Boulevard, Unit 0444, Houston, TX 77030, USA
* Corresponding author. Department of Melanoma Medical Oncology, The University of Texas MD Anderson Cancer Center, 7455 Fannin, 1SCRB2.3019, Unit 0904, Houston, TX 77054.
E-mail address: mdavies@mdanderson.org

cells, most affect certain signaling pathways and functions. Cancer cells are subsequently often critically dependent on these pathways for survival, a phenomenon termed *oncogene addiction*. This reliance on pathways that are hyperactivated by genetic events occurring specifically in cancer cells presents a therapeutic opportunity to block those targets to inhibit the growth and survival of the cancer while sparing the normal cells of the body. This approach, termed *targeted therapy*, has been shown to be effective and is approved by the U.S. Food and Drug Administration (FDA) for treating several cancers, including chronic myelogenous leukemia, gastrointestinal stromal tumors (GISTs), and renal cell carcinoma.[6] Targeted therapies have also been effective in treating specific subpopulations of patients with other cancers, such as trastuzumab (Herceptin) for treating HER2/neu-amplified breast cancer.[7] For each of these examples, successful implementation of a targeted therapeutic approach was critically dependent on the identification of activating genetic events and the affected pathways that were present for each specific tumor type.

Evidence now shows that most melanomas harbor one or more mutations in critical kinase signaling pathways. Accumulating data support that the prevalence of these events varies greatly among the melanoma subtypes that have been defined by clinical and pathologic characteristics.[8] Most *cutaneous melanomas* (CMs) arise from melanocytes on sun-exposed skin. Exposure to ultraviolet radiation is thought to play a major causative role in these tumors. However, the role of ultraviolet radiation is less clear for cutaneous melanomas arising from relatively sun-protected sites. Examples of these melanomas include those arising on the palms and soles, termed *acral lentiginous melanomas* (ALMs). Melanomas may also arise from melanocytes in the mucosa of the head and neck, the gastrointestinal tract, and the genitourinary tract. Melanomas arising in these sites are classified as *mucosal melanomas*, and clearly arise in the absence of exposure to ultraviolet radiation. Consistent with the hypothesis that these melanoma subtypes are caused by different factors, comparative genomic hybridization (CGH) analysis has shown that these clinically defined groups of tumors have markedly different patterns of DNA copy number changes, including subtype-specific gene amplifications and deletions.[9] CMs that arise in areas with chronic sun exposure and that have histologic evidence of chronic sun damage (CSD) also exhibit markedly different chromosomal and gene copy number changes compared with cutaneous melanomas without chronic sun damage. Melanomas may also arise from melanocytes in the uveal tract of the eye (iris, ciliary body, and choroid) and are referred to as *uveal melanomas*. These tumors are also characterized by chromosomal changes that are distinct from cutaneous, acral lentiginous, and mucosal melanomas.[10,11]

The identification of activating mutations in melanoma, combined with a growing appreciation of the different pattern of genetic changes in the anatomically defined melanoma subtypes, has become the focus of a concerted effort to translate these discoveries into personalized therapeutic approaches for this disease. This article reviews the known mutations, amplifications, and deletions in kinase signaling pathways that have been implicated in melanoma; the prevalence of these genetic events in clinicopathologically defined melanoma subtypes; and the results of clinical trials that use targeted therapy approaches to block aberrantly activated pathways resulting from these mutations. The challenges that must be overcome to achieve improved outcomes with targeted therapies in melanoma in the future are also discussed.

BRAF

The RAS-RAF-MEK-MAPK signaling pathway is a critical regulator of cellular growth and survival (**Fig. 1**).[12,13] The first components of the pathway are the RAS-family

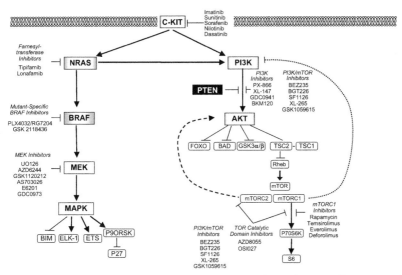

Fig. 1. Kinase signaling pathways and targeted therapies for melanoma. Illustration of key proteins in the RAS-RAF-MEK-MAPK and the PI3K-AKT kinase cascades. Arrows represent activation, whereas bars represent inhibition. Genes that are affected by activating mutations in melanoma (*BRAF, NRAS, PI3K, C-KIT,* and *AKT*) are shaded; the degree of shading reflects the relative prevalence of these mutations in cutaneous melanomas. Genes that are affected by genetic inactivation (*PTEN*) are shown with white type against a black background. The feedback regulation of PI3K and AKT by mTORC1 and mTORC2, respectively, is shown by the dashed lines. Classes and examples of targeted therapies against various effectors in the pathways are shown as free text beside the pathways.

GTP-ases. The RAS family members (HRAS, KRAS, NRAS) are guanine-nucleotide binding proteins that are embedded in the inner surface of the cell membrane. Normally, the RAS proteins are GDP-bound and inactive. Various activating signals result in the exchange of GTP for GDP, which activates RAS. RAS family members are also frequently affected by mutations in cancer that result in constitutive GTP-binding. The activated RAS members physically interact with the RAF family of serine-threonine protein kinases (ARAF, BRAF, CRAF) downstream of RAS. This interaction activates the RAF proteins, which then translocate to the cytoplasm and phosphorylate the MEK protein kinases (MEK1, MEK2). The MEK proteins are activated by this phosphorylation, and subsequently phosphorylate the P44/42 MAPK serine-threonine kinases (ERK1, ERK2). The activated MAPKs phosphorylate various transcription factors and cytosolic proteins to promote proliferation and survival.

In 2002, an experimental screen for mutations in RAF family members in cancer cell lines and tumors identified point mutations in *BRAF* in approximately half of the melanomas that were examined in the study, and occasional (3%–18%) colon, lung, breast, and ovarian cancer specimens.[14] Since this sentinel observation, the high frequency of point mutations in *BRAF* in melanoma has been confirmed in multiple studies. A recent meta-analysis of more than 200 published studies reported an overall mutation rate of 65% in melanoma cell lines and 42% in tumors.[15] The higher frequency of mutations in cell lines likely reflects a positive selection for cells with the *BRAF* mutation to propagate in vitro. Analysis of anatomic subtypes showed that *BRAF* mutations are common in cutaneous (42.5%) but uncommon in mucosal melanomas (5.6%) and rare in uveal melanomas (<1%) (**Table 1**). Among cutaneous

Table 1
Patterns of gene mutations and amplifications in melanoma

Melanoma Subtype	BRAF Mutation	NRAS Mutation	c-KIT Mutation	c-KIT Amplification	GNαQ Mutation
Sun-exposed cutaneous	43%	26%	Non-CSD: <2% CSD: 2%–17%	Non-CSD: 0%–7% CSD: 6%	<1%
Acral	18%	4%	18%	24%	<1%
Mucosal	6%	14%	24%	26%	<1%
Uveal	<1%	<1%	<1%	<1%	45%

Abbreviation: CSD, chronic-sun damaged.
The prevalence of the listed genetic events in melanoma clinical specimens.

melanomas, *BRAF* mutations are common in superficial spreading melanomas (53%) but less prevalent in acral lentiginous (18%) and lentigo maligna melanomas (9%).[15] Lentigo maligna melanomas are associated with CSD, and often originate in the head and neck region. The low prevalence of *BRAF* mutations in these tumors is consistent with the different patterns of DNA copy number gains and losses observed in the CGH analysis of cutaneous melanomas with or without CSD. *BRAF* mutations are also detectable in up to 80% of common acquired nevi.[16–18] However, *BRAF* mutation rates are lower in several of the less-common nevi types, including congenital, Spitz, and blue nevi.[18–20]

Approximately 50 different point mutations in *BRAF* have been identified in cancer.[21] A single substitution, the *BRAF V600E* mutation, comprises approximately 85% of the *BRAF* mutations detected in melanoma.[15] The *V600E* mutation increases the in vitro kinase activity of the BRAF protein more than 400-fold.[21] Most of the other reported somatic *BRAF* mutations, particularly other changes involving the V600 residue, also increase BRAF's catalytic activity (5- to 700-fold). A few *BRAF* mutations that have been detected in cancer cells (*G466E, G466V, G596R, D594V*) decrease the catalytic activity of the BRAF protein.[21,22] Because *BRAF V600E* is the predominant mutation identified in tumors, including melanoma, most functional studies have examined the function of the protein encoded by this change. Expression of the BRAF V600E protein results in constitutive phosphorylation and activation of MEK and MAPK.[14,21] Inhibition of BRAF V600E with small interfering RNA (siRNA, shRNA) inhibits MAPK activation, growth, and survival of human melanoma cell lines with this mutation.[23,24] These data support that melanomas with the *BRAF V600E* mutation depend on it for survival, and thus implicated this mutation as a therapeutic target.

Sorafenib was the first BRAF inhibitor to be used in clinical trials in melanoma. Sorafenib is a small molecule inhibitor of multiple tyrosine kinases, including BRAF, CRAF, c-KIT, vascular endothelial growth factor receptor (VEGFR), and platelet-derived growth factor receptor (PDGFR).[25] In preclinical studies, sorafenib slowed the growth of melanoma xenografts in nude mice, but it did not cause tumor regression.[26] Among 34 evaluable patients with metastatic melanoma in a phase II trial, only one partial response was observed.[27] Subsequently, more promising results were reported in a phase I/II clinical trial of sorafenib combined with paclitaxel and carboplatin.[28] Although the trial enrolled patients with multiple tumor types, all of the clinical responses were achieved in patients with melanoma; among these patients, the response rate was 42% and the median progression-free survival was approximately 10 months. These results were encouraging when compared with previous trials in melanoma with paclitaxel and carboplatin alone (response rates of <10%–20%)[29,30]; however, a subsequent randomized phase III trial showed that sorafenib did not improve the response rate or progression-free survival compared with the doublet of paclitaxel and carboplatin alone.[31]

These results raised the possibility that mutant *BRAF* was not a good therapeutic target in melanoma. The observation that activating *BRAF* mutations are present in up to 80% of benign nevi—indolent lesions with almost no malignant potential—is certainly consistent with the hypothesis that this genetic alteration alone cannot fully explain the aggressive biology of melanoma.[16] Similarly, introduction of the *BRAF V600E* mutation alone was not sufficient to transform melanocytes into invasive lesions in multiple models, but rather required complementation by other genetic events to transform cells.[32–34] An alternative explanation for the failure of sorafenib is that mutant *BRAF* is actually a good therapeutic target, but that the drug did not inhibit BRAF effectively. Sorafenib has shown marked clinical efficacy in renal cell carcinoma, a tumor characterized by dependence on VEGFR signaling but not BRAF.[35,36] In the phase II trial of paclitaxel, carboplatin, and sorafenib, no association was noted between the presence of *BRAF* mutations and clinical responses, but a positive association was seen with expression of the VEGFR2 protein and clinical response.[28,37]

The potential of the BRAF V600E protein as a therapeutic target for melanoma has now been validated by clinical trials with second-generation BRAF inhibitors. PLX4032 (also known as RG7204) is a more potent BRAF inhibitor than sorafenib, and it is selective for the V600E mutant form of the protein. PLX4032 inhibits the catalytic activity of the BRAF V600E protein at an IC50 of 13 nM, which is more than 10-fold lower than the dose that inhibits the wild-type protein.[38] In contrast to sorafenib, an inhibitor of multiple protein kinases at therapeutic drug levels, PLX4032 has minimal activity against most other protein kinases, with an IC50 greater than 1000 nM for many related proteins. Preclinical studies showed that PLX4032 inhibited the growth of melanoma cells with a *BRAF* mutation at 10 to 100 times lower concentrations than melanoma cell lines without a mutant *BRAF*.[39] PLX4032 also caused the regression of *BRAF*-mutant melanoma xenografts in mouse models.[39]

Recently, the results of a phase I clinical trial with PLX4032 were reported.[40,41] In the initial phase of the trial, the drug was well tolerated but no clinical responses were observed. However, the serum levels achieved were below those that correlated with antitumor activity in vitro. The drug was then reformulated from a crystalline compound to a microprecipitated bulk powder. Subsequently, linear dose-dependent increases in serum levels were observed, as were clinical responses. In the phase I trial dose expansion cohort of 32 patients with *BRAF V600E*–mutant melanoma treated with 960 mg twice daily (the dose selected for further testing), 2 complete and 24 partial responses were observed, for an overall response rate of 81%.[41] The major toxicity was the development of cutaneous squamous cell carcinomas, mostly keratoacanthomas, which developed in 31% of patients. These lesions were treated with surgical resection and did not result in any patient coming off study. No squamous cell carcinomas were observed at noncutaneous sites. Although this high overall response rate is unprecedented for a single agent in melanoma, several patients developed secondary resistance after their initial response, noted by tumor recurrence or progression. The median duration of response to PLX4032 in the initial trial report was approximately 7 months.[41]

The efficacy of targeting mutant *BRAF* is also supported by early results from the phase I trial of GSK2118436, another potent, mutant-specific BRAF inhibitor.[42] Although the maximum tolerated dose has yet to be reached, patients with *BRAF*-mutant melanoma treated with 150 to 200 mg twice daily had a 63% response rate, and 39% of patients treated with lower doses had also experienced a response.

The duration of these responses is currently unknown. Similar to the PLX4032 trial, cutaneous squamous cell carcinomas were the major toxicity observed in the GSK2118436 trial.

The reported activities of PLX4032 and GSK2118436 in patients with *BRAF V600E*–mutant melanoma suggest that a new standard of care likely will soon exist for these patients. However, it is also apparent that these agents should not be used in unselected patients with melanoma. In the phase I trial of PLX4032, five patients were included who did not have a *BRAF* mutation. None of these patients experienced a response; in fact, four experienced tumor progression in the first 2 months of treatment.[41] The lack of clinical response, and possible rapid progression, in patients not harboring a *BRAF* mutation is consistent with observations in preclinical models by four different groups, suggesting potential promotion of tumor growth when mutant-selective BRAF inhibitors are used to treat *BRAF* wild-type melanomas.[22,43–45] In these experiments, inhibition of BRAF in melanoma cell lines expressing wild-type *BRAF* resulted in the hyperactivation of the MAPK pathway. Although the results varied somewhat among the groups, the BRAF inhibitors promoted the formation of heterodimers of BRAF and CRAF that potently activate MEK in cells without a *BRAF* mutation. The cells were then dependent on CRAF for MAPK pathway activation and survival. Low–catalytic-activity BRAF mutants seem to activate MAPK similarly, and preclinical evidence suggests that melanoma cells with these mutations are sensitive to CRAF inhibition, including treatment with sorafenib.[22,46] Thus, although sorafenib failed to show activity in unselected patients, it may be effective for certain genetic subtypes of melanoma.

NRAS

Mutations in the members of the RAS family of GTP-ases are one of the most frequent events in cancer.[47] Although mutations of *HRAS* and *KRAS* are common in many cancer types, they are rare in melanoma. However, *NRAS* mutations have been reported in 14% of human melanoma cell lines and 15% to 25% of melanoma clinical specimens.[15,48–50] The mutations affecting *NRAS* are highly conserved; mutations affecting codons 12, 13, and 61 constitute approximately 90% of the mutations reported in melanoma.[15] The prevalence of *NRAS* mutations varies across the different anatomically defined melanoma subgroups, although not as dramatically as observed with *BRAF* mutations (see **Table 1**). *NRAS* mutations are detected in approximately 26% of cutaneous, 14% of mucosal, and fewer than 1% of uveal melanomas.[15] Among cutaneous melanomas, 22% of superficial spreading melanomas and 28% of nodular melanomas have *NRAS* mutations, whereas significantly lower rates are observed in acral lentiginous (4%), spitzoid (10%), and lentigo maligna melanomas (0%).[49–51] *NRAS* mutations are also present in common acquired nevi (6%–20%) at a similar rate as has been detected in melanomas, and potentially at an even higher rate in congenital nevi.[17–20] Although rare in melanoma and other types of melanocytic nevi, *HRAS* mutations have been reported in 12 to 29% of Spitz nevi.[51,52]

With rare exceptions, the common activating *BRAF* and *NRAS* mutations are mutually exclusive in melanoma tumor and cell lines,[48,49,53] probably because both of these mutations potentially activate the MAPK pathway, and the presence of both would be functionally redundant. In contrast, approximately 10% of melanomas with *BRAF* mutations that are catalytically inactive (ie, D594V) also have activating *NRAS* mutations.[22] Although the activated mutant forms of BRAF and NRAS both activate MEK and MAPK, the activation of these downstream elements is CRAF-dependent in melanomas with *NRAS* mutations, whereas it is BRAF-dependent in *BRAF*-mutant cells.[54]

The development of direct RAS inhibitors, a priority in several cancer types, has been challenging.[55] One approach has involved the development of farnesyl transferase inhibitors (FTIs), because RAS proteins must be farnesylated to translocate to the plasma membrane and activate their related signaling pathways. However, when farnesylation is inhibited, both NRAS and KRAS undergo an alternative modification, geranylgeranylation, that allows the proteins to be recruited to the plasma membrane.[56] In addition, because more than 60 cellular proteins have been shown to be farnesylated, FTIs will likely have off-target effects (and potentially dose-limiting toxicities) that compromise the ability to reach levels that effectively inhibit RAS. This lack of specificity also makes the role of RAS in both the activity and toxicity of FTIs challenging to determine.

An alternative strategy to treat *NRAS*-mutant tumors is to inhibit pathways that are downstream of the mutant RAS protein. Experiments in multiple tumor types have shown that mutant RAS activates multiple prosurvival and proliferative pathways in addition to the RAF-MEK-MAPK cascade.[57] Other RAS effectors include PI3K, RALGDS, and PKCε. Among these, PI3K has gained particular attention, because the PI3K-AKT pathway has been implicated in melanoma by other genetic events, and is the target of aggressive drug development (see **Fig. 1**).[58,59]

PI3K-AKT PATHWAY

The PI3K-AKT pathway is one of the most important signaling networks in cancer.[60] PI3K is a lipid kinase that consists of a regulatory subunit (*PIK3R*; p85) and a catalytic subunit (*PIK3C;* p110). PI3K's catalytic activity is activated by several different signals, including growth factor tyrosine kinase receptors and activated RAS proteins. Activation of PI3K results in the phosphorylation of the 3'-OH of phosphatidylinositols (PI) in the plasma membrane, generating $PI(3,4)P_2$ and $PI(3,4,5)P_3$. These 3'-phospholipids recruit proteins to the cell membrane that have a pleckstrin homology domain, such as AKT and PDK1. AKT, a serine-threonine kinase that normally exists in an inactive state in the cytoplasm, has been extensively studied as one of the key molecules regulated by PI3K. On recruitment to the plasma membrane, AKT is phosphorylated at two critical residues, Ser473 (by the mTORC2 complex) and Thr308 (by PDK1), which activates its serine–threonine kinase activity. The activated AKT molecule translocates to the cytoplasm where it phosphorylates various substrates, including FOXO, GSK3α/β, BAD, TSC2, and MDM2 (see **Fig. 1**). Through these and other substrates, AKT activation regulates several processes that contribute to the malignant phenotype, including proliferation, survival, invasion, and angiogenesis.[60]

The PI3K-AKT pathway is affected by mutations that activate it more than any other signaling pathway in cancer.[61] The PI3K-AKT pathway was initially implicated in melanoma through the identification of activating *NRAS* mutations. In addition, loss of function of PTEN, a critical negative regulator of the pathway, is a frequent event in melanoma. PTEN inhibits the activation of AKT by dephosphorylating PIs at the 3' position, thereby antagonizing PI3K-mediated signaling (see **Fig. 1**).[62] Loss of PTEN results in constitutive activation of AKT in multiple cancer types, including melanoma.[63] Loss of PTEN, through both genetic and epigenetic mechanisms, has been reported in 10% to 30% of melanomas.[64–66] The prevalence of PTEN loss has been defined predominantly in cutaneous melanomas, and therefore the relative prevalence in anatomically defined subtypes is unknown. Nonetheless, loss of PTEN is frequently detected in melanoma tumors and cell lines with a concurrent *BRAF* mutation, but it appears to be mutually exclusive with *NRAS* mutations.[50,67–69] Although this pattern of mutations suggests that PTEN loss and *NRAS* mutations may have functional redundancy, quantitative analysis of AKT activation in melanoma tumors and cell lines showed that loss of PTEN correlated with much higher levels of activated AKT.[70] This finding is similar to those of previous studies that showed nonequivalent activation of, and functional dependence on, different PI3K-AKT pathway effectors by PTEN loss and *PIK3CA* mutations.[71] *PIK3CA* mutations are relatively common in breast and colon cancer, but have been detected in only 2–3% of melanomas.[72,73] Activating mutations of *AKT*, initially identified in breast, colon, and ovarian cancers, have also been detected as rare events in melanoma (2%).[74,75] Each melanoma with an *AKT* mutation also had a *BRAF* mutation. Although activating mutations of *AKT* in other cancers all involved the *AKT1* isoform, some mutations in melanoma affected the *AKT3* gene. A role for AKT3 in melanoma is supported by previous studies that showed a frequent switch from AKT1 to AKT3 expression and dependence in metastatic melanomas.[76,77]

Inhibitors against multiple components of the PI3K-AKT pathway have been developed and are in various stages of clinical testing (see **Fig. 1**).[58] Initial clinical trials were performed with mTOR (mammalian target of rapamycin) inhibitors, partly because the safety of these agents was previously established by the use of rapamycin (an mTOR inhibitor) in patients who underwent transplantation. Similar to the experience in several other cancers, mTOR inhibitors have shown little activity in melanoma. In a phase II clinical trial, the rapamycin analog (rapalog) CCI-779 produced only one short-lived partial response among 33 patients with metastatic melanoma.[78] In contrast to at least some other targeted therapies, in which drug levels sufficient to significantly inhibit their intended target are not attained, mTOR inhibitors seem to reach levels that significantly inhibit their target in vivo.[79,80] However, studies in both clinical specimens and cell lines have shown that rapalogs activate AKT, thus contributing to their lack of efficacy.[80,81]

The mTOR protein participates in two different complexes, referred to as *mTORC1* and *mTORC2*. The mTORC1 complex, which is inhibited by rapalogs, regulates the activation of protein translational machinery through activating P70S6K. However, it also negatively regulates PI3K as part of a feedback regulatory loop of the PI3K-AKT pathway. The mTORC2 complex, which is not inhibited by the rapalogs, phosphorylates and activates AKT.[82] In preclinical models, combined inhibition of the mTORC1 and mTORC2 complexes blocked the activation of P70S6K and AKT, and more effectively inhibited growth and survival of cancer cells, than inhibition of mTORC1 alone.[83] Clinical testing has yet to be reported for this agent. Similarly, clinical trials of PI3K and AKT inhibitors are ongoing. However, preclinical experiments with RAS-mutant tumors, including melanomas, showed synergistic inhibition of tumor growth and survival when inhibitors against the RAS-RAF-MEK-MAPK and PI3K-AKT pathways were combined.[84,85] The high frequency of *BRAF* mutations in melanomas with PTEN loss suggests that combinatorial regimens also may be necessary in other melanoma genotypes.[86]

C-KIT

Although most sun-exposed cutaneous melanomas harbor an activating mutation in *BRAF* or *NRAS* in the MAPK signaling pathway, these changes are relatively rare in noncutaneous melanomas. This disparity led to investigations that attempted to identify other genetic changes that could activate the same or other kinase signaling pathways in these tumors. In the CGH analysis of melanoma subtypes, the chromosomal region 4q12 was selectively amplified in acral lentiginous and mucosal melanomas.[9]

This region harbors several candidate genes, but detailed analysis showed that the *c-KIT* gene was the focal target of copy number gain in this region.[87] Extra copies of *c-KIT* were identified in 8% of mucosal and 7% of acral lentiginous melanomas. The *c-KIT* gene was also amplified in 6% of cutaneous melanomas with evidence of CSD, whereas no amplifications were detected in cutaneous melanomas without CSD. In addition, sequencing of *c-KIT* identified missense mutations in 21% of the mucosal, 11% of the acral, and 17% of the CSD cutaneous melanomas, but 0% of the non-CSD cutaneous melanomas.[87] Subsequent studies reported similar rates of *c-KIT* mutations in mucosal and acral melanomas, but lower rates of mutations in CSD cutaneous tumors, and different rates of gene copy number gain across the subtypes (see **Table 1**).[88–90]

The *c-KIT* gene encodes a membrane tyrosine kinase receptor. Mutations of *c-KIT* are the most common mutation detected in GISTs.[91] These mutations result in constitutive activation of the c-KIT tyrosine kinase and activation of multiple prosurvival signaling pathways, including the MAPK and PI3K-AKT pathways (see **Fig. 1**). GISTs exhibit oncogene addiction to the mutant c-KIT proteins, and c-KIT inhibitors (eg, imatinib) have become the standard treatment for this disease.[92,93]

The mutations that affect *c-KIT* in melanoma occur in the same regions of the gene as are observed in GIST. The finding of activating mutations of *c-KIT* in melanoma was surprising, because previous studies showed that c-KIT protein expression is frequently lost in melanoma progression.[94] Although c-KIT is required for normal melanocyte development, enforced expression of c-KIT in melanoma cells lines resulted in decreased growth and tumorigenicity.[94] Perhaps most importantly, in three phase II clinical trials of imatinib in patients with melanoma, the clinical response rate was only 1.5%.[90] However, these clinical trials were overwhelmingly composed of patients with cutaneous primary melanomas, and thus probably did not include patients with *c-KIT* mutations or amplifications. There are now multiple case reports of metastatic melanoma patients with *c-KIT* mutations achieving dramatic clinical responses to various c-KIT inhibitors.[95–97] Clinical trials restricted to patients with metastatic melanoma with *c-KIT* mutations or amplifications are ongoing.

GNαQ

Mutations in *BRAF, NRAS,* and *c-KIT* are detected in fewer than 1% of uveal melanomas (see **Table 1**). Recently, two different groups reported point mutations in the gene encoding the stimulatory α-subunit of G-protein coupled receptors, GNαQ.[98,99] The mutations were detected in approximately 45% of uveal melanoma clinical specimens and cell lines. The mutations were highly conserved, affecting the *RAS*-like domain of the protein, and specifically occur at the Q209 residue that is analogous to the Q61 residue frequently mutated in *NRAS*.[99] Expression of the mutant GNαQ protein in melanocytes cooperated efficiently with other genes to induce both anchorage-independent growth and tumor formation in mice. Although the pathways that are activated by and critical to the function of the GNαQ protein remain to be fully elucidated, the RAS-RAF-MEK-MAPK pathway seems to be one of its effectors.[99] This finding suggests that inhibitors of this pathway, which were previously believed to be indicated only for cutaneous melanomas, may also have a role in uveal melanoma.

SUMMARY

More than 10 years have passed since the FDA approved a systemic therapy for the treatment of metastatic melanoma. After years of negative clinical trials, melanoma now seems to be entering a new era in which multiple new therapeutic options will be available. The identification of clinically active targeted therapy approaches has been a gradual process, built upon an improved understanding of the appropriate use of these agents. Although the recent results described in this article have generated great enthusiasm in the melanoma community, many critical challenges remain.

The development of effective BRAF inhibitors, associated with unprecedented clinical response rates in appropriately selected patients, is both exciting and informative. The initial negative clinical trials with sorafenib have been followed by promising studies with PLX4032 and GSK2118436. In retrospect, the failure of sorafenib was likely from insufficient inhibition of the MAPK pathway. Indeed, PLX4032 initially failed to show clinical activity, and only achieved clinical responses when its formulation was changed, increasing drug exposure to levels that correlated with efficacy in vitro. Thus, the successful development of this highly active therapy for BRAF-mutant melanomas depended on not only detailed evaluation beyond simply the measurement of clinical efficacy, but also studies to determine if the drug was being appropriately dosed. Going forward, the evaluation of other experimental therapies must include assessment of the drug levels and on-target effects to determine if failures are from the selection of a poor target or the pharmacodynamic failure of the therapy. Melanoma presents the rare opportunity to evaluate easily accessible tumor tissue in many patients because of the frequent spread of this disease to cutaneous, subcutaneous, and lymphatic sites, and thus may be an ideal clinical venue for evaluating new therapies against important targets.

Although targeted therapies against both BRAF and c-KIT have shown marked activity in patients with mutations in these genes, secondary resistance has rapidly developed in many patients.[41,96] If the mutations or pathways that cause this resistance can be identified, rational targeted therapy combinations to overcome or prevent relapses may be identified. Alternatively, targeted therapies may need to be combined with other therapeutic modalities to improve outcomes. For example, while targeted therapies are seemingly characterized by high response rates but relatively short duration of response, immunotherapies are characterized by infrequent responses that are often durable. It is reasonable to hope that combining these modalities may lead to treatments with high rates of durable responses. Evidence exists that targeting activated pathways in melanoma may enhance the immunologic response to the tumors,[100] suggesting that evaluating the effects of new therapies on the interaction of tumor cells with, and their effects on, the immune response may be important to study.[101]

The discovery of BRAF, NRAS, PTEN, and c-KIT alterations in melanoma has supported the development of various rational therapeutic approaches. Although tremendous effort is being focused on optimizing targeted therapies against these proteins and related pathways, approximately 30% of patients with melanoma have no detectable abnormality in these genes. To improve outcomes in these patients, it will be critical to determine whether the tumors are activating similar pathways through as yet unidentified genetic alterations, or if they are characterized by dependence on completely separate and heretofore underappreciated signaling cascades in this disease.

Recently, the first whole-genome sequence of a melanoma was published.[102] This study identified more than 33,000 changes in the melanoma genome compared with the germline, including almost 200 nonsynonymous coding region substitutions. A second high-throughput study to identify mutations in protein tyrosine kinase family members identified somatic mutations in 19 members of this family alone.[103] These initial findings suggest that identifying critical mutational events will require the sequencing of many melanomas to identify recurrent events that are most likely to be functional, which will then need to be investigated further. However, as the identification of *c-KIT* mutations has shown, these analyses will need to incorporate the recognition of the possible molecular diversity of melanomas arising from different anatomic sites. As the recent experiences with targeted therapies have shown, this investment in the understanding of the molecular biology of this disease may rapidly translate into improved outcomes in patients with this highly aggressive disease.

REFERENCES

1. Tsao H, Atkins MB, Sober AJ. Management of cutaneous melanoma. N Engl J Med 2004;351(10):998–1012.
2. Atkins MB, Kunkel L, Sznol M, et al. High-dose recombinant interleukin-2 therapy in patients with metastatic melanoma: long-term survival update. Cancer J Sci Am 2000;6(Suppl 1):S11–14.
3. Phan GQ, Attia P, Steinberg SM, et al. Factors associated with response to high-dose interleukin-2 in patients with metastatic melanoma. J Clin Oncol 2001; 19(15):3477–82.
4. Hodi FS, O 'Day SJ, McDermott DF, et al. Improved survival with ipilimumab in patients with metastatic melanoma. N Engl J Med 2010;363(8):711–23.
5. Atkins MB, Lotze MT, Dutcher JP, et al. High-dose recombinant interleukin 2 therapy for patients with metastatic melanoma: analysis of 270 patients treated between 1985 and 1993. J Clin Oncol 1999;17(7):2105.
6. Davies M, Hennessy B, Mills GB. Point mutations of protein kinases and individualised cancer therapy. Expert Opin Pharmacother 2006;7(16):2243–61.
7. Mass RD, Press MF, Anderson S, et al. Evaluation of clinical outcomes according to HER2 detection by fluorescence in situ hybridization in women with metastatic breast cancer treated with trastuzumab. Clin Breast Cancer 2005;6(3): 240–6.
8. Miller AJ, Mihm MC Jr. Melanoma. N Engl J Med 2006;355(1):51–65.
9. Curtin JA, Fridlyand J, Kageshita T, et al. Distinct sets of genetic alterations in melanoma. N Engl J Med 2005;353(20):2135–47.
10. Harbour JW. Molecular prognostic testing and individualized patient care in uveal melanoma. Am J Ophthalmol 2009;148(6):823–9 e821.
11. Landreville S, Agapova OA, Harbour JW. Emerging insights into the molecular pathogenesis of uveal melanoma. Future Oncol 2008;4(5):629–36.
12. Colicelli J. Human RAS superfamily proteins and related GTPases. Sci STKE 2004;2004(250):RE13.
13. Rubinfeld H, Seger R. The ERK cascade: a prototype of MAPK signaling. Mol Biotechnol 2005;31(2):151–74.
14. Davies H, Bignell GR, Cox C, et al. Mutations of the BRAF gene in human cancer. Nature 2002;417(6892):949–54.
15. Hocker T, Tsao H. Ultraviolet radiation and melanoma: a systematic review and analysis of reported sequence variants. Hum Mutat 2007;28(6):578–88.
16. Pollock PM, Harper UL, Hansen KS, et al. High frequency of BRAF mutations in nevi. Nat Genet 2003;33(1):19–20.
17. Poynter JN, Elder JT, Fullen DR, et al. BRAF and NRAS mutations in melanoma and melanocytic nevi. Melanoma Res 2006;16(4):267–73.
18. Indsto JO, Kumar S, Wang L, et al. Low prevalence of RAS-RAF-activating mutations in Spitz melanocytic nevi compared with other melanocytic lesions. J Cutan Pathol 2007;34(6):448–55.

19. Bauer J, Curtin JA, Pinkel D, et al. Congenital melanocytic nevi frequently harbor NRAS mutations but no BRAF mutations. J Invest Dermatol 2007;127(1):179–82.

20. Saldanha G, Purnell D, Fletcher A, et al. High BRAF mutation frequency does not characterize all melanocytic tumor types. Int J Cancer 2004;111(5):705–10.

21. Garnett MJ, Rana S, Paterson H, et al. Wild-type and mutant B-RAF activate C-RAF through distinct mechanisms involving heterodimerization. Mol Cell 2005;20(6):963–9.

22. Heidorn SJ, Milagre C, Whittaker S, et al. Kinase-Dead BRAF and oncogenic RAS cooperate to drive tumor progression through CRAF. Cell 2010;140(2):209–21.

23. Hingorani SR, Jacobetz MA, Robertson GP, et al. Suppression of BRAF(V599E) in human melanoma abrogates transformation. Cancer Res 2003;63(17): 5198–202.

24. Sumimoto H, Miyagishi M, Miyoshi H, et al. Inhibition of growth and invasive ability of melanoma by inactivation of mutated BRAF with lentivirus-mediated RNA interference. Oncogene 2004;23(36):6031–9.

25. Strumberg D. Preclinical and clinical development of the oral multikinase inhibitor sorafenib in cancer treatment. Drugs Today (Barc) 2005;41(12):773–84.

26. Karasarides M, Chiloeches A, Hayward R, et al. B-RAF is a therapeutic target in melanoma. Oncogene 2004;23(37):6292–8.

27. Eisen T, Ahmad T, Flaherty KT, et al. Sorafenib in advanced melanoma: a phase II randomised discontinuation trial analysis. Br J Cancer 2006;95(5):581–6.

28. Flaherty KT, Schiller J, Schuchter LM, et al. A phase I trial of the oral, multikinase inhibitor sorafenib in combination with carboplatin and paclitaxel. Clin Cancer Res 2008;14(15):4836–42.

29. Hodi FS, Soiffer RJ, Clark J, et al. Phase II study of paclitaxel and carboplatin for malignant melanoma. Am J Clin Oncol 2002;25(3):283–6.

30. Zimpfer-Rechner C, Hofmann U, Figl R, et al. Randomized phase II study of weekly paclitaxel versus paclitaxel and carboplatin as second-line therapy in disseminated melanoma: a multicentre trial of the Dermatologic Co-operative Oncology Group (DeCOG). Melanoma Res 2003;13(5):531–6.

31. Hauschild A, Agarwala SS, Trefzer U, et al. Results of a phase III, randomized, placebo-controlled study of sorafenib in combination with carboplatin and paclitaxel as second-line treatment in patients with unresectable stage iii or stage iv melanoma. J Clin Oncol 2009;27(17):2823–30.

32. Dankort D, Curley DP, Cartlidge RA, et al. Braf(V600E) cooperates with Pten loss to induce metastatic melanoma. Nat Genet 2009;41(5):544–52.

33. Michaloglou C, Vredeveld LC, Soengas MS, et al. BRAFE600-associated senescence-like cell cycle arrest of human naevi. Nature 2005;436(7051):720–4.

34. Patton EE, Widlund HR, Kutok JL, et al. BRAF mutations are sufficient to promote nevi formation and cooperate with p53 in the genesis of melanoma. Curr Biol 2005;15(3):249–54.

35. Escudier B, Szczylik C, Eisen T, et-al. Randomized phase III trial of the Raf kinase and VEGFR inhibitor sorafenib (BAY 43-9006) in patients with advanced renal cell carcinoma (RCC). Presented at: ASCO Annual Meeting 2005. Orlando (FL), May 13–17, 2005.

36. Ratain MJ, Eisen T, Stadler WM, et al. Phase II placebo-controlled randomized discontinuation trial of sorafenib in patients with metastatic renal cell carcinoma. J Clin Oncol 2006;24(16):2505–12.

37. Jilaveanu L, Zito C, Lee SJ, et al. Expression of sorafenib targets in melanoma patients treated with carboplatin, paclitaxel and sorafenib. Clin Cancer Res 2009;15(3):1076–85.

38. Tsai J, Lee JT, Wang W, et al. Discovery of a selective inhibitor of oncogenic B-Raf kinase with potent antimelanoma activity. Proc Natl Acad Sci U S A 2008;105(8):3041–6.

39. Yang H, Higgins B, Kolinsky K, et al. RG7204 (PLX4032), a selective BRAFV600E inhibitor, displays potent antitumor activity in preclinical melanoma models. Cancer Res 2010;70(13):5518–27.

40. Flaherty KT, Puzanov J, Sosman J, et al. Phase I study of PLX4032: proof of concept for V600E BRAF mutation as a therapeutic target in human cancer. J Clin Oncol 2009;27(15s):9000.

41. Flaherty KT, Puzanov I, Kim KB, et al. Inhibition of mutated, activated braf in metastatic melanoma. N Engl J Med 2010;363(9):809–19.

42. Kefford RF, Arkenau H, Brown MP, et al. Phase I/II study of GSK2118436, a selective inhibitor of oncogenic mutant BRAF kinase, in patients with metastatic melanoma and other solid tumors. J Clin Oncol 2010;28(15s):8503.

43. Halaban R, Zhang W, Bacchiocchi A, et al. PLX4032, a selective BRAF V600E kinase inhibitor, activates the erk pathway and enhances cell migration and proliferation of braf wt melanoma cells. Pigment Cell Melanoma Res 2010; 23(2):190–200.

44. Poulikakos PI, Zhang C, Bollag G, et al. RAF inhibitors transactivate RAF dimers and ERK signalling in cells with wild-type BRAF. Nature 2010; 464(7287):427–30.

45. Hatzivassiliou G, Song K, Yen I, et al. RAF inhibitors prime wild-type RAF to activate the MAPK pathway and enhance growth. Nature 2010;464(7287):431–5.

46. Smalley KS, Xiao M, Villanueva J, et al. CRAF inhibition induces apoptosis in melanoma cells with non-V600E BRAF mutations. Oncogene 2009;28(1):85–94.

47. Giehl K. Oncogenic Ras in tumour progression and metastasis. Biol Chem 2005; 386(3):193–205.

48. Edlundh-Rose EA, Egyhazi SB, Omholt KB, et al. NRAS and BRAF mutations in melanoma tumours in relation to clinical characteristics: a study based on mutation screening by pyrosequencing. Melanoma Res 2006;16(6):471–8.

49. Omholt K, Platz A, Kanter L, et al. NRAS and BRAF mutations arise early during melanoma pathogenesis and are preserved throughout tumor progression. Clin Cancer Res 2003;9(17):6483–8.

50. Tsao H, Goel V, Wu H, et al. Genetic interaction between nras and braf mutations and pten//mmac1 inactivation in melanoma. J Invest Dermatol 2004;122(2): 337–41.

51. Bastian BC, LeBoit PE, Pinkel D. Mutations and copy number increase of HRAS in Spitz nevi with distinctive histopathological features. Am J Pathol 2000;157(3): 967–72.

52. van Dijk MC, Bernsen MR, Ruiter DJP. Analysis of mutations in b-raf, n-ras, and h-ras genes in the differential diagnosis of Spitz nevus and spitzoid melanoma. Am J Surg Pathol 2005;29(9):1145–51.

53. Greene VR, Johnson MM, Grimm EA, et al. Frequencies of NRAS and BRAF mutations increase from the radial to the vertical growth phase in cutaneous melanoma. J Invest Dermatol 2009;129(6):1483–8.

54. Dumaz N, Hayward R, Martin J, et al. In Melanoma, RAS mutations are accompanied by switching signaling from BRAF to CRAF and disrupted cyclic AMP Signaling. Cancer Res 2006;66(19):9483–91.

55. Konstantinopoulos PA, Karamouzis MV, Papavassiliou AG. Post-translational modifications and regulation of the RAS superfamily of GTPases as anticancer targets. Nat Rev Drug Discov 2007;6(7):541–55.

56. Zhang FL, Kirschmeier P, Carr D, et al. Characterization of Ha-ras, N-ras, Ki-Ras4A, and Ki-Ras4B as in vitro substrates for farnesyl protein transferase and geranylgeranyl protein transferase type I. J Biol Chem 1997;272(15):10232–9.

57. Downward J. PI 3-kinase, Akt and cell survival. Semin Cell Dev Biol 2004;15(2): 177–82.

58. Courtney KD, Corcoran RB, Engelman JA. The PI3K pathway as drug target in human cancer. J Clin Oncol 2010;28(6):1075–83.

59. Hennessy BT, Smith DL, Ram PT, et al. Exploiting the PI3K/AKT pathway for cancer drug discovery. Nat Rev Drug Discov 2005;4(12):988–1004.

60. Vivanco I, Sawyers CL. The phosphatidylinositol 3-Kinase AKT pathway in human cancer. Nat Rev Cancer 2002;2(7):489–501.

61. Yuan TL, Cantley LC. PI3K pathway alterations in cancer: variations on a theme. Oncogene 2008;27(41):5497–510.

62. Maehama T, Dixon JE. The tumor suppressor, PTEN/MMAC1, dephosphorylates the lipid second messenger, phosphatidylinositol 3,4,5-trisphosphate. J Biol Chem 1998;273(22):13375–8.

63. Stahl JM, Cheung M, Sharma A, et al. Loss of PTEN promotes tumor development in malignant melanoma. Cancer Res 2003;63(11):2881–90.

64. Mirmohammadsadegh A, Marini A, Nambiar S, et al. Epigenetic silencing of the PTEN gene in melanoma. Cancer Res 2006;66(13):6546–52.

65. Wu H, Goel V, Haluska FG. PTEN signaling pathways in melanoma. Oncogene 2003;22(20):3113–22.

66. Zhou XP, Gimm O, Hampel H, et al. Epigenetic PTEN silencing in malignant melanomas without PTEN mutation. Am J Pathol 2000;157(4):1123–8.

67. Goel VK, Lazar AJ, Warneke CL, et al. Examination of mutations in BRAF, NRAS, and PTEN in primary cutaneous melanoma. J Invest Dermatol 2006;126(1): 154–60.

68. Tsao H, Zhang X, Benoit E, et al. Identification of PTEN/MMAC1 alterations in uncultured melanomas and melanoma cell lines. Oncogene 1998;16(26): 3397–402.

69. Tsao H, Zhang X, Fowlkes K, et al. Relative reciprocity of NRAS and PTEN/MMAC1 alterations in cutaneous melanoma cell lines. Cancer Res 2000;60(7): 1800–4.

70. Davies MA, Stemke-Hale K, Lin E, et al. Integrated molecular and clinical analysis of AKT activation in metastatic melanoma. Clin Cancer Res 2009;15(24): 7538–46.

71. Vasudevan KM, Barbie DA, Davies MA, et al. AKT-independent signaling downstream of oncogenic PIK3CA mutations in human cancer. Cancer Cell 2009; 16(1):21–32.

72. Omholt K, Krockel D, Ringborg U, et al. Mutations of PIK3CA are rare in cutaneous melanoma. Melanoma Res 2006;16(2):197–200.

73. Curtin JA, Stark MS, Pinkel D, et al. PI3-kinase subunits are infrequent somatic targets in melanoma. J Invest Dermatol 2006;126(7):1660–3.

74. Carpten JD, Faber AL, Horn C, et al. A transforming mutation in the pleckstrin homology domain of AKT1 in cancer. Nature 2007;448(7152):439–44.

75. Davies MA, Stemke-Hale K, Tellez C, et al. A novel AKT3 mutation in melanoma tumours and cell lines. Br J Cancer 2008;99(8):1265–8.

76. Robertson GP. Functional and therapeutic significance of Akt deregulation in malignant melanoma. Cancer Metastasis Rev 2005;24(2):273–85.

77. Stahl JM, Sharma A, Cheung M, et al. Deregulated Akt3 activity promotes development of malignant melanoma. Cancer Res 2004;64(19):7002–10.

78. Margolin K, Longmate J, Baratta T, et al. CCI-779 in metastatic melanoma: a phase II trial of the California Cancer Consortium. Cancer 2005;104(5):1045–8.
79. Kim KB, Davies MA, Papadopoulos N, et al. Phase I/II study of the combination of sorafenib and temsirolimus in patients with metastatic melanoma. J Clin Oncol 2009;27(15s):9026.
80. Tabernero J, Rojo F, Calvo E, et al. Dose- and schedule-dependent inhibition of the mammalian target of rapamycin pathway with everolimus: a phase I tumor pharmacodynamic study in patients with advanced solid tumors. J Clin Oncol 2008;26(10):1603–10.
81. O 'Reilly KE, Rojo F, She QB, et al. mTOR inhibition induces upstream receptor tyrosine kinase signaling and activates Akt. Cancer Res 2006;66(3):1500–8.
82. Sarbassov DD, Ali SM, Sengupta S, et al. Prolonged rapamycin treatment inhibits mTORC2 assembly and Akt/PKB. Mol Cell 2006;22(2):159–68.
83. Chresta CM, Davies BR, Hickson I, et al. AZD8055 Is a potent, selective, and orally bioavailable ATP-competitive mammalian target of rapamycin kinase inhibitor with in vitro and in vivo antitumor activity. Cancer Res 2010;70(1):288–98.
84. Engelman JA, Chen L, Tan X, et al. Effective use of PI3K and MEK inhibitors to treat mutant Kras G12D and PIK3CA H1047R murine lung cancers. Nat Med 2008;14(12):1351–6.
85. Jaiswal BS, Janakiraman V, Kljavin NM, et al. Combined targeting of BRAF and CRAF or BRAF and PI3K effector pathways is required for efficacy in NRAS mutant tumors. PLoS One 2009;4(5):e5717.
86. Tran MA, Gowda R, Sharma A, et al. Targeting V600EB-Raf and Akt3 using nanoliposomal-small interfering RNA inhibits cutaneous melanocytic lesion development. Cancer Res 2008;68(18):7638–49.
87. Curtin JA, Busam K, Pinkel D, et al. Somatic activation of KIT in distinct subtypes of melanoma. J Clin Oncol 2006;24(26):4340–6.
88. Beadling C, Jacobson-Dunlop E, Hodi FS, et al. KIT gene mutations and copy number in melanoma subtypes. Clin Cancer Res 2008;14(21):6821–8.
89. Handolias D, Salemi R, Murray W, et al. Mutations in KIT occur at low frequency in melanomas arising from anatomical sites associated with chronic and intermittent sun exposure. Pigment Cell Melanoma Res 2010;23:210–5.
90. Woodman SE, Davies MA. Targeting KIT in melanoma: a paradigm of molecular medicine and targeted therapeutics. Biochem Pharmacol 2010;80(5):568–74.
91. Hirota S, Isozaki K, Moriyama Y, et al. Gain-of-function mutations of c-kit in human gastrointestinal stromal tumors. Science 1998;279(5350):577–80.
92. Blanke CD, Demetri GD, von Mehren M, et al. Long-term results from a randomized phase II trial of standard- versus higher-dose imatinib mesylate for patients with unresectable or metastatic gastrointestinal stromal tumors expressing KIT. J Clin Oncol 2008;26(4):620–5.
93. Demetri GD, von Mehren M, Blanke CD, et al. Efficacy and safety of imatinib mesylate in advanced gastrointestinal stromal tumors. N Engl J Med 2002;347(7):472–80.
94. Huang S, Luca M, Gutman M, et al. Enforced c-KIT expression renders highly metastatic human melanoma cells susceptible to stem cell factor-induced apoptosis and inhibits their tumorigenic and metastatic potential. Oncogene 1996;13(11):2339–47.
95. Hodi FS, Friedlander P, Corless CL, et al. Major response to imatinib mesylate in KIT-mutated melanoma. J Clin Oncol 2008;26(12):2046–51.
96. Woodman SE, Trent JC, Stemke-Hale K, et al. Activity of dasatinib against L576P KIT mutant melanoma: molecular, cellular, and clinical correlates. Mol Cancer Ther 2009;8(8):2079–85.

97. Quintas-Cardama A, Lazar AJ, Woodman SE, et al. Complete response of stage IV anal mucosal melanoma expressing KIT Val560Asp to the multikinase inhibitor sorafenib. Nat Clin Pract Oncol 2008;5(12):737–40.

98. Onken MD, Worley LA, Long MD, et al. Oncogenic mutations in GNAQ occur early in uveal melanoma. Invest Ophthalmol Vis Sci 2008;49(12):5230–4.

99. Van Raamsdonk CD, Bezrookove V, Green G, et al. Frequent somatic mutations of GNAQ in uveal melanoma and blue naevi. Nature 2009;457(7229):599–602.

100. Boni A, Cogdill AP, Dang P, et al. Selective BRAFV600E inhibition enhances T-Cell recognition of melanoma without affecting lymphocyte function. Cancer Res 2010;70(13):5213–9.

101. López-Fauqued M, Gil R, Grueso J, et al. The dual PI3K/mTOR inhibitor PI-103 promotes immunosuppression, in vivo tumor growth and increases survival of sorafenib-treated melanoma cells. Int J Cancer 2010;126(7):1549–61.

102. Pleasance ED, Cheetham RK, Stephens PJ, et al. A comprehensive catalogue of somatic mutations from a human cancer genome. Nature 2010;463(7278):191–6.

103. Prickett TD, Agrawal NS, Wei X, et al. Analysis of the tyrosine kinome in melanoma reveals recurrent mutations in ERBB4. Nat Genet 2009;41(10):1127–32.

Evidence-Based Follow-up for the Patient with Melanoma

Ryan C. Fields, MD[a], Daniel G. Coit, MD[b],*

KEYWORDS

• Melanoma • Evidence-based follow-up • Outcomes

When a patient with a solid tumor has been found to have no evidence of disease (NED) by a combination of surgery, chemotherapy, and/or radiation, they are entered into a follow-up program that entails a combination of clinical visits with history and physical examination, laboratory and radiographic investigations, and psychosocial support. The frequency and intensity of visits and choice of studies are generally based on the timing and patterns of recurrence for that particular malignancy. The primary goal of a follow-up program is early detection of recurrent disease, and is based on the premise that earlier detection of tumor recurrence allows for treatment and potential cure of recurrent disease. A secondary goal of a follow-up program is detection of second primary tumors, which is based on the observation in many solid malignancies that patients are at higher risk for developing secondary malignancies compared with the general population. Tertiary goals of follow-up programs include psychosocial support for the surviving patient and systematic recording of outcomes to track the efficacy of treatment regimens.

Conceptually, if early detection of recurrence and/or new primary lesions can lead to improved survival, the surface location, locoregional recurrence patterns, and increased rates of secondary tumors make melanoma ideal for a program of intensive follow-up. Overall, among patients whose melanoma recurs, 20% to 28% first recur with local or in-transit disease, 26% to 60% with regional nodal disease, and 15% to 50% with distant metastases.[1] When melanoma recurs locally, in-transit, or in regional nodal basins, approximately one-third of patients can be cured with additional treatment.[2] In contrast, patients with distant metastases have a more dismal prognosis,

---

The authors have nothing to disclose.

[a] Department of Surgery, Memorial Sloan-Kettering Cancer Center, 1275 York Avenue, New York, NY 10065, USA

[b] Gastric & Mixed Tumor Service, Department of Surgery, Memorial Sloan-Kettering Cancer Center, 1275 York Avenue, New York, NY 10065, USA

* Corresponding author.

E-mail address: coitd@mskcc.org

Surg Oncol Clin N Am 20 (2011) 181–200

doi:10.1016/j.soc.2010.09.009

surgonc.theclinics.com

with 5-year survival less than 10%. However, there is a small, highly selected subset of patients with resectable stage IV tumors who can achieve 5-year survival of 20%.[3]

On the one hand, a physician who treats patients with melanoma could argue that intensive follow-up identifies patients with early recurrences who could be effectively treated to positively affect survival. On the other hand, with decades of experience with intensive follow-up programs, there is no level 1 evidence (and scant level 2–4 evidence) to support the hypothesis that more intensive follow-up of the patient with melanoma (consisting of combinations of history, physical examination, laboratory tests, and radiographic studies) has any effect on survival. Furthermore, both the rising prevalence of melanoma[4] and the fact that most patients with melanoma are rendered NED after initial treatment, have led to more patients who need to be enrolled in follow-up programs for longer periods, creating a scenario in which providers of melanoma care could be overwhelmed with cured patients in follow-up programs. Even the basic premise of early detection of recurrence leading to improved outcomes is questionable, because there is no effective treatment that leads to improved survival in patients with recurrent systemic melanoma.[5] All of these factors, along with the need for cost-effective health care, have led many to question the need for and usefulness of intensive follow-up in patients with melanoma[1,2,6] and to stress the importance of better prospective studies to evaluate the benefit of follow-up.[7]

There are no universally accepted guidelines for the follow-up of patients with melanoma. Most follow-up schedules are based on timing and patterns of recurrence derived from large retrospective reviews. Patient-related features, such as the definition of a patient-detected recurrence, clinician-detected recurrence, and the breakdown of symptomatic and asymptomatic recurrences and their corresponding definitions, limits comparisons of these studies. There is significant variability in follow-up recommendations from various organizations (**Table 1**) across all continents. The efficacy and outcomes of these follow-up programs are also retrospective in nature. Thus, the evidence for and against various types of follow-up is weak (level 3 and lower). Only one prospective study in the literature addresses melanoma follow-up,[8] and this was methodologically limited by the inclusion of patients with known metastatic disease. To date, the most methodologically complete data on follow-up of patients with melanoma come from 2 comprehensive literature reviews.[1,2]

This article reviews the best evidence available to guide the follow-up of patients with melanoma, focusing on incidence and detection of melanoma recurrence, frequency of follow-up visits, yield of laboratory and radiographic tests, outcomes of patients with recurrent melanoma based on method of detection, detection of secondary melanomas, and stage-specific follow-up.

INCIDENCE OF MELANOMA RECURRENCE DURING FOLLOW-UP

Of all patients with stage I to III completely resected melanomas, 30% develop a recurrence,[2,9,10] and approximately 80% of these occur within 3 years of diagnosis of their primary melanoma.[11] Although it is rare for a melanoma to recur after 10 years of follow-up, there are case reports of recurrent melanoma up to 46 years after treatment of a primary melanoma.[12] Late recurrence of melanoma (>10 years after treatment) is largely an observation limited to patients who initially present with early, node-negative primary tumors.

The probability of recurrence is clearly stage dependent. In an analysis of 4748 patients with stage I and II melanoma, melanoma recurred in 18.9% of patients: 5.2% for stage IA, 18.4% for stage IB, 28.7% for stage IIA, 40.6% for stage IIB, and 44.3% for stage IIC.[13]

Table 1
Comparison of follow-up recommendations for patients with melanoma from the NCCN guidelines (United States), the clinical practice guidelines for the management of melanoma in Australia and New Zealand, and the German Cancer Society

Follow-up Category	Consensus Group Recommendations		
	NCCN (United States)[23]	Australia/New Zealand[27]	Germany[26]
Self-examination Recommended?	Yes	Yes	Not stated
Follow-up Interval			
Stage I	3–12 mo × 5 years[a]	6 mo × 5 years[b]	6 mo × 5 years[c]
Stage II and III	3 – 6 mo × 2 years[a] 3–12 months × 3 years[a]	3–4 mo × 5 years[b]	3 mo × 5 years[d]
Routine Imaging?			
Stage I	No	No	No
Stage II and III	Consider[e]	No	Yes[f]
Routine Blood Work?	No	No	Yes[g]

Abbreviations: CT, computed tomography; CXR, chest radiograph; MRI, magnetic resonance imaging; PET, positron emission tomography; US, ultrasound.
[a] Annual follow-up after 5 years as clinically indicated.
[b] Annual follow-up after 5 years.
[c] 6- to 12-month follow-up in years 6 to 10.
[d] 6-month follow-up in years 6 to 10.
[e] Consider CXR, CT, and/or PET-CT scans to screen for recurrent/metastatic disease. Consider brain MRI annually. Routine imaging is not recommended after 5 years.
[f] Regional lymph node US for stage II (every 6 months) and III (every 3 months) melanomas for 5 years. Abdominal US and CXR or CT, MRI, or PET scan at each visit for 5 years.
[g] Serum S-100B protein levels every 3 to 6 months for stage II and III melanomas.

PATTERNS OF MELANOMA RECURRENCE DURING FOLLOW-UP

In their comprehensive literature review in 2005, Francken and colleagues[1] identified 8 studies that reported the incidence of recurrence in patients with melanoma in follow-up programs. In all patients, most of whom were stage I or II, the rates of recurrence were 3% to 5% for local or in-transit, 5% to 13% for regional nodal, and 3% to 10% for distant recurrence. Among patients whose melanoma recurred, 20% to 28% first present with local or in-transit recurrences, 26% to 60% with regional nodal recurrences, and 15% to 50% with distant recurrences. The wide variation in recurrence rates and patterns can likely be explained by the different proportion of stage I, II, and III patients, as well as how they were staged in these studies. For example, Baughan and colleagues[14] included only stage I patients in their analysis, whereas Hoffman and colleagues[15] included all completely resected stage I, II, and III patients in their series. Most recently, Francken and colleagues[16] from the Sydney Melanoma Unit showed that the site of first recurrence in 211 patients with stage I to III melanoma was local in 13% of patients, in-transit in 17%, regional in 46%, and distant in 24% of patients.

DETECTION OF MELANOMA RECURRENCE

In general, melanoma recurrences are detected more often by patients than by health care professionals at scheduled follow-up visits.[14,16–20] Numerous reports in the literature indicate that three-quarters of all recurrences are detected by patients, whereas one-quarter are detected by clinicians. However, some series have found the opposite, with increased rates of recurrences detected by health care professionals.[15,21] Overall, the rate of first recurrences detected by patients from all reports in the literature is 33% to 99%. Even in stage III patients, who could be considered at highest risk for systemic recurrence and might benefit most from physician-directed follow-up examination and studies, 62% of local and in-transit recurrences, 49% of nodal recurrences, and 37% of systemic recurrences were initially detected by the patients.[22] The retrospective nature of these reports and varied methods of detection of recurrence make comparisons difficult. For example, some studies used questionnaires that were mailed out to all patients whose melanoma recurred and asked them to recall who detected the recurrence, whereas other studies audited the medical record to determine who detected the first recurrence. Yet others based definition of a patient-detected recurrence as one found on an unscheduled clinic visit. In the single prospective study evaluating follow-up of patients with melanoma, only 17% of recurrences were detected by the patients.[8] However, this study captured all recurrences (first and subsequent), so it is difficult to compare with the other retrospective analyses.

A logical question is whether method of detection of recurrence has any effect on survival: no study has ever randomized patients to follow-up versus no follow-up, so level I evidence to address this question is lacking and only indirect observations can be made. Two studies have specifically addressed this question. Mooney and colleagues[20] did not find any difference in overall survival between patients with asymptomatic (recurrences detected by clinicians on physical examination and/or laboratory/imaging investigations) versus symptomatic (patient-detected) recurrences. In their study, 72% of recurrences were detected by patients. Similarly, Francken and colleagues[16] found no difference in survival in recurrences detected by patients versus recurrences detected by physicians. In their report, 73% of recurrences were detected by the patients, and most were symptomatic. In contrast, Poo-Hwu and colleagues[21] reported a 5.8% improvement in overall survival for patients with asymptomatic recurrences discovered at routine follow-up, compared with symptomatic recurrences discovered by patients. However, biases in lead time (earlier detection that increases the time between diagnosis and death artificially) and length time (slow-progressing lesions with less aggressive potential are preferably detected), differences in the biologic nature of tumors discovered by patients versus health care providers, and differences in patients included in these analyses could account for these differences. In their prospective evaluation of melanoma recurrence, Garbe and colleagues[8] stratified first recurrences as either early (asymptomatic) or late (symptomatic) and found a higher survival rate for patients with early versus late recurrences (76% vs 38% overall survival after 3 years). In this analysis, recurrences were not stratified based on who detected them (patient vs health care professional), and patients with all types of recurrences (first or subsequent) were included in their study and evaluation, once again limiting the ability to compare these results with other studies. Romano and colleagues[22] specifically addressed site and timing for first relapse in stage III patients with melanoma. Their evaluation of 340 patients with a median follow-up of 77 months found overall recurrence-free survival rates for stage IIIA, IIIB, and IIIC of 63%, 32%, and 11%, respectively. Site of first relapse was local/in-transit in 28% of patients, regional nodal in 21% of patients, and systemic in 51% of patients. First relapses were detected by the patient in 47% of cases, clinically by the physician in 21% of patients, and by screening radiologic tests in 32% of patients. Multivariate analysis found that improved survival was associated with younger age, local/in-transit or nodal recurrence, asymptomatic recurrences, or resectable systemic recurrences. The investigators concluded that, based on the timing and site of relapse, routine physical examinations beyond 3 years for stage IIIA, 2 years for stage IIIB, and 1 year for stage IIIC and routine radiologic imaging beyond 3 years for stages IIIA and IIIB and 2 years for stage IIIC patients was of low yield and that published guidelines should strongly consider whether or not they should be included in recommendations for long-term follow-up.

FREQUENCY OF FOLLOW-UP

Guidelines from most countries, melanoma cooperative groups, and consensus guidelines recommend follow-up visits with a physician who specializes in melanoma (surgical oncologist, dermatologist, or medical oncologist) with a complete history, physical examination (including skin and regional lymph node examination) every 3 to 12 months for the first 5 years after treatment of melanoma.[23–27] Generally, follow-up is spaced out to every 6 to 12 months for 5 more years, with stage-specific frequency of visits. **Table 1** summarizes the recommendations from 3 major multidisciplinary groups with expertise in melanoma (the National Comprehensive Cancer Network [NCCN, United States], the Clinical Practice Guidelines for the Management of Melanoma in Australia and New Zealand, and the German Cancer Society) across 3 continents. The variability in follow-up frequency in these 3 recommendations is representative of other national and professional organizations.

Based on the consistent observations that most recurrences are detected by patients and that patient- versus clinician-detected recurrences do not affect survival, the concluding remarks from many studies suggest less frequent follow-up, although a specific time course outside major published guidelines is rarely suggested. For example, Francken and colleagues[16] conclude that "the frequency of follow-up visits in an earlier SMU (Sydney Melanoma Unit) study and by other groups could be reduced for most patients." They go on to remark, "However, individual patient-related factors such as physical and mental health, travel distance, and personal preferences will always need to be considered, and the extent of resources available to conduct follow-up programs may also be of relevance." This statement summarizes the sentiment that many melanoma providers instinctually feel: that increased frequency follow-up does not affect survival and in the era of burgeoning practices and cost constraints, it is difficult to justify. A follow-up article recommends annual follow-up for stage I patients, 6-month follow-up for 2 years, followed by annual visits for stage IIA patients, and 4-month follow-up for 2 years, 6-month follow-up in year 3, and annual follow-up thereafter for stage IIB and IIC patients.[13] As discussed in the preceding section, follow-up examinations and imaging tests were found to be of low yield beyond 3 years in patients with resected stage III melanoma.[22]

In their prospective evaluation of follow-up, Garbe and colleagues[8] adhered to the guidelines published by the German Society of Dermatology, which recommended follow-up examinations every 3 months in the first 5 years, with continued follow-up every 6 months until the 10th year. Based on the results of their study, the German Cancer Society adopted the guidelines presented in **Table 1**, which slightly increased the follow-up intervals for early-stage melanoma.

One strategy to continue high-frequency follow-up, but relieve the burden of the melanoma specialist provider, is to transition patients to their primary care physician (general practitioner [GP]) for follow-up. A randomized trial of GP-led melanoma follow-up in the United Kingdom showed that such a strategy is safe, feasible, engenders greater patient satisfaction, permits closer adherence to guidelines, and does not result in adverse effects on health status or anxiety.[28] There were 142 patients enrolled in this study over a 1-year period. Participating GPs were educated with a 4-hour training session and comprehensive literature for follow-up care, which focused on presentation of new and recurrent melanomas. Although the numbers are small, this study indicates that melanoma follow-up can be safely provided by any clinician, including physician extenders (such as nurse practitioners or physician assistants) educated in the timing and patterns of melanoma recurrence. This finding should not be surprising given the high likelihood that most recurrences are detected by patients.

USEFULNESS OF LABORATORY AND RADIOGRAPHIC TESTS IN THE FOLLOW-UP OF THE PATIENT WITH MELANOMA

In the preceding sections, it seems that patient versus clinician detection of melanoma recurrences, along with the timing and frequency of follow-up visits, does not have an effect on survival. A logical question, then, is whether the addition of laboratory or imaging tests to clinic visits may be able to detect subclinical recurrences, which could then be treated with a combination of surgery, chemotherapy, and/or radiation therapy to improve outcomes. A central premise to this question is that earlier detection of recurrence improves survival. Although intuitively, oncologists often believe this hypothesis to be the case, there is no high-level evidence in melanoma to support it. Intensive follow-up with frequent laboratory and imaging studies, which have a significant false-positive rate, may be detrimental in terms of cost and patient-related anxiety.[2,7,19] The next section reviews the evidence for inclusion of such studies in melanoma follow-up programs.

Laboratory Tests

As **Table 1** indicates, the inclusion of laboratory studies during routine follow-up of the patient with melanoma varies across national guidelines. Historically, a complete laboratory panel (blood count, chemistry, liver enzymes, and lactate dehydrogenase [LDH]) was recommended in the follow-up of all patients with melanoma, but was not based on any evidence.[29,30] The usefulness of this type of shotgun approach to the use of laboratory studies can be summarized as useless in the detection of recurrences,[6,20,31] and detrimental in terms of cost and false-positive results, leading to subsequent futile tests.[20] Even the usefulness of LDH, which has prognostic relevance in stage IV patients, and is incorporated into the staging classification for melanoma, does not have a role in the routine follow-up of stage I to III patients with melanoma.[30,32,33]

The S-100B protein is currently used as a routine immunohistochemical marker in the diagnosis of melanoma and melanoma metastases,[34] and serum levels of S-100B have been shown to be increased in patients with metastatic melanoma.[35,36] Serum levels of S-100B have also been evaluated as a method of early detection of recurrent melanoma. In 141 patients followed for 15 months after complete resection of localized (stage I–II) melanoma, 7 patients experienced a recurrence, and in 6 of these 7 patients, rising serum S-100B levels preceded clinical or radiographic detection of metastases by 4 to 21 months.[37] Similarly, Garbe and colleagues[38] found that in patients with stage II to III resected melanoma, serum S-100B levels enabled earlier detection of distant metastases. In this study, 411 consecutive high-risk patients with melanoma were screened with S-100B serum levels. There were 41 recurrences and 13 (32%) of these patients had an increased S-100B serum level and in 8 (20%) of these, S-100B was the first sign of recurrence. This finding corresponds to a sensitivity and specificity of 32% and 96%, respectively, for the detection of metastases in this study group. A subsequent study by the same group found that S-100B had a sensitivity, specificity, and overall diagnostic accuracy for melanoma recurrence of 29%, 93%, and 84%, respectively.[38] This finding was comparable with another serologic marker, melanoma-inhibitory activity (MIA) protein, which had a sensitivity, specificity, and overall diagnostic accuracy of 22%, 97%, and 86%, respectively. Both S-100B and MIA were superior to LDH and alkaline phosphatase, which had overall accuracy rates of 77% to 79%. In their prospective trial of melanoma follow-up, Garbe and colleagues obtained annual and biannual blood testing in the follow-up of stage I to II and stage III patients, respectively, which included blood counts, erythrocyte sedimentation rate, blood chemistries, liver enzymes, LDH, and S-100B (for the second half of the study, 1996–1998). They found that blood tests were rarely the first sign of metastases, and a first diagnosis was made in only 3 patients after further investigation after the detection of an increased LDH value. S-100B was increased in approximately half of patients with distant metastases and was the first sign of metastases in 25% of patients. However, S-100B was rarely increased in patients with locoregional recurrences and levels did not correlate with survival. Based on these results, the German Cancer Society guidelines recommend the measurement of serum S-100B levels in stage II and III patients with melanoma every 3 to 6 months during follow-up. These are the only major guidelines that recommend routine blood testing in follow-up of patients with melanoma. There is limited experience with S-100B outside Europe; thus, comparison studies are lacking.

The routine use of blood tests in the asymptomatic patient during follow-up for resected melanoma is not warranted. The low sensitivity, specificity, and accuracy for general laboratory profiles make them futile in the detection of subclinical recurrence. There may be a role for melanoma-specific markers (S-100B, MIA) in the follow-up of patients with melanoma, but this is not clearly defined. The lack of increase of these markers in locoregional recurrences, which may be treated for cure, further limits their usefulness.

Radiographic Tests

The role of routine radiographic testing as an adjunct to scheduled clinical visits to detect early recurrences follows the aforementioned unproven hypothesis that earlier detection of melanoma recurrences leads to improved survival. Although effective treatment of local, in-transit, and regional node metastases offers the possibility of cure, long-term survival after resection of systemic metastases is less frequent, but is possible. There are reports using chest radiograph (CXR), regional/nodal ultrasound (US), abdominal US, and computed tomography (CT) and magnetic resonance imaging (MRI) scans in the follow-up of patients with melanoma. Similar to studies mentioned earlier, the comparison of these studies is difficult given the heterogenicity of the patient cohorts, time frames of analysis, and definitions of recurrences. Further, with the exception of the single prospective study by Garbe and colleagues, all of these studies are retrospective in nature. However, the following studies represent the best data to date to guide our clinical practice. Each imaging modality is discussed in the following sections.

CXR and chest CT to detect pulmonary metastases

Screening for pulmonary metastases with CXR and CT scans in patients with melanoma is based on the observation that the lungs are the most common visceral site of metastases.[39] Of patients with pulmonary involvement, 12% to 25% are eligible for surgical resection,[40,41] with 80% to 90% of these patients undergoing complete (R0) resection.[39,42] The 5-year survival in this highly selected group can be as high as 30%.[39,42] Thus, the goal of radiographic screening tests to detect pulmonary metastases is to detect asymptomatic lesions at an earlier stage that are amenable to an R0 resection. Ideally, a randomized trial of routine pulmonary imaging versus no imaging could answer the question of whether these tests improve survival; however, these studies do not exist. CXR is the most studied test to date. In terms of detection of pulmonary metastases, there are mixed findings in the published literature concluding that CXR is able[6,15,20,31,43,44] or unable[45–47] to detect asymptomatic pulmonary metastases from melanoma. In the studies that found that CXR was able to detect pulmonary recurrences, the rate was 0.5% to 6.2% of patients. The wide variability reported in these studies can be explained by the wide range of patients included and the differing length of follow-up. For example Kittler and colleagues[46] and Bassères and colleagues[43] specifically analyzed patients with thin melanomas, whereas studies by Kersey and colleagues, Goerz and colleagues, and Mooney and colleagues [31,44,48] each included more high-risk stage II and III patients in their analyses. No study has shown that the early detection of pulmonary metastases by routine imaging is associated with improved survival. Taso and colleagues[49] examined 994 patients at the Massachusetts General Hospital and found that 75 (8%) patients had pulmonary metastases detected by CXR (1937 total CXRs). In addition, there were 63 (6% of patients) with false-positive results. In 41 patients (4%), CXR was the initial evidence of metastases. Survival after identification of pulmonary metastases did not differ between patients with asymptomatically detected pulmonary metastases versus those with symptomatic or pulmonary metastases found in the setting of other metastatic sites. Meyers and colleagues[19] found that in 118 patients with stage II or III melanoma followed with routine clinical examinations and imaging tests over at least 2 years, only 2 of 43 recurrences (5%) were detected by CXR. At the SMU, Morton and colleagues[50] enrolled 108 patients with stage III patients in a prospective monitoring schedule of CXR every 6 months for 5 years. Patients were followed for a median of 52.5 months, and 23 (21%) developed pulmonary metastases, of which 11 (48% of recurrences) were detected by CXR. Three of the 23 patients with pulmonary recurrences detected by CXR (13% of total) went on to resection. Further, abnormal CXRs were found in 19 additional patients, but not because of recurrence (false-positive result). Median survival did not differ between recurrences detected by CXR and those not detected by CXR. The investigators concluded that because routine CXRs detected only half of pulmonary recurrences, infrequently identified patients for potentially curative surgery, had a high rate of false positivity, and did not affect survival, their use was not justified. In Garbe and colleagues[8] prospective study of melanoma follow-up, CXR detected metastases in 2 patients (11.1%) with stage I melanoma, 11 patients (22.4%) with stage II melanoma, and 13 patients (9.5%) with stage III melanoma. Overall, 0.6% of all CXRs were responsible for the detection of metastases, and as many as 75% of recurrences detected by CXR were first discovered at an advanced phase. These investigators concluded that the routine CXR was of little benefit for stage I and II patients and should be restricted to follow-up of patients with more advanced stages of disease.

Mooney and colleagues[48] performed a cost-effectiveness analysis using data from the Roswell Park Cancer Institute and the National Cancer Institute's Surveillance, Epidemiology, and End Results (SEER) program. They found that the cost of CXR screening per nonquality-adjusted life year and quality-adjusted life year were $150,000 and $165,000, respectively, in 1996 US dollars. This amount accounted for 80% of program costs. Based on these findings, the investigators suggested reducing the frequency of screening CXR.

In an effort to improve the usefulness of CXR in detecting pulmonary recurrences of melanoma, 3 studies have evaluated the use of chest CT scans.[43,45,47] Only one identified metastases, but in only 3 of 364 patients with stage I to III melanoma, 2 of whom had distant metastases elsewhere.[45] However, these studies are limited; the study by Bassères and colleagues[43] evaluated only patients with stage I melanoma, whereas the study by Mijnhout and colleagues[47] comprised only 67 patients with resected stage I to III melanoma, 51 of whom (76%) underwent screening CT scans. Given these results, along with the inability of screening CT scans to readily detect primary lung cancers in heavy smokers without an unacceptable rate of false-positive results,[51] this modality does not seem appropriate for general use in the follow-up of the patient with melanoma.

The overall sensitivity, specificity, false-positive, and false-negative rates of studies examining screening CXR in the follow-up of patients with melanoma is presented in **Table 2**. The inability of this testing modality to detect recurrences and affect survival has led to the omission of routine CXR in the NCCN and Australia/New Zealand guidelines and the limited use of CXR only in stage II and III patients in the German guidelines (see **Table 1**).

Lymph node US to detect regional recurrences

The clinical scenario of isolated local, in-transit, or regional nodal recurrence of melanoma is best suited for intervention for cure. However, a subset of patients presenting with a clinically evident recurrence of this nature, including pathologically enlarged (and thus palpable) regional lymph nodes, also have subclinical stage IV disease and cannot be effectively treated with regional modalities. Thus, earlier detection of regional nodal recurrences, where the recurrence may be limited to the regional nodal basin and can be cured with complete resection, may positively affect survival. All such studies are limited by biases in lead time and length time, as well as differences in biologic growth dynamics of tumors discovered by US versus palpation,[1,2] so the results of these retrospective studies must be taken in this context. Several retrospective studies have evaluated the usefulness of regional/nodal US to detect subclinical nodal metastases. They are summarized in **Table 3** and discussed later.

Tregnaghi and colleagues[52] assessed the diagnostic accuracy of US in 87 patients with resected stage I to III melanomas over a 3-year period. They found a sensitivity, specificity, and accuracy of 86.6%, 94.6%, and 93.3%, with false-positive and false-negative rates of 4.5% and 3.2%. They established several ultrasonographic criteria for determining a positive node on US to improve the overall usefulness of the test in patients with melanoma. These parameters include round shape without striae, localized alteration of the cortex and/or medulla, and expression of nodular formation. Binder and colleagues[53] reported on US versus palpation for detecting regionally recurrent melanoma in 264 patients. They found that US had a sensitivity, specificity, and accuracy of 90.0%, 98.9%, and 97.8%, respectively, with false-positive and false-negative rates of 1.0% and 0.2%, respectively. This finding did not differ significantly with the results of palpation and the investigators concluded that patients with a negative clinical examination did not require further sonography for verification. However, the follow-up length in their study is not stated, thus limiting the interpretation of this conclusion, because it may take time for a melanoma recurrence detected by US to manifest clinically. Blum and colleagues[54] reported on the only prospective study evaluating US compared with palpation for detection of regionally recurrent melanoma. They found that US had a sensitivity and specificity of 89.2% and 99.79%, with a false-positive rate of 9.1%. The sensitivity of US was superior to that of palpation (71.4%). The rates of sensitivity, specificity, and false-positive results in this study, compared with the others in **Table 3**, may be more accurate and a reflection of the prospective nature of this study. Nevertheless, this study clearly shows an advantage

Table 2
Usefulness of CXRs for detection of pulmonary metastases in patients with melanoma

Study	n	Sensitivity (%)	Specificity (%)	False-positive (%)	False-negative (%)	F/U (mo)	Notes
Mooney et al[48] 1997	See footnote[a]	97	54	NR	NR	NR	Cost-effectiveness analysis concluded decreasing screening frequency of CXR
Hoffman et al[15] 2002	661	NR	NR	Stage I/II: 19 Stage III: 12	NR	Stage I/II: 49 Stage III: 18	Detection rates: 7.4% Stage I/II 5% Stage III
Tsao et al[49] 2004	994	NR	48	41%	NR	NR	7.5% of patients identified with pulmonary metastases, 55% of which were asymptomatic
Morton et al[50] 2009	108[b]	48%	78%	52	14	52.5	6- to 12-mo surveillance CXR program

Abbreviations: F/U, follow-up; NR, not reported.
[a] Multiple data sources, including SEER (n = 37,276), Institutional database (n = 1004).
[b] Stage IIIA/B.

Table 3
Recent series evaluating the use of US for nodal recurrences in melanoma

Study	n	Sensitivity (%)	Specificity (%)	Accuracy (%)	False-positive (%)	False-negative (%)	F/U (mo)	Notes
Tregnaghi et al[52] 1996	87	86.6	94.6	93.3	4.5	2.2	36	Shape, central zone US features used to define (+) lymph node
Binder et al[53] 1997	264	90.0	98.9	97.8	1.0	0.2	NR	US compared with PE every 3 months, median examinations/patient = 8 US = PE
Blum et al[54] 2000	1288	89.2	99.7	NR	9.1	NR	42	Prospective study US > PE[a]
Voit et al[55] 2001	829	99.2	98.3	99.3	1.7	0.1	NR	US compared with PE over 4-year period, median examinations/patient = 8 US > PE[b]
Hofmann et al[15] 2002	661	NR	NR	NR	9.3	NR	Stage I/II: 48 Stage III: 18	Part of German melanoma F/U study Reported as detection rate[c] PE > US
Brountzos et al[56] 2003	148	98	98	NR	0.9	2.3	NR	Cervical and axillary more sensitive than inguinal US > PE

Abbreviations: F/U, follow-up; NR, not reported; PE, physical examination.
[a] Sensitivity and specificity of PE 71.4% and 99.7%, respectively.
[b] Sensitivity and specificity of PE 25.2% and 98.4%, respectively.
[c] Detection rate of 12.5% and 10% for stage I/II and stage III, respectively.

of US over palpation in the early detection of regional/nodal melanoma recurrences. No survival analysis was performed in this evaluation. Voit and colleagues[55] compared US B-scan with palpation in 829 patients with resected stage I to III melanoma. These investigators found that US had a sensitivity, specificity, and accuracy of 99.2%, 98.3%, and 99.3%, respectively, with false-positive and false-negative rates of 1.7% and 0.1%, respectively. This finding was significantly better than the sensitivity (25.2%) of palpation. Overall survival was affected by diameter of the largest metastasis ($P = .001$) and the number of metastatic lesions ($P = .012$), but not by method of detection (palpation vs US). The investigators concluded that US B-scanning was highly effective in early detection of regional melanoma metastases compared with palpation. Further, the investigators comment that, based on the fact that fewer and smaller recurrences in regional lymph nodes were associated with improved survival, earlier detection using US may result in improved survival. However, their results do not directly support this conclusion. Brountzos and colleagues[56] compared US with palpation in 148 patients with stage II and III melanomas. They reported 98% sensitivity and specificity, with a false-positive rate of 0.9% and a false-negative rate of 2.3% and found US superior to palpation in determining melanoma metastases (sensitivity and specificity of 72.7% and 97%, respectively). The investigators concluded that regional US should be included in the follow-up of this patient group. They also found that US had increased sensitivity in the cervical and axillary nodal basins when compared with the inguinal region. Only one study found that palpation was superior to US in the detection of regional nodal metastases. Hoffman and colleagues[15] reported on 661 patients and reported that palpation detected first recurrences in 47% of patients, whereas regional lymph node US detected such recurrences in 13% of cases, but comprised 24% of total follow-up costs. Furthermore, there was a 9.3% rate of false positivity with US. They did not report sensitivity, specificity, accuracy, or false-negative rates in their reports. In the prospective study of melanoma follow-up by Garbe and colleagues,[8] metastases were detected by regional nodal US in 0 patients with stage I melanoma, 1 patient (2.0%) with stage II melanoma, and 6 patients (4.4%) with stage III melanoma. A total of 3490 US examinations were performed, with a suspicion of metastasis arising in 5% of examinations, with an increase in positive examinations for higher-stage disease (15.5% in stage III and IV disease). These investigators found this study to have the highest yield for early detection of metastases (71% vs 48% on average for other detection methods). They conclude that lymph node US should be included as part of a regular follow-up protocol in patients with primary melanomas of higher tumor thickness and in patients with regional metastases, which is incorporated in the German Cancer Society guidelines presented in **Table 1**.

A meta-analysis comparing US versus palpation for detection of melanoma invasion was performed by Bafounta and colleagues[57] in 2004. This meta-analysis comprised 12 studies, including 6642 patients and 18,610 paired palpation and US examinations. These investigators concluded that US had a higher discriminatory power compared with palpation (odds ratio = 1755, 95% confidence interval [CI] 726–4238, $P = .0001$). Positive-likelihood ratios were 42.9 (95% CI 29–75) for US and 4.55 (95% CI 2–18) for palpation and negative-likelihood ratios were 0.024 (95% CI 0.01–0.03) for US and 0.22 (95% CI 0.06–0.31) for palpation. The investigators concluded that US detects lymph node invasion more accurately than palpation and should be used routinely in patients with melanoma. However, no study has shown a survival advantage in earlier detection of nodal recurrence using US. A direct randomized trial designed to answer this question would require more than 3000 patients[58] and is unlikely to be performed. The design of the Multicenter Selective Lymphadenectomy Trial II

(MSLT-II) will provide some insight into the effect of US on survival.[59] The trial random-izes patients with a positive sentinel node biopsy to nodal observation with US eval-uation of the at-risk nodal basin every 4 months for 2 years and every 6 months thereafter versus immediate completion lymph node dissection. This trial seeks to accrue 4200 patients and results will be available in 2017.

There are several limitations of the studies discussed earlier addressing the use of US in the detection of regional nodal recurrences. First, comparisons between these studies are difficult, if not impossible, because they comprised different patient pop-ulations. For example, Tregnaghi and colleagues[52] and Blum and colleagues[54] included 97 and 235 patients, respectively, with surgically resected melanoma, but there was no further mention of primary tumor characteristics in either of these studies. Binder and colleagues[53] studied 264 patients with surgically resected mela-nomas more than 0.75 mm thick (median tumor thickness, 1.80 mm); 33% of patients had melanomas more than 3.0 mm in thickness. Voit and colleagues[55] included 829 patients in their analysis with a median tumor thickness of 1.50 mm. All of these studies were performed before the routine use of sentinel lymph node biopsy. This point is particularly relevant to modern practice, because the sentinel lymph node biopsy procedure by definition removes the most likely site of first recurrence of mela-noma. Thus, the usefulness of US in following patients is altered by this technique and, based on the previous era in which they were performed, the studies described earlier are not able to specifically address this issue. In general, the yield of US in follow-up of patients after sentinel lymph node biopsy is not known. The yield would be expected to be low in the sentinel lymph node-negative patient. As mentioned earlier, the best data we can expect to address this issue will come from the MSLT-II trial.

In patients who undergo surgical resection for melanoma without clinically involved lymph nodes, regional lymph node US has high sensitivity, specificity, and overall accuracy in detecting regional nodal metastases during follow-up. This finding, combined with its low rate of false-positive and false-negative results, makes it an excellent modality for diagnosing early regional recurrent melanoma. Whether early detection of residual nodal recurrence leads to improved outcomes remains to be seen and will be partially addressed by the results of the MSLT-II trial.

Other imaging modalities
After the lungs, melanoma next most commonly metastasizes to intraabdominal organs, including the liver, brain, small bowel, and adrenal glands. Such spread confers a dismal prognosis. Rose and colleagues[60] described a series of 1750 patients with hepatic metastases from melanoma. Only 34 patients (2%) underwent exploration, with complete resection in 18 patients (1%). Seven of these 18 (0.4%) were alive at 5 years. Median survival with small bowel metastases is 9 months.[61] The routine use of abdominal US was not found to improve the detection of resectable lesions, nor affect survival.[43] False-positive results occurred in 9% of cases. Other studies have reported false-positive rates as high as 20% and have failed to show a benefit for the use of routine abdominal US in the follow-up of patients with mela-noma.[44–47] In the prospective study by Garbe and colleagues, abdominal US showed metastasis in 0 patients with stage I melanoma, 1 patient (2%) with stage II melanoma, and 6 patients (4.4%) with stage III melanoma, and 6 patients (4.4%) with stage IV melanoma. A total of 2464 abdominal US examinations were performed, with a subse-quent suspicion of metastasis in 0.8% of investigations. The value was highest at 4% for pooled stage III and IV patients. The investigators felt that abdominal US should be omitted in stage I and II patients, but continued to be used in stage III and IV patients, which is the current recommendation of the German Cancer Society (see **Table 1**).

Routine imaging (CT or MRI) for the detection of asymptomatic brain metastases is not of sufficient yield to be justified, because these patients nearly always have synchronous extracranial metastases and/or neurologic symptoms that initiate a metastatic workup.[62] The exception to this are patients with stage IIIC melanoma, in whom Romano and colleagues[22] found a risk greater than 5% for first relapse in the brain within the first 13 months of follow-up, and 36% of these patients presented with seizures. Because early detection of brain metastases may spare patients from experiencing a seizure, it is reasonable for stage IIIC patients to have brain imaging during the first year of follow-up.

Melanoma does not spread to bones as often as other solitary malignancies. A single study investigating the value of bone scintigraphy showed abnormal scans in 7 of 116 (6%) patients with resected stage I to III melanoma (80% stage I/II, 20% stage III), but none was caused by melanoma. Further, one patient with a normal bone scintigram had bone metastases.[31] Thus, the role of routine bone imaging is not justified.

DIFFERENCES IN OUTCOMES BASED ON METHOD OF DETECTION OF MELANOMA RECURRENCE

When considering the frequency and extent of follow-up for patients with melanoma, a central question is whether method of detection (patient vs clinician, symptomatic vs asymptomatic, clinically detected vs radiographically or laboratory test-detected recurrence) affects survival. For example, if radiographically detected recurrences led to improved survival, one could strongly argue for more frequent clinic visits with use of that particular radiographic test. However, in the absence of such findings, frequent clinic visits using many screening tests could be considered frivolous and a poor allocation of resources.

Francken and colleagues[16] prospectively evaluated 211 patients with resected stage I to III melanoma and found that there was no statistically significant difference in survival between patient- and clinician-detected recurrences. Mooney and colleagues[20] reported similar findings in 1004 patients with stage I or II resected melanoma. In both of these studies, approximately 75% of recurrences were detected by patients, with other recurrences detected by clinicians on physical examination (~12%) and blood tests or radiographic examinations (~12%). Similarly, Meyers and colleagues[19] reported on a prospective study of 118 patients with resected stage II and III melanoma, showing no differences in survival based on method of detection. Two-thirds of recurrences were detected by a patient or were symptomatic, with most of the remainder of recurrences detected during routine physical examination. Taken together, these data suggest that there is no difference in outcomes in patients with recurrent melanoma based on detection methods. As has been discussed previously, most recurrences are detected by patients, and the addition of more investigations (laboratory, radiographic) in the asymptomatic patient in melanoma follow-up has not been shown to improve survival. Further, such investigations have not been found to be cost-effective.[48] In their prospective study, Garbe and colleagues[8] failed to show a survival advantage in the use of increased frequency of physical examination, CXR, abdominal US, CT scanning, blood tests, or whole-body scintigraphy on survival in patients with stage I to IV melanoma. They did find an improvement in survival in the 21% of recurrences detected with regional lymph node US detected at an early stage (48% of total). This finding held true for both stage I/II and stage III patients. The 3-year overall survival for recurrences detected early versus late was 76% versus 38%, respectively, for stage I/II disease and 60% versus 18%, respectively, for stage III disease.

DETECTION OF A SUBSEQUENT PRIMARY MELANOMA DURING FOLLOW-UP

Patients with a first primary melanoma have an increased risk compared with the general population of developing a subsequent primary melanoma. This risk is reported from 2% to 8% in large series of patients without a known genetic syndrome predisposing them to melanoma (presence of multiple atypical nevi, positive family history of melanoma, or the rarely seen presence of a p16 mutation) in the literature.[1,2,63] In structured follow-up, the incidence of discovery of a second invasive melanoma is 2%[46] and does not vary based on the stage of the first melanoma.[18] It is highest in the first 2 years, then decreases to approximately 0.3%/y.[63] The risk for development of a subsequent in situ (noninvasive) melanoma is 6%, which is approximately 5 times higher than the general population.[11] Most series do not recommend follow-up, per se, after treatment of an in situ melanoma other than continued dermatologic surveillance for a subsequent melanoma.[64] Similar to recurrences of a first melanoma, most subsequent primary melanomas are detected by patients.[31] Their tumor characteristics are generally less advanced than their first melanoma. For example, the Breslow thickness is approximately half of the first melanoma.[1,46] Findings on the interval between the initial and subsequent primary melanomas are inconsistent. For example, Goggins and Tsao[65] found that most subsequent primary melanomas develop within 2 years after the initial melanoma. In contrast, Johnson and colleagues[66] found that 40% of subsequent primary melanomas were diagnosed after 7 years of follow-up, and up to 31 years later. In their prospective evaluation of melanoma follow-up, Garbe and colleagues detected 62 (3.1%) second primary melanomas in 46 patients (2.3%) in a total of 3800 clinical examinations and 12,398 imaging techniques. Three of the 62 lesions (4.8%) were detected by patients, with the remainder detected by clinicians. Forty-four (71%) were stage IA, 7 (11.3%) were stage IB, 7 (11.3%) were stage IIA, and 4 (6.4%) were stage III.

The risk of developing a subsequent primary melanoma is much the same as the risk for recurrence for melanoma for stage I patients.[1] No specific investigations, other than clinical dermatologic examinations, are warranted. The time course for development of a subsequent melanoma varies widely and most new primary melanomas are detected by clinicians. Thus, after treatment of any stage of primary melanoma, patients should be followed for development of a second primary melanoma with complete skin and regional nodal examinations. This follow-up can be performed in conjunction with any other stage-specific follow-up visits and tests based on the characteristics of that patient's primary melanoma. These visits also give the opportunity for the provider of melanoma care to stress the importance of patient education and self-examination, both for melanoma recurrences and detection of second primary melanomas. As was discussed earlier, such follow-up programs could be incorporated into the annual primary care physician/GP clinic visit without sacrificing detection rates and patient satisfaction.[28]

PATIENT EDUCATION AND SATISFACTION IN RELATION TO FOLLOW-UP

After diagnosis and treatment of primary melanoma, patients generally have a vast amount of conflicting information at their disposal regarding their prognosis. This situation is even more evident in the Internet era. Patients rely on their treating physician(s) for guidance, education, and satisfaction. Thus, alleviation of undue anxiety is an important secondary goal of follow-up. Patients generally want to know what they can do to detect a recurrence or subsequent primary melanoma.[2] An individual patient's ability to detect a recurrence or subsequent primary varies greatly, with some individuals consistently and correctly identifying recurrences not detectable by clinicians, whereas others are unable to detect subcutaneous metastases greater than 5 cm in size.[2]

Baughan and colleagues[14] assessed the value of follow-up from the patient's perspective using a questionnaire. They concluded that 86% of patients believed follow-up was worthwhile, with only 5% indicating they believed follow-up was a waste of time. However, more than half of the patients in the study reported anxiety before the follow-up visit. Longman and Graham[67] found similar results, whereas Brandberg and colleagues[68] found that regular follow-up was neutral in producing negative or positive psychological or psychosomatic effects. Schofield and colleagues[69] found that 63% of patients in follow-up valued the extra information provided and 75% took advantage of the option of discussing their disease with a counselor.

Most patients in follow-up programs for melanoma are satisfied and find some, if not all, aspects of the follow-up program beneficial. Most patients appreciate the additional information given and the answers to unclear questions, but a significant percentage may find routine follow-up anxiety-provoking, outweighing the benefits mentioned earlier.[70,71] However, these reasons alone are not enough to justify rigorous clinical follow-up in this era of cost-conscious delivery of health care. The combination of melanoma follow-up and education as part of a patient's annual examination with their primary care physician may be the best way to achieve patient satisfaction without unduly stressing the health care system, and such a program is well accepted by patients and clinicians alike.[28] It may be that, as we address patient concerns, one schedule for melanoma follow-up may not be correct for all patients.

SUMMARY

The most concrete statement that one can make regarding follow-up of the patient with melanoma is that there is no level 1 evidence evaluating the effect of various follow-up regimens on outcomes (survival) in patients with completely resected stage I to III melanoma. This observation includes the question of frequency of follow-up visits, length of time that patients should be followed, laboratory and radiographic tests to be used as adjuncts to physical examination at clinic visits, the appropriate care provider to perform melanoma follow-up (melanoma specialist vs primary care physician), and the effect of follow-up on the length and quality of a patient's life. No convincing evidence exists that regional control, survival, and quality of life improve through surveillance. The guidelines from consensus groups and national cancer organizations (see **Table 1**) vary widely. In light of the few prospective and multiple retrospective studies evaluating all of the issues addressed in this article, some summary statements can be made:

- Most melanoma recurrences are detected by patients.
- There is no clear improvement in survival if melanoma recurrence is detected by a patient or a clinician.
- There is no clear improvement in survival if melanoma recurrence is symptomatic or asymptomatic.
- There is no clear improvement in survival if melanoma recurrence is detected clinically or by laboratory or radiographic testing. Thus, there is no evidence to support the routine use of laboratory and radiographic studies in the follow-up of patients with melanoma.
- Regional/nodal US seems to have the highest accuracy to detect asymptomatic, early regional recurrences, but further evaluation is required to determine if earlier detection positively affects survival.

- The incidence of subsequent primary melanomas is 5% to 8%, and is heavily weighted by in situ lesions. Because these lesions are largely curable, ongoing lifetime dermatologic surveillance is reasonable.
- Melanoma follow-up may be effectively provided by melanoma specialists or well-educated primary care physicians and physician extenders, with equal rates of recurrence detection and patient satisfaction.

REFERENCES

1. Francken AB, Bastiaannet E, Hoekstra HJ. Follow-up in patients with localised primary cutaneous melanoma. Lancet Oncol 2005;6(8):608–21.
2. Nieweg OE, Kroon BB. The conundrum of follow-up: should it be abandoned? Surg Oncol Clin N Am 2006;15(2):319–30.
3. Wong JH, Skinner KA, Kim KA, et al. The role of surgery in the treatment of non-regionally recurrent melanoma. Surgery 1993;113(4):389–94.
4. Soong SJ, Ding S, Coit D, et al. Predicting survival outcome of localized melanoma: an electronic prediction tool based on the AJCC melanoma database. Ann Surg Oncol 2010;17(8):2006–14.
5. Eigentler TK, Caroli UM, Radny P, et al. Palliative therapy of disseminated malignant melanoma: a systematic review of 41 randomised clinical trials. Lancet Oncol 2003;4(12):748–59.
6. Weiss M, Loprinzi CL, Creagan ET, et al. Utility of follow-up tests for detecting recurrent disease in patients with malignant melanomas. JAMA 1995;274(21):1703–5.
7. Francken AB, Hoekstra HJ. Follow-up of melanoma patients: the need for evidence-based protocols. Ann Surg Oncol 2009;16(4):804–5.
8. Garbe C, Paul A, Kohler-Spath H, et al. Prospective evaluation of a follow-up schedule in cutaneous melanoma patients: recommendations for an effective follow-up strategy. J Clin Oncol 2003;21(3):520–9.
9. McCarthy WH, Shaw HM, Thompson JF, et al. Time and frequency of recurrence of cutaneous stage I malignant melanoma with guidelines for follow-up study. Surg Gynecol Obstet 1988;166(6):497–502.
10. Martini L, Brandani P, Chiarugi C, et al. First recurrence analysis of 840 cutaneous melanomas: a proposal for a follow-up schedule. Tumori 1994;80(3):188–97.
11. Dicker TJ, Kavanagh GM, Herd RM, et al. A rational approach to melanoma follow-up in patients with primary cutaneous melanoma. Scottish Melanoma Group. Br J Dermatol 1999;140(2):249–54.
12. Rosenkranz L, Schroeder C. Recurrent malignant melanoma following a 46-year disease-free interval. N Y State J Med 1985;85(3):95.
13. Francken AB, Accortt NA, Shaw HM, et al. Follow-up schedules after treatment for malignant melanoma. Br J Surg 2008;95(11):1401–7.
14. Baughan CA, Hall VL, Leppard BJ, et al. Follow-up in stage I cutaneous malignant melanoma: an audit. Clin Oncol (R Coll Radiol) 1993;5(3):174–80.
15. Hofmann U, Szedlak M, Rittgen W, et al. Primary staging and follow-up in melanoma patients–monocenter evaluation of methods, costs and patient survival. Br J Cancer 2002;87(2):151–7.
16. Francken AB, Shaw HM, Accortt NA, et al. Detection of first relapse in cutaneous melanoma patients: implications for the formulation of evidence-based follow-up guidelines. Ann Surg Oncol 2007;14(6):1924–33.
17. Francken AB, Thompson JF, Bastiaannet E, et al. [Detection of the first recurrence in patients with melanoma: three quarters by the patient, one quarter during outpatient follow-up]. Ned Tijdschr Geneeskd 2008;152(10):557–62 [in Dutch].

18. Einwachter-Thompson J, MacKie RM. An evidence base for reconsidering current follow-up guidelines for patients with cutaneous melanoma less than 0.5 mm thick at diagnosis. Br J Dermatol 2008;159(2):337–41.

19. Meyers MO, Yeh JJ, Frank J, et al. Method of detection of initial recurrence of stage II/III cutaneous melanoma: analysis of the utility of follow-up staging. Ann Surg Oncol 2009;16(4):941–7.

20. Mooney MM, Kulas M, McKinley B, et al. Impact on survival by method of recurrence detection in stage I and II cutaneous melanoma. Ann Surg Oncol 1998; 5(1):54–63.

21. Poo-Hwu WJ, Ariyan S, Lamb L, et al. Follow-up recommendations for patients with American Joint Committee on cancer stages I-III malignant melanoma. Cancer 1999;86(11):2252–8.

22. Romano E, Scordo M, Dusza SW, et al. Site and timing of first relapse in stage III melanoma patients: implications for follow-up guidelines. J Clin Oncol 2010; 28(18):3042–7.

23. NCCN Clinical Practice Guidelines in Oncology: Melanoma. 2010. Available at: http://www.nccn.org/professionals/physician_gls/PDF/melanoma.pdf. Accessed July 26, 2010.

24. Dummer R, Bosch U, Panizzon R, et al. Swiss guidelines for the treatment and follow-up of cutaneous melanoma. Dermatology 2001;203(1):75–80.

25. Dummer R, Hauschild A, Guggenheim M, et al. Melanoma: ESMO clinical practice guidelines for diagnosis, treatment and follow-up. Ann Oncol 2010; 21(Suppl 5):v194–7.

26. Garbe C, Hauschild A, Volkenandt M, et al. Evidence and interdisciplinary consense-based German guidelines: diagnosis and surveillance of melanoma. Melanoma Res 2007;17(6):393–9.

27. Clinical Practice Guidelines for the Management of Melanoma in Australia and New Zealand. 2008. Available at: http://www.nhmrc.gov.au/_files_nhmrc/file/publications/synopses/cp111.pdf. Accessed July 26, 2010.

28. Murchie P, Nicolson MC, Hannaford PC, et al. Patient satisfaction with GP-led melanoma follow-up: a randomised controlled trial. Br J Cancer 2010;102(10): 1447–55.

29. Provost N, Marghoob AA, Kopf AW, et al. Laboratory tests and imaging studies in patients with cutaneous malignant melanomas: a survey of experienced physicians. J Am Acad Dermatol 1997;36(5 Pt 1):711–20.

30. Huang CL, Provost N, Marghoob AA, et al. Laboratory tests and imaging studies in patients with cutaneous malignant melanoma. J Am Acad Dermatol 1998; 39(3):451–63.

31. Kersey PA, Iscoe NA, Gapski JA, et al. The value of staging and serial follow-up investigations in patients with completely resected, primary, cutaneous malignant melanoma. Br J Surg 1985;72(8):614–7.

32. Campora E, Repetto L, Giuntini P, et al. LDH in the follow-up of stage I malignant melanoma. Eur J Cancer Clin Oncol 1988;24(2):277–8.

33. Balch CM, Soong SJ, Atkins MB, et al. An evidence-based staging system for cutaneous melanoma. CA Cancer J Clin 2004;54(3):131–49 [quiz: 182–4].

34. Cochran AJ, Wen DR, Herschman HR, et al. Detection of S-100 protein as an aid to the identification of melanocytic tumors. Int J Cancer 1982;30(3):295–7.

35. Bonfrer JM, Korse CM, Nieweg OE, et al. The luminescence immunoassay S-100: a sensitive test to measure circulating S-100B: its prognostic value in malignant melanoma. Br J Cancer 1998;77(12):2210–4.

36. Guo HB, Stoffel-Wagner B, Bierwirth T, et al. Clinical significance of serum S100 in metastatic malignant melanoma. Eur J Cancer Am 1995;31(11):1898–902.
37. Jury CS, McAllister EJ, MacKie RM. Rising levels of serum S100 protein precede other evidence of disease progression in patients with malignant melanoma. Br J Dermatol 2000;143(2):269–74.
38. Garbe C, Leiter U, Ellwanger U, et al. Diagnostic value and prognostic significance of protein S-100beta, melanoma-inhibitory activity, and tyrosinase/MART-1 reverse transcription-polymerase chain reaction in the follow-up of high-risk melanoma patients. Cancer 2003;97(7):1737–45.
39. Harpole DH Jr, Johnson CM, Wolfe WG, et al. Analysis of 945 cases of pulmonary metastatic melanoma. J Thorac Cardiovasc Surg 1992;103(4):743–8 [discussion: 748–50].
40. Coit DG. Role of surgery for metastatic malignant melanoma: a review. Semin Surg Oncol 1993;9(3):239–45.
41. Allen PJ, Coit DG. The role of surgery for patients with metastatic melanoma. Curr Opin Oncol 2002;14(2):221–6.
42. Wong JH, Euhus DM, Morton DL. Surgical resection for metastatic melanoma to the lung. Arch Surg 1988;123(9):1091–5.
43. Bassères N, Grob JJ, Richard MA, et al. Cost-effectiveness of surveillance of stage I melanoma. A retrospective appraisal based on a 10-year experience in a dermatology department in France. Dermatology 1995;191(3):199–203.
44. Goerz G, Schulte-Beerbuhl R, Roder K, et al. [Malignant melanoma: which examinations are useful in staging and follow-up?]. Dtsch Med Wochenschr 1986; 111(33):1230–3 [in German].
45. Bastien M, Tessier MH, Legoux B, et al. Usefulness of paraclinical follow-up in stage I melanoma. Arch Dermatol 1997;133(11):1462–3.
46. Kittler H, Weitzdorfer R, Pehamberger H, et al. Compliance with follow-up and prognosis among patients with thin melanomas. Eur J Cancer 2001;37(12): 1504–9.
47. Mijnhout GS, Teule GJ, Hoekstra OS, et al. [Follow-up after melanoma resection is more extensive than recommended in the practice guidelines, primarily for reassurance of the patient]. Ned Tijdschr Geneeskd 1999;143(19):997–1001 [in Dutch].
48. Mooney MM, Mettlin C, Michalek AM, et al. Life-long screening of patients with intermediate-thickness cutaneous melanoma for asymptomatic pulmonary recurrences: a cost-effectiveness analysis. Cancer 1997;80(6):1052–64.
49. Tsao H, Feldman M, Fullerton JE, et al. Early detection of asymptomatic pulmonary melanoma metastases by routine chest radiographs is not associated with improved survival. Arch Dermatol 2004;140(1):67–70.
50. Morton RL, Craig JC, Thompson JF. The role of surveillance chest X-rays in the follow-up of high-risk melanoma patients. Ann Surg Oncol 2009;16(3):571–7.
51. Toyoda Y, Nakayama T, Kusunoki Y, et al. Sensitivity and specificity of lung cancer screening using chest low-dose computed tomography. Br J Cancer 2008; 98(10):1602–7.
52. Tregnaghi A, De Candia A, Calderone M, et al. Ultrasonographic evaluation of superficial lymph node metastases in melanoma. Eur J Radiol 1997;24(3): 216–21.
53. Binder M, Kittler H, Steiner A, et al. Lymph node sonography versus palpation for detecting recurrent disease in patients with malignant melanoma. Eur J Cancer 1997;33(11):1805–8.

54. Blum A, Schlagenhauff B, Stroebel W, et al. Ultrasound examination of regional lymph nodes significantly improves early detection of locoregional metastases during the follow-up of patients with cutaneous melanoma: results of a prospective study of 1288 patients. Cancer 2000;88(11):2534–9.

55. Voit C, Mayer T, Kron M, et al. Efficacy of ultrasound B-scan compared with physical examination in follow-up of melanoma patients. Cancer 2001;91(12):2409–16.

56. Brountzos EN, Panagiotou IE, Bafaloukos DI, et al. Ultrasonographic detection of regional lymph node metastases in patients with intermediate or thick malignant melanoma. Oncol Rep 2003;10(2):505–10.

57. Bafounta ML, Beauchet A, Chagnon S, et al. Ultrasonography or palpation for detection of melanoma nodal invasion: a meta-analysis. Lancet Oncol 2004; 5(11):673–80.

58. Machet L, Perrinaud A, Giraudeau B. Routine ultrasonography in melanoma follow-up? Lancet Oncol 2005;6(1):2 [discussion: 3].

59. Complete lymph node dissection or observation in treating patients with localized melanoma and sentinel node metastasis who have undergone sentinel lymphadenectomy. Available at: http://clinicaltrials.gov/ct2/show/NCT00389571?term=mslt&rank=8. Accessed August 6, 2010.

60. Rose DM, Essner R, Hughes TM, et al. Surgical resection for metastatic melanoma to the liver: the John Wayne Cancer Institute and Sydney Melanoma Unit experience. Arch Surg 2001;136(8):950–5.

61. Berger AC, Buell JF, Venzon D, et al. Management of symptomatic malignant melanoma of the gastrointestinal tract. Ann Surg Oncol 1999;6(2):155–60.

62. Saha S, Meyer M, Krementz ET, et al. Prognostic evaluation of intracranial metastasis in malignant melanoma. Ann Surg Oncol 1994;1(1):38–44.

63. Ferrone CR, Ben Porat L, Panageas KS, et al. Clinicopathological features of and risk factors for multiple primary melanomas. JAMA 2005;294(13):1647–54.

64. Roberts DL, Anstey AV, Barlow RJ, et al. U.K. guidelines for the management of cutaneous melanoma. Br J Dermatol 2002;146(1):7–17.

65. Goggins WB, Tsao H. A population-based analysis of risk factors for a second primary cutaneous melanoma among melanoma survivors. Cancer 2003;97(3): 639–43.

66. Johnson TM, Hamilton T, Lowe L. Multiple primary melanomas. J Am Acad Dermatol 1998;39(3):422–7.

67. Longman AJ, Graham KY. Living with melanoma: content analysis of interviews. Oncol Nurs Forum 1986;13(4):58–64.

68. Brandberg Y, Mansson-Brahme E, Ringborg U, et al. Psychological reactions in patients with malignant melanoma. Eur J Cancer 1995;31A(2):157–62.

69. Schofield PE, Butow PN, Thompson JF, et al. Psychological responses of patients receiving a diagnosis of cancer. Ann Oncol 2003;14(1):48–56.

70. Dancey A, Rayatt S, Courthold J, et al. Views of UK melanoma patients on routine follow-up care. Br J Plast Surg 2005;58(2):245–50.

71. Fawzy FI, Canada AL, Fawzy NW. Malignant melanoma: effects of a brief, structured psychiatric intervention on survival and recurrence at 10-year follow-up. Arch Gen Psychiatry 2003;60(1):100–3.

Assessment of Patient-Reported Outcomes in Patients with Melanoma

Janice N. Cormier, MD, MPH*, Robert L. Askew, MPH

KEYWORDS

- Melanoma • Patient-reported outcomes
- Health-related quality of life • Preferences • Utilities • Cancer

Traditional outcome measures for patients with cancer have been expressed in terms of survival and recurrence, as these represent familiar domains of treatment effectiveness. Although other treatment-related measures, such as morbidity and toxicity, are commonly evaluated, few would argue that these primarily quantitative measures represent the entirety of the disease experience. A recent systematic review of health-related quality of life (HRQOL) in cutaneous melanoma recognized that about one-third of patients with melanoma report clinically significant levels of distress, particularly around the time of diagnosis and immediately after treatment.[1] It is now clear that patient-reported outcomes (PROs) have emerged as a means of capturing important clinical information related to disease treatment and management, namely, the patient experience.[2] PROs have been defined in general as patient indicators of "well-being," which can be expressed as single or multidimensional measures, and HRQOL is the most commonly assessed PRO. PROs provide distinct prognostic information and have been found to be associated with survival in patients with cancer,[3,4] including those with melanoma.[5–7]

INSTRUMENTS

There are numerous instruments available for assessing general HRQOL in addition to others targeting specific diseases or conditions. An inherent strength of generic instruments is that they facilitate comparisons of scores across populations and conditions,

Part of the work presented was supported by Grant No. 5-K12-CA088084 from the National Institutes of Health.

The authors have no disclosures.

Department of Surgical Oncology, Unit 444, University of Texas MD Anderson Cancer Center, 1515 Holcombe Boulevard, Houston, TX 77030, USA

* Corresponding author.

E-mail address: jcormier@mdanderson.org

but they have been criticized for their lack of sensitivity to change for specific conditions.[8,9] Conversely, disease-specific instruments have increased sensitivity for detecting predicted differences among various subgroups of patients (eg, according to disease stage) and demonstrating change over time but lack the comparability of more generalized instruments.[10,11] It has been suggested that the most informative instruments for longitudinal assessments of PROs, therefore, would be a combination that includes both generic and disease-specific items to capitalize on the strengths of each.[12] Whether measurement is performed with generalized or disease-specific items or instruments or both combined, accurate assessment of PROs has been shown to provide important clinical information to assist with decisions regarding treatment protocols and other factors related to disease management.[1] This is particularly important when modest differences in treatment outcomes (ie, survival, recurrence, morbidity) are expected.

Despite the increasing burden of melanoma as a public health problem, to date there have been only a limited number of studies examining HRQOL in patients with melanoma. Among the available studies, most have used generic instruments of HRQOL, such as the Medical Outcomes Study Short Form 36 (SF-36)[13-17] and cancer-specific HRQOL instruments such as the Functional Assessment of Cancer Therapy-General (FACT-G),[10,18] and, more frequently, the European Organization for Research and Treatment of Cancer Quality of Life Questionnaire (EORTC-QLQ).[6,19-23] Both the FACT-G and the EORTC-QLQ are validated instruments designed to assess HRQOL in patients with cancer, but they do not address uniquely relevant melanoma-specific constructs. There are no items in the FACT-G or the EORTC-QLQ related to surgical scarring, nor are there any items pertaining to lymphedema (eg, postoperative extremity swelling), a common consequence of treatment for patients undergoing the surgical treatment of stage III melanoma. Although the overall incidence of cancer-related lymphedema and its impact on HRQOL are poorly defined for patients with melanoma, the consequences of this condition are known to have a significant decremental impact. In addition, scarring and the cosmetic impact of surgery are important constructs for the assessment of HRQOL in melanoma patient populations, as has been shown in patients with early-stage melanoma.[24]

In 2003, an 11-item melanoma-specific HRQOL instrument was reported in the literature as a companion scale to the 36-item quality-of-life questionnaire from the EORTC-QLQ.[25] This instrument was validated in patients with advanced-stage (stage IV) melanoma and reported that these patients experienced sensory dysfunction, dyspnea, and pain after 9 weeks of chemotherapy.[26] This melanoma-specific instrument contains 2 items assessing extremity numbness and swelling but does not include any items to assess perceptions related to scarring—a particularly relevant concern of early-stage patients. Thus, the sensitivity of the instrument (often defined as the minimal change considered to be important by the persons with the health condition, their significant others, or their providers[27]) may be inadequate in discriminating between patients at different melanoma disease stages.

FACT-MELANOMA

The Functional Assessment of Chronic Illness Therapy is a well-known catalog of HRQOL assessment instruments that share a common core set of items representing patient well-being in the physical, functional, emotional, and social/family domains.[8] In the context of cancer disease management, physical well-being refers to symptoms related to disease (eg, pain, fatigue, and nausea) and side effects of treatment. Functional well-being assesses the ability to carry out daily living activities (eg, walking, bathing, and dressing oneself) and performing social roles and tasks. Emotional well-being refers to patients' coping abilities and reflects their experience of emotions ranging from enjoyment to distress. Last, social well-being reflects the quality of relationships with family and friends and serves as a measure of social interaction.[28] These common core items facilitate comparisons among patients with different types of malignancies, but they are supplemented with disease-specific modules that increase the instrument's sensitivity with items addressing concerns most relevant to disease-specific subpopulations. For patients with cancer, the common core items representing the physical, functional, social/family, and emotional domains are collectively known as the Functional Assessment of Cancer Therapy–General (FACT-G). A number of supplementary disease-specific FACT subscales have been developed,[29] including cancers of the breast,[30] colon and rectum,[31] and lung.[32]

A melanoma-specific module has also been developed to accompany the FACT-G to address limitations related to instrument sensitivity and discriminatory power for patients with all stages of melanoma.[33] When the melanoma-specific items are combined with the FACT-G, the expanded questionnaire is known as the FACT-Melanoma (FACT-M). The instrument was developed according to standardized methodology used for all of the Functional Assessment of Chronic Illness Therapy (FACIT) including subscales of the FACT-G with 3 distinct phases: item generation, item review and reduction, and scale construction.[8,28,33] Following an extensive review of data gathered from 4 primary sources (the literature, the FACIT item bank, health care providers, and patients with melanoma), a total of 23 items distinct from the FACT-G were identified for consideration. Additional items were generated through questionnaires seeking expert opinion from 20 melanoma researcher/health care providers at the Melanoma and Skin Center at the University of Texas MD Anderson Cancer Center. With institutional review board approval, a pilot study of 40 patients diagnosed within the previous 3 years with stages I, II, III, and IV melanoma was performed to evaluate the relevance of the items using semi-structured interviews to assess item comprehension, relevance, and overall content. Additional content and linguistic revisions were made based on reviews of the linguistic team at the Center on Outcomes, Research, and Education of Evanston Northwestern Healthcare. The FACT-M supplements version 4 of the FACT-G with 24 items (**Box 1**) representing 3 of the 4 HRQOL domains of the FACT-G.

Additional studies have been performed to establish the FACT-M as a valid and reliable measure of patient-reported HRQOL.[10] Specifically, the psychometric properties of the FACT-M have been examined with respect to the following properties[10,28,34]:

- *Face validity* reflecting how well the items represent the specific construct of interest
- *Construct validity* demonstrating the relationships between FACT-M scores and other related PRO variables
- *Criterion validity* examining the ability of the FACT-M to reflect known differences between disease subgroups
- *Convergent and Divergent validity* demonstrated as positive and negative associations between FACT-M scores and scores from related constructs
- *Internal consistency* demonstrating the extent to which scale items assess a single underlying concept
- *Discrimination* representing the ability of the scale to differentiate between known subgroups (eg, different stages of disease or according to treatment status—active treatment vs surveillance).

Box 1
Melanoma-specific items of the FACT-M

Melanoma Subscale

I have pain at my melanoma site or surgical site

I have noticed new changes in my skin (lumps, bumps, color)

I worry about the appearance of surgical scars

I have been short of breath

I have to limit my physical activity because of my condition

I have had headaches

I have had fevers

I have swelling or cramps in my stomach area

I have a good appetite

I have aches and pains in my bones

I have noticed blood in my stool

I have to limit my social activity because of my condition

I feel overwhelmed by my condition

I isolate myself from others because of my condition

I have difficulty thinking clearly (remembering, concentrating)

I feel fatigued

Melanoma Surgery Subscale

I have swelling at my melanoma site

I have swelling as a result of surgery

I am bothered by the amount of swelling

Movement of my swollen area is painful

Swelling keeps me from doing the things I want to do

Swelling keeps me from wearing the clothes or shoes that I want to wear

I feel numbness at my surgical site

I have good range of motion in my arm or leg

Data from Cormier JN, Davidson L, Xing Y, et al. Measuring quality of life in patients with melanoma: development of the FACT-melanoma subscale. J Support Oncol 2005;3:139; and Cormier JN, Ross MI, Gershenwald JE, et al. Prospective assessment of the reliability, validity, and sensitivity to change of the Functional Assessment of Cancer Therapy-Melanoma questionnaire. Cancer 2008;112:2249.

Significant differences in FACT-M scores were found between disease stage subgroups with decrements in HRQOL for patients with advanced (stage III and IV) melanoma (**Fig. 1**).[10] FACT-M responsiveness and sensitivity to change were also examined and confirmed through longitudinal comparisons of patient disease stage according to American Joint Committee on Cancer melanoma staging criteria[35] and performance status as rated by patients and providers using the Eastern Cooperative Oncology Group Performance Status Rating (ECOG-PSR)[36] and the Karnofsky Performance Scale (KPS).[37]

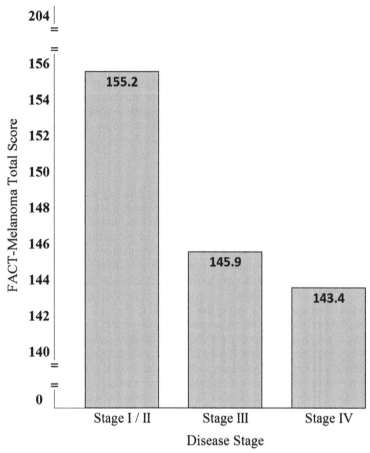

Fig. 1. Stage-specific FACT-Melanoma total scores. (*Data from* Cormier JN, Ross MI, Gershenwald JE, et al. Prospective assessment of the reliability, validity, and sensitivity to change of the Functional Assessment of Cancer Therapy-Melanoma questionnaire. Cancer 2008;112:2249.)

MINIMAL IMPORTANT DIFFERENCES

In longitudinal assessments of patient HRQOL, it is important to determine which changes in questionnaire scores can be considered clinically meaningful. This is particularly so in the context of clinical trial research in terms of defining benchmarks of change (eg, for responder analysis) and in the clinical setting for medical decision making. Multiple statistical techniques have been used to assess minimal important differences (MIDs) in HRQOL, including distribution-based methods,[38,39] anchor-based methods,[40] mixed modeling procedures,[41] or combinations of methods.[42,43] Distribution-based methods make use of distributional measures to establish minimum thresholds of change. Although distributional measures such as the Standard Error of Measurement (SEM) and effect-size correlates of one-half and one-third standard deviation have been shown to approximate the MID,[39,44,45] it is important to note that these methods provide no direct information about the clinical meaning of change-score thresholds.[46,47] In contrast, anchor-based methods make use of known clinically relevant indicators of patient change, such as functional performance status. With anchor-based methods, relevant differences in performance status scores are used to create patient groups, and the differences in HRQOL scores between groups is used to quantify an MID. Mixed modeling procedures facilitate visit-level analysis (vs patient-level) and often use clinical anchors as independent variables and HRQOL scales scores as dependent variables. A particular advantage to this technique is that it allows statistical control of known covariates in the model. Whichever techniques are chosen, a comprehensive assessment of MIDs makes use of multiple approaches to triangulate on the minimum score or range of scores to be considered clinically meaningful thresh-olds of change.[47] MIDs have been determined for a number cancer-specific HRQOL instruments.[48–50] MIDs for the FACT-M have been reported as 4 to 6 points.[44]

RESPONSE BURDEN

HRQOL instruments are often used when studying the very young, elderly, and those with advanced disease, and the burden associated with completing prolonged assessments can be difficult to tolerate in these populations.[51] Respondent burden has been defined as "the time, effort, and other demands placed on those to whom the instrument is administered,"[52] and excessive instrument burden can reduce both response rates and data quality.[53] Particularly for oncology research, instruments with fewer items are highly desirable to minimize the biases associated with respon-dent burden,[53,54] and for melanoma in particular investigations are currently under way to reduce respondent burden of the FACT-M.

Multiple psychometric methods have been developed and applied to various HRQOL instruments in an attempt to reduce respondent burden while maintaining instrument validity, including item response theory and computer adaptive testing.[51,52,54,55] The Patient-Reported Outcomes Measurement Information System (PROMIS) is a National Institutes of Health–funded project designed to create a publically available set of stan-dardized instruments that capitalize on the advantages of these techniques to reduce respondent burden and accomplish other related measurement objectives.[56,57] By developing an extensive item bank, researchers in the PROMIS network have been able to create multiple HRQOL instruments that include short forms, long forms, and computer-adapted tests for many domains, including pain, fatigue, emotional distress, physical functioning, and social role participation.[58] Instruments from the PROMIS network are field tested and calibrated such that patient scores from all items for a particular domain are represented on a single unidimensional scale (eg, difficulty getting out of bed vs difficulty running for long distances).[58] These scales are then stan-dardized to the US population (mean score = 0, standard deviation = 1) to facilitate broad comparisons across disease, condition, and other population-specific subsets. There are a number of advantages associated with the PROMIS system, and expansion into other HRQOL domains is expected to continue.[56,59,60]

HEALTH UTILITIES

Health utilities are distinct yet related measures of HRQOL that assess patient and population preferences for specific health states.[61] In the context of cancer care, cura-tive treatment can often be accompanied by serious decrements in patient HRQOL, and health state preferences help quantify the value associated with these and other compromised health states.[62] Health utilities are particularly important in the context of cost-benefit and comparative effectiveness analyses, as they facilitate the calcula-tion of quality-adjusted life years (QALY), a measure created by multiplying years of survival by the value (percentage) associated with the health states experienced during those years.[63] The health utility coefficients and the subsequent measures of

QALY facilitate comparisons of the costs and benefits associated with treatment protocols and can often inform policy decisions regarding resource allocation.[63]

There are multiple methods available to derive health utility coefficients, including use of a visual analog scale, standard gamble techniques, and time-tradeoff evaluations.[64] The visual analog scale is one of the most commonly used methods of preference elicitation, in which respondents are asked to visually rank multiple states of compromised health on a 0 (worst) to 100 (best) -point line scale.[63] With this method,

Table 1
Summary of melanoma-specific studies eliciting patient-derived health utilities

Author, Year	Melanoma Population	Source/Elicitation Techniques	Health State[a]	Utility[b]
Beusterien et al,[78] 2009	Advanced melanoma	Standard gamble	*Clinical response states*	
			Partial response	0.88
			Stable disease	0.80
			Progressive disease	0.52
			Best supportive care	0.52
Dixon et al,[21] 2006	Stage III	EQ-5D	Treatment with Interferon	0.76
			Controls	0.79
Crott et al,[73] 2004	Stage III	Time trade-off	Treatment with Interferon	0.52
			Recurrence	0.23
Kilbridge et al,[79] 2001	Early stage melanoma	Standard gamble	Interferon with no side effects	0.92
			Interferon with mild-moderate side effects	0.88
			Interferon with laboratory side effects	0.86
			Interferon with severe side effects	0.81
			Interferon, recurrence	0.62
			Recurrence	0.61
			Disease-free survival	0.96
Chen et al,[80] 2004	Stages I, II, III	Time trade-off	Stage I (Actual/ Hypothetical)	0.93/0.94
			Stage II (Actual/ Hypothetical)	0.97/0.73
			Stage III (Actual/ Hypothetical)	0.52/0.50
FACT-M validation study		EQ-5D	Stage I	0.90
			Stage II	0.87
			Stage III	0.82
			Stage IV	0.82

Abbreviations: EQ-5D, EuroQol EQ-5D; FACT-M, Functional Assessment of Cancer Therapy-Melanoma.
[a] The health states presented in this table do not reflect the entirety of health states estimated in these studies.
[b] When separate utility coefficients were estimated for multiple time points, the earliest time point was presented.

the rank-order of states is established along with strength of preference for given health states.[63] The standard gamble is a choice-based technique of eliciting health utilities where the respondent is asked to hypothetically choose between a certain health state for a specific number of years and a *given* probability of achieving a preferred health state (from a presumed treatment or decision) for the same number of years.[65] Similar choices are presented in series with varying probability for the preferred state until the respondent is indifferent to the choice (ie, when the options are of equal value to the respondent). This final probability value represents the respondent's preference for the health state under consideration.[65] For the time-tradeoff method, respondents are asked to sequentially compare a specific period of time in a compromised health state with an increasingly shorter span of time in a perfect health state.[62] When the respondent is indifferent to the choice, the percentage of time in perfect health in relation to its initial value represents the preference value for the health state.[62]

Multiattribute utility measures assess preferences for health states covering multiple HRQOL domains. The EuroQol EQ-5D (EQ-5D) is a well-known multiattribute utility measure used to assess quality of life and has been used for cost-benefit analyses.[66] For the EQ-5D, the utility function is derived from large population-based samples of respondents, and the scores represent summary utility coefficients ranging from 0 (death) to 1 (perfect health).[67] Health utilities like the EQ-5D have been positively associated with relevant clinical factors such as symptom burden in patients with cancer.[68,69]

Melanoma-specific utilities have been reported for a number of health states using techniques involving standard gamble, time-tradeoff estimation, and visual analog scales. Most of the reported studies have used these utilities to estimate the cost-effectiveness of treatment strategies by incorporating measures of cost, survival, and quality-adjusted life years, among other factors.[21,70–77] Directly elicited utilities ranged from 0.52 to 0.97 for patients with stages I to IV melanoma and included a number of health states ranging from disease-free to advanced disease under treatment. Stage-specific melanoma utilities have also been collected using the EQ-5D in the context of a longitudinal study designed to validate the FACT-M.[10] The results are summarized in **Table 1**.

SUMMARY

Melanoma-specific HRQOL instruments are important for characterizing melanoma patient populations and in evaluating the effects of psychosocial and medical interventions. The FACT-M is a melanoma-specific module that has been validated to assess HRQOL for patients with all stages of melanoma. Stage-specific differences in FACT-M scores have been shown with statistically significant decrements in HRQOL for patients with advanced (stages III and IV) disease. Melanoma-specific utilities have also been published for a number of health states and are available for calculating quality-adjusted life years and performing cost-effectiveness studies. Current PRO research is focused on using publicly available item banks and reducing respondent burden by using computer-adaptive testing. PROs should be incorporated into routine clinical practice to inform clinicians and researchers of the patient perspective for clinical decision making.

REFERENCES

1. Cornish D, Holterhues C, van de Poll-Franse LV, et al. A systematic review of health-related quality of life in cutaneous melanoma. Ann Oncol 2009; 20(Suppl 6):vi51–8.

2. Oliver A, Greenberg CC. Measuring outcomes in oncology treatment: the importance of patient-centered outcomes. Surg Clin North Am 2009;89:17–25, vii.

3. Gotay CC, Kawamoto CT, Bottomley A, et al. The prognostic significance of patient-reported outcomes in cancer clinical trials. J Clin Oncol 2008;26: 1355–63.

4. Montazeri A. Quality of life data as prognostic indicators of survival in cancer patients: an overview of the literature from 1982 to 2008. Health Qual Life Outcomes 2009;7:102.

5. Butow PN, Coates AS, Dunn SM. Psychosocial predictors of survival in metastatic melanoma. J Clin Oncol 1999;17:2256–63.

6. Lehto US, Ojanen M, Dyba T, et al. Baseline psychosocial predictors of survival in localized melanoma. J Psychosom Res 2007;63:9–15.

7. Chiarion-Sileni V, Del Bianco P, De Salvo GL, et al. Quality of life evaluation in a randomised trial of chemotherapy versus bio-chemotherapy in advanced melanoma patients. Eur J Cancer 2003;39:1577–85.

8. Cella DF, Tulsky DS. Quality of life in cancer: definition, purpose, and method of measurement. Cancer Invest 1993;11:327–36.

9. Langenhoff BS, Krabbe PF, Wobbes T, et al. Quality of life as an outcome measure in surgical oncology. Br J Surg 2001;88:643–52.

10. Cormier JN, Ross MI, Gershenwald JE, et al. Prospective assessment of the reliability, validity, and sensitivity to change of the Functional Assessment of Cancer Therapy-Melanoma questionnaire. Cancer 2008;112:2249–57.

11. Lipscomb J, Gotay CC, Snyder C. Outcomes assessment in cancer: measures, methods, and applications. Cambridge (UK); New York: Cambridge University Press; 2005.

12. Both H, Essink-Bot ML, Busschbach J, et al. Critical review of generic and dermatology-specific health-related quality of life instruments. J Invest Dermatol 2007; 127:2726–39.

13. Devine D, Parker PA, Fouladi RT, et al. The association between social support, intrusive thoughts, avoidance, and adjustment following an experimental cancer treatment. Psychooncology 2003;12:453–62.

14. McHorney CA, Ware JE Jr, Rogers W, et al. The validity and relative precision of MOS short- and long-form health status scales and Dartmouth COOP charts. Results from the Medical Outcomes Study. Med Care 1992;30: MS253–65.

15. Trask PC, Griffith KA. The identification of empirically derived cancer patient subgroups using psychosocial variables. J Psychosom Res 2004;57:287–95.

16. Trask PC, Paterson AG, Griffith KA, et al. Cognitive-behavioral intervention for distress in patients with melanoma: comparison with standard medical care and impact on quality of life. Cancer 2003;98:854–64.

17. Trask PC, Paterson AG, Hayasaka S, et al. Psychosocial characteristics of individuals with non-stage IV melanoma. J Clin Oncol 2001;19:2844–50.

18. Cella DF, Tulsky DS, Gray G, et al. The Functional Assessment of Cancer Therapy scale: development and validation of the general measure. J Clin Oncol 1993;11: 570–9.

19. Al-Shakhli H, Harcourt D, Kenealy J. Psychological distress surrounding diagnosis of malignant and nonmalignant skin lesions at a pigmented lesion clinic. J Plast Reconstr Aesthet Surg 2006;59:479–86.

20. Avril MF, Aamdal S, Grob JJ, et al. Fotemustine compared with dacarbazine in patients with disseminated malignant melanoma: a phase III study. J Clin Oncol 2004;22:1118–25.

21. Dixon S, Walters SJ, Turner L, et al. Quality of life and cost-effectiveness of interferon-alpha in malignant melanoma: results from randomised trial. Br J Cancer 2006;94:492–8.

22. Rataj D, Jankowiak B, Krajewska-Kulak E, et al. Quality-of-life evaluation in an interferon therapy after radical surgery in cutaneous melanoma patients. Cancer Nurs 2005;28:172–8.

23. Lehto US, Ojanen M, Kellokumpu-Lehtinen P. Predictors of quality of life in newly diagnosed melanoma and breast cancer patients. Ann Oncol 2005;16: 805–16.

24. Cassileth BR, Lusk EJ, Tenaglia AN. Patients' perceptions of the cosmetic impact of melanoma resection. Plast Reconstr Surg 1983;71:73–5.

25. Sigurdardottir V, Bolund C, Brandberg Y, et al. The impact of generalized malignant melanoma on quality of life evaluated by the EORTC questionnaire technique. Qual Life Res 1993;2:193–203.

26. Sigurdardottir V, Bolund C, Sullivan M. Quality of life evaluation by the EORTC questionnaire technique in patients with generalized malignant melanoma on chemotherapy. Acta Oncol 1996;35:149–58.

27. Lohr K, Aaronson NK, Alonso J, et al. Scientific Advisory Committee: instrument review criteria. Boston (MA): Medical Outcomes Trust; 1997. p.1–5.

28. Cella D, Nowinski CJ. Measuring quality of life in chronic illness: the functional assessment of chronic illness therapy measurement system. Arch Phys Med Rehabil 2002;83:S10–7.

29. Webster K, Cella D, Yost K. The Functional Assessment of Chronic Illness Therapy (FACIT) Measurement System: properties, applications, and interpretation. Health Qual Life Outcomes 2003;1:79.

30. Brady MJ, Cella DF, Mo F, et al. Reliability and validity of the Functional Assessment of Cancer Therapy-Breast quality-of-life instrument. J Clin Oncol 1997;15: 974–86.

31. Ward WL, Hahn EA, Mo F, et al. Reliability and validity of the Functional Assessment of Cancer Therapy-Colorectal (FACT-C) quality of life instrument. Qual Life Res 1999;8:181–95.

32. Cella DF, Bonomi AE, Lloyd SR, et al. Reliability and validity of the Functional Assessment of Cancer Therapy-Lung (FACT-L) quality of life instrument. Lung Cancer 1995;12:199–220.

33. Cormier JN, Davidson L, Xing Y, et al. Measuring quality of life in patients with melanoma: development of the FACT-melanoma subscale. J Support Oncol 2005;3:139–45.

34. Doward LC, McKenna SP. Defining patient-reported outcomes. Value Health 2004;7(Suppl 1):S4–8.

35. Balch CM, Buzaid AC, Soong SJ, et al. Final version of the American Joint Committee on Cancer staging system for cutaneous melanoma. J Clin Oncol 2001;19:3635–48.

36. Oken MM, Creech RH, Tormey DC, et al. Toxicity and response criteria of the Eastern Cooperative Oncology Group. Am J Clin Oncol 1982;5:649–55.

37. Karnofsky DA, Burchenal JH. The clinical evaluation of chemotherapeutic agents in cancer. In: Macleod CM, editor. Evaluation of chemotherapeutic agents in cancer. New York: Columbia University Press; 1949. p. 191–205.

38. Rejas J, Pardo A, Ruiz MA. Standard error of measurement as a valid alternative to minimally important difference for evaluating the magnitude of changes in patient-reported outcomes measures. J Clin Epidemiol 2008;61: 350–6.

39. Wyrwich KW, Tierney WM, Wolinsky FD. Further evidence supporting an SEM-based criterion for identifying meaningful intra-individual changes in health-related quality of life. J Clin Epidemiol 1999;52:861–73.
40. Juniper EF, Guyatt GH, Willan A, et al. Determining a minimal important change in a disease-specific Quality of Life Questionnaire. J Clin Epidemiol 1994;47:81–7.
41. Brant R, Sutherland L, Hilsden R. Examining the minimum important difference. Stat Med 1999;18:2593–603.
42. Barrett B, Brown R, Mundt M. Comparison of anchor-based and distributional approaches in estimating important difference in common cold. Qual Life Res 2008;17:75–85.
43. Kulkarni AV. Distribution-based and anchor-based approaches provided different interpretability estimates for the Hydrocephalus Outcome Questionnaire. J Clin Epidemiol 2006;59:176–84.
44. Askew RL, Xing Y, Palmer JL, et al. Evaluating minimal important differences for the FACT-melanoma quality of life questionnaire. Value Health 2009;12:1144–50.
45. Cohen J. Statistical power analysis for the behavioral sciences. New York: Academic Press; 1977.
46. Hays RD, Farivar SS, Liu H. Approaches and recommendations for estimating minimally important differences for health-related quality of life measures. COPD 2005;2:63–7.
47. Revicki D, Hays RD, Cella D, et al. Recommended methods for determining responsiveness and minimally important differences for patient-reported outcomes. J Clin Epidemiol 2008;61:102–9.
48. Eton DT, Cella D, Yost KJ, et al. A combination of distribution- and anchor-based approaches determined minimally important differences (MIDs) for four endpoints in a breast cancer scale. J Clin Epidemiol 2004;57:898–910.
49. Pickard AS, Neary MP, Cella D. Estimation of minimally important differences in EQ-5D utility and VAS scores in cancer. Health Qual Life Outcomes 2007;5:70.
50. Yost KJ, Cella D, Chawla A, et al. Minimally important differences were estimated for the Functional Assessment of Cancer Therapy-Colorectal (FACT-C) instrument using a combination of distribution- and anchor-based approaches. J Clin Epidemiol 2005;58:1241–51.
51. Bjorner JB, Chang CH, Thissen D, et al. Developing tailored instruments: item banking and computerized adaptive assessment. Qual Life Res 2007;16(Suppl 1):95–108.
52. Science Advisory Committee of the Medical Outcomes Trust. Assessing health status and quality-of-life instruments: attributes and review criteria. Qual Life Res 2002;11:193–205.
53. Bernhard J, Cella DF, Coates AS, et al. Missing quality of life data in cancer clinical trials: serious problems and challenges. Stat Med 1998;17:517–32.
54. Ballatori E. Unsolved problems in evaluating the quality of life of cancer patients. Ann Oncol 2001;12(Suppl 3):S11–3.
55. Coste J, Guillemin F, Pouchot J, et al. Methodological approaches to shortening composite measurement scales. J Clin Epidemiol 1997;50:247–52.
56. Cella D, Yount S, Rothrock N, et al. The Patient-Reported Outcomes Measurement Information System (PROMIS): progress of an NIH Roadmap cooperative group during its first two years. Med Care 2007;45:S3–11.
57. Garcia SF, Cella D, Clauser SB, et al. Standardizing patient-reported outcomes assessment in cancer clinical trials: a patient-reported outcomes measurement information system initiative. J Clin Oncol 2007;25:5106–12.

58. Reeve BB, Hays RD, Bjorner JB, et al. Psychometric evaluation and calibration of health-related quality of life item banks: plans for the Patient-Reported Outcomes Measurement Information System (PROMIS). Med Care 2007;45: S22–31.

59. Gershon R, Rothrock NE, Hanrahan RT, et al. The development of a clinical outcomes survey research application: assessment center. Qual Life Res 2010; 19:677–85.

60. McNeil C. Quality of life researchers have new tool and new focus on measurement. J Natl Cancer Inst 2008;100:234–6.

61. Brauer CA, Rosen AB, Greenberg D, et al. Trends in the measurement of health utilities in published cost-utility analyses. Value Health 2006;9:213–8.

62. Fayers PM, Machin D. Quality of life: the assessment, analysis, and interpretation of patient-reported outcomes. Chichester (UK); Hoboken (NJ): John Wiley 2007.

63. Feeny D. Preference-based measures: utility and quality adjusted life years. In: Fayers PM, Hays RD, editors. Assessing quality of life in clinical trials. 2nd edition. New York: Oxford University Press; 2005. p. 405–29.

64. Stiggelbout AM, de Haes JC. Patient preference for cancer therapy: an overview of measurement approaches. J Clin Oncol 2001;19:220–30.

65. Feeny DH. The roles for preference-based measures in support of cancer research and policy. In: Lipscomb J, Gotay CC, Snyder CF, editors. Outcomes assessment in cancer. Cambridge (UK): Cambridge University Press; 2005. p. 69–92.

66. Rabin R, de Charro F. EQ-5D: a measure of health status from the EuroQol Group. Ann Med 2001;33:337–43.

67. Shaw JW, Johnson JA, Coons SJ. US valuation of the EQ-5D health states: development and testing of the D1 valuation model. Med Care 2005;43:203–20.

68. Cantor SB, Volk RJ, Cass AR, et al. Psychological benefits of prostate cancer screening: the role of reassurance. Health Expect 2002;5:104–13.

69. Shih YC, Wang XS, Cantor SB, et al. The association between symptom burdens and utility in Chinese cancer patients. Qual Life Res 2006;15:1427–38.

70. Morton RL, Howard K, Thompson JF. The cost-effectiveness of sentinel node biopsy in patients with intermediate thickness primary cutaneous melanoma. Ann Surg Oncol 2009;16:929–40.

71. Cashin RP, Lui P, Machado M, et al. Advanced cutaneous malignant melanoma: a systematic review of economic and quality-of-life studies. Value Health 2008;11: 259–71.

72. Cormier JN, Xing Y, Ding M, et al. Cost effectiveness of adjuvant interferon in node-positive melanoma. J Clin Oncol 2007;25:2442–8.

73. Crott R, Ali F, Burdette-Radoux S. Cost-utility of adjuvant high-dose interferon alpha therapy in stage III cutaneous melanoma in Quebec. Value Health 2004; 7:423–32.

74. Hengge UR, Wallerand A, Stutzki A, et al. Cost-effectiveness of reduced follow-up in malignant melanoma. J Dtsch Dermatol Ges 2007;5:898–907.

75. Lafuma A, Dreno B, Delaunay M, et al. Economic analysis of adjuvant therapy with interferon alpha-2a in stage II malignant melanoma. Eur J Cancer 2001;37: 369–75.

76. Losina E, Walensky RP, Geller A, et al. Visual screening for malignant melanoma: a cost-effectiveness analysis. Arch Dermatol 2007;143:21–8.

77. Wilson LS, Reyes CM, Lu C, et al. Modelling the cost-effectiveness of sentinel lymph node mapping and adjuvant interferon treatment for stage II melanoma. Melanoma Res 2002;12:607–17.

78. Beusterien KM, Szabo SM, Kotapati S, et al. Societal preference values for advanced melanoma health states in the United Kingdom and Australia. Br J Cancer 2009;101:387–9.
79. Kilbridge KL, Weeks JC, Sober AJ, et al. Patient preferences for adjuvant interferon alfa-2b treatment. J Clin Oncol 2001;19:812–23.
80. Chen S, Bendeck S, Hadley J, et al. Can melanoma patients predict the quality of life impact of an alternate melanoma stage? In 26th Annual Meeting of the Society for Medical Decision Making Edition. Atlanta (GA), October 17–20, 2004.

Index

Note: Page numbers of article titles are in **boldface** type.

A

ADH-1, for in-transit melanoma metastases, 90–91
Adjuvant therapy, for melanoma, surgical perspective on, **105–114**
 future prospects for, 111
 immunotherapy with interferon, 107–108
 risk assessment, 106–107
  after resection of oligometastatic melanoma, 107
  lymph node status, 106–107
 to reduce disease recurrence and death, 107–110
  immunotherapy with interferon, 107–108
  investigations with new vaccines and immunotherapies, 109
  lack of efficacy of chemotherapy and nonspecific immunotherapies, 107
  neoadjuvant, 109–110
  pegylated interferon as alternative to standard interferon, 108–109
 to reduce local, regional nodal, and in-transit recurrence, 110–111
  intra-arterial infusion or perfusion, 110–111
 radiotherapy to the primary site in desmoplastic melanoma, 116
 radiotherapy to the regional lymph node basin in melanoma, 117–122
  after lymph node dissection, 117–119
  dose and fractionation, 122–123
  in absence of complete dissection, 119
  with concurrent chemotherapy, 121
  with concurrent interferon, 119–121
  with hyperthermia, 121–122
Adoptive cell therapy, for melanoma, 150–153
Adverse events, of lymph node biopsy for melanoma, 72
AJCC Cancer Staging Manual, updates in 7th edition, 2
Apoptotic threshold, strategies for altering, for in-transit melanoma metastases, 91–93
 dasatinib, 92–93
 sorafenib, 91–92

B

Bevacizumab, for in-transit melanoma metastases, 91
Biochemotherapy, for melanoma, 147–149
Biomarkers, for cutaneous melanoma, 13
Biopsy, of suspicious pigmented lesions, 20–21
 sentinel lymph node, 46–47, **57–78**
Biotherapy, for melanoma, 149
Borderline melanocytic tumors, pathologic analysis of, 26–27
BRAF, in targeted therapy for melanoma, 166–170
Brain metastasis, of melanoma, 123–128

Surg Oncol Clin N Am 20 (2011) 215–227
doi:10.1016/S1055-3207(10)00110-9
1055-3207/11/$ – see front matter © 2011 Elsevier Inc. All rights reserved.

surgonc.theclinics.com

Moving?

Make sure your subscription moves with you!

To notify us of your new address, find your **Clinics Account Number** (located on your mailing label above your name), and contact customer service at:

Email: journalscustomerservice-usa@elsevier.com

800-654-2452 (subscribers in the U.S. & Canada)
314-447-8871 (subscribers outside of the U.S. & Canada)

Fax number: 314-447-8029

Elsevier Health Sciences Division
Subscription Customer Service
3251 Riverport Lane
Maryland Heights, MO 63043

ELSEVIER

Printed and bound by CPI Group (UK) Ltd, Croydon, CR0 4YY

03/10/2024

01040446-0008